The Human Pursuit of Well-Being

Ingrid Brdar
Editor

The Human Pursuit of Well-Being

A Cultural Approach

Springer

Editor
Ingrid Brdar
Department of Psychology
Faculty of Humanities and Social Sciences
University of Rijeka
Slavka Krautzeka bb
51000 Rijeka
Croatia
ibrdar@ffri.hr

ISBN 978-94-007-1374-1 e-ISBN 978-94-007-1375-8
DOI 10.1007/978-94-007-1375-8
Springer Dordrecht Heidelberg London New York

Library of Congress Control Number: 2011930750

Cover design: SPi Publisher Services

Printed on acid-free paper

Springer is part of Springer Science+Business Media (www.springer.com)

Preface

The contributions in this book are based on selected papers presented at the 4th European Conference on Positive Psychology held in Opatija, Croatia in 2008. Conferences offer opportunities to bring out research from different cultures and to discuss new theoretical perspectives. The broad range of positive psychology topics was addressed during the conference. At this conference the number of presentations nearly doubled compared to previous conferences in Italy and Portugal (from 173 to 324), showing that positive psychology is swiftly growing field of research. About 500 conference attendees came from 39 countries, predominantly from Europe, but also from other parts of the world – United States, Australia, South Africa, etc. This was an excellent opportunity to learn about studies from many different cultures.

The book brings together the latest research on positive psychology from an international cast of researchers, mostly from Europe. Why Europe? This world's second-smallest continent with approximately 50 countries is placed at the crossroad of cultures. Living together in such a cultural diversity needs mutual understanding and appreciation. Dialogue between cultures and making the most of differences is an opportunity to research all three pillars of positive psychology: the subjective level, the individual level, and the group level.

So far, only few books brought together European researchers in positive psychology. One of the goals of this book is to fill this gap. Europe offers great opportunities for research into various areas of positive psychology through cultural approach. The book describes research from 11 different cultures: nine European countries, Egypt and South Africa. Selection of studies from different cultures aims at broadening our understanding of those aspects of human experience that make life worth living in diverse cultural conditions.

A great number of contributions were submitted for publication. Regretfully, not all of them could be included in this book. Carefully chosen chapters describe research and practice from diverse fields of positive psychology. The book includes work of some distinguished authors, but it also includes valuable studies of less well known authors, thus giving insight into studies of growing body of European researchers in positive psychology. This book is the result of work done by 52 contributors and presents research that has been conducted in the last few years.

The chapters are diverse in many ways, yet they all deal with the human pursuit of well-being. 22 chapters are grouped into six parts: happiness and well-being, motivation and goals, personality, academic performance and coping, measurement and intervention.

In Part I different aspects of *Happiness and Well-Being* are explored, beginning with an intriguing question: "Can We Get Happier Than We Are?" Other contributions analyze and discuss how several phenomena are related to well-being: self-serving attributional bias, affect specificity, leisure activities, the quality of subjective experience throughout daily life, benefits of positive emotions and predictors of post-traumatic growth in patients.

Part II deals with *Motivation and Goals*. It starts with a review of the relationship between goals and well-being and continues with a study of adolescent life goals. The last paper explores meaning, personal growth and motivation toward therapy.

Part III, *Personality*, has two chapters about character strengths and well-being. The first is focused on biological origins of well-being, and the second analyses gender differences.

Part IV includes research on *Academic Performance and Coping*. The studies are focused on optimistic attributional style, patterns of self-regulated learning and burnout in secondary school context.

Part V is focused on *Measurement* and comprises three chapters which analyze psychometric characteristics of five different instruments: Ryff's Psychological Well-Being Scales, Children Hope Scale, Students' Life Satisfaction Scale, Keyes' Mental Health Continuum and Vitality Scale.

Finally, Part VI describes and evaluates *Interventions*. The first contribution analyzes the effects of school interventions for promoting psychological well-being in adolescence. Other two interventions are aimed for specific groups: obese individuals and male disadvantaged adolescents.

Acknowledgments

This book is the product of a common project of 52 authors, who invested a lot of time and work to write the chapters. I would like to express my sincere thanks to the contributing authors. Special thanks to Esther Otten for her valuable editorial assistance in organizing this book. The assistance provided by my young colleagues Petra and Marko has been greatly appreciated. Finally, my sincere thanks go to my family for their support and for allowing me the necessary time to devote to this project.

Contents

Part V Measurement

Contributors

Elisa Albieri Department of Psychology, University of Bologna, Bologna, Italy

Petra Anić Department of Psychology, Faculty of Humanities and Social Sciences, University of Rijeka, Rijeka, Croatia

Sandro Barni Hospital of Treviglio, Treviglio (BG), Italy

Carlotta Belaise Department of Psychology, University of Bologna, Bologna, Italy

Maria Luisa Bonetti Hospital of Treviglio, Treviglio (BG), Italy

Ingrid Brdar Department of Psychology, Faculty of Humanities and Social Sciences, University of Rijeka, Rijeka, Croatia

Tihana Brkljačić Institute of Social Sciences Ivo Pilar, Zagreb, Croatia

Ernesto Caffo Mother-Infant Department, University of Modena and Reggio Emilia, Modena, Italy

Gabriele Covotta Institute for Advanced Study "Donald J. Ottenberg", Modena, Italy

Giovanni A. Fava Department of Psychology, University of Bologna, Bologna, Italy

Teresa Freire School of Psychology, University of Minho, Portugal

Tamara O. Gordeeva Moscow State University, Moscow, Russia

Rodolfo Gordillo Department of Personality Psychology, School of Psychology, Universidad Nacional de Educación a Distancia (UNED), Madrid, Spain

Jamin Halberstadt University of Otago, Dunedin, New Zealand

Ann-Marie K. Hutchinson University of Johannesburg, Johannesburg, South Africa

Amany Ismaïl Laboratory of Sociology and Anthropology, Department of Sociology, Rennes II University, Rennes, France

Ljiljana Kaliterna Lipovčan Institute of Social Sciences Ivo Pilar, Zagreb, Croatia

Darko Lončarić Faculty of Teacher Education, University of Rijeka, Rijeka, Croatia

Shane J. Lopez The Clifton Strengths School and Gallup, Omaha, USA

Alejandro Magallares Department of Social Psychology, School of Psychology, Universidad Nacional de Educación a Distancia (UNED), Madrid, Spain

Maria Elena Magrin Department of Psychology, University of Studies of Milan-Bicocca, Milan, Italy

Susana C. Marques Faculty of Psychology and Educational Sciences, University of Porto, Porto, Portugal

Charles Martin-Krumm CREAD EA 3875, IUFM de Bretagne, Ecole Interne UBO, Rennes, France
and
IFEPSA, Les Ponts de Cé, France

Marina Merkaš Ivo Pilar Institute of Social Sciences, Zagreb, Croatia

Sónia Mestre Faculty of Psychology and Educational Sciences, University of Porto, Porto, Portugal

Dubravka Miljković Faculty of Teacher Education, University of Zagreb, Zagreb, Croatia

Ali Montazeri Iranian Institute for Health Sciences Research, ACECR, Tehran, Iran

Jeroen Nawijn NHTV Breda University of Applied Sciences & Faculty of Social Sciences, Erasmus University, Rotterdam, The Netherlands

Emanuela Offidani Department of Psychology, University of Bologna, Bologna, Italy

Marie Oger Université Lille Nord de France, Faculté des Sciences du Sport et de l'Education Physique, EA 4488, F-59000 Lille , France

Evgeny N. Osin State University, Higher School of Economics, Moscow, Russia

Fedra Ottolini Department of Psychology, University of Bologna, Bologna, Italy

José Pais-Ribeiro Faculty of Psychology and Educational Sciences, University of Porto, Porto, Portugal

Patrick Pelayo Université Lille Nord de France, Faculté des Sciences du Sport et de l'Education Physique, EA 4488, F-59000 Lille, France

Lesley Powell Applied Research Centre in Health and Lifestyle Interventions, University of Oxford, UK

Hester G. Pretorius University of Johannesburg, Johannesburg, South Africa

Zvjezdana Prizmić-Larsen Washington University in St. Louis, St. Louis, USA

Zora Raboteg-Šarić Ivo Pilar Institute of Social Sciences, Zagreb, Croatia

Majda Rijavec Faculty of Teacher Education, University of Zagreb, Zagreb, Croatia

Charles Roncin Laboratory of Sociology and Anthropology, Department of Sociology, Rennes II University, Rennes, France

Chiara Ruini Department of Psychology, University of Bologna, Bologna, Italy

Mareï Salama-Younes Psychology Department, European University of Brittany, Rennes, France
and
Sport Psychology Department, Helwan University, Helwan, Egypt

Pilar Sanjuán Department of Personality Psychology, School of Psychology, Universidad Nacional de Educación a Distancia (UNED), Madrid, Spain

Philippe Sarrazin SENS, University Joseph Fourier, Grenoble 1, Grenoble, France

Marta Scrignaro Department of Psychology, University of Studies of Milan-Bicocca, Milan, Italy

Elin Strand Oslo University Hospital, Oslo, Norway

Anita D. Stuart University of Johannesburg, Johannesburg, South Africa

Krzysztof Szadejko Institute for Advanced Study "Donald J. Ottenberg", Modena, Italy

Elena Tomba Department of Psychology, University of Bologna, Bologna, Italy

Ruut Veenhoven Faculty of Social Sciences, Erasmus University, Rotterdam, The Netherlands

Dalila Visani Department of Psychology, University of Bologna, Bologna, Italy

Mami Yamaguchi University of Otago, Dunedin, New Zealand

Introduction

The Human Pursuit of Well-Being: A Cultural Approach

Positive psychology emphasizes the key role of individuals' resources and potentials, which have been neglected in previous research in psychology. The study of the conditions and processes that contribute to the flourishing or optimal functioning of people, groups and institutions can integrate research findings from different fields and give a more global perspective to study of life worth living.

Positive psychology is rapidly growing field of psychology with the aim to bring solid empirical research into areas of well-being, personal strengths and resources and positive groups and institutions. Literally hundreds of articles published on the topics of positive psychology since 1998 show the rapid growth of this field of psychology. "It is wonderful to see what has happened in such a short period of time in this emerging field of Positive Psychology", says Mihaly Csikszentmihalyi (2009, p. 203).

The three pillars proposed by Seligman (2002) that serve as guides to positive psychology include valued experiences at the subjective level, positive characteristics at the individual level, and positive institutions and communities at the group level. By far the most positive psychology research was conducted on the first two areas, while much less investigations were done into the third (Gable & Haidt, 2005).

Positive Psychology and Culture

Many pathways lead to a better life. The meaning of what is positive or good is shaped by culture. People rely on the information that are emphasized in their culture. Ideals, values and philosophical traditions influence the conceptions of a life well-lived. Lately, cultural influences on positive psychology research and practice attracted more interest as well as in other fields of psychological research. Studies from different cultures aim at broadening our understanding of those aspects of human experience that make life worth living in diverse cultural conditions. Because meanings and concepts are molded by culture, it is necessary to explore conceptions of happiness construed by a unique cultural tradition. People from different cultures differ in the way they make judgments about their happiness (Suh, Diener, Oishi, & Triandis, 1998). In individualist nations the judgments are more strongly based on emotions, while in collectivist nations the judgments are based on both emotions and social cues.

Culture generally refers to social norms, roles, values and life way practices that are shared by a social group and are transmitted across age generations (Betancourt & Lopez, 1993). Culture must be integrated in theory and research of human behavior. Matsumoto (2007) identifies three major sources of influence on behavior: (1) basic human nature (via universal psychological processes), (2) culture (via social roles), and (3) personality (via individual role identities). Individual behaviors are the products of the interaction between these influences, but situational context moderates the relative contributions of these sources.

So far, the majority of research in positive psychology has been conducted in Western cultures. But to what extend are these research findings applicable to all cultures? Positive psychology must search for invariant as well as for variant features of human functioning. Mainstream theories in psychology often ignore culture and therefore lack universality. Because happiness and well-being are significantly grounded in socio-cultural modes of being a person and interacting with others, it is important to expand the research to Non-Western cultures. Most of cross-cultural studies compare Western and Eastern cultures. Some of the differences between these two cultures concern individualism and collectivism are values, orientation to time and thought processes (Snyder & Lopez, 2007). However, there are also considerable differences between Eastern and Western cultures. For example, Americans and Canadians to a greater extent over report social desirable behavior like religious service attendance than people in European Catholic countries (Brenner, 2011).

Studies from diverse cultural backgrounds find both commonalities and differences in people's conceptions of a good life. For example, character strengths are universal. There is a considerable cross-cultural similarity in VIA character strengths (Park, Peterson, & Seligman, 2006). As for differences, substantial cultural variations in cultural meanings of happiness, motivations underlying happiness, and predictors of happiness were identified (Uchida, Norasakkunkit, & Kitayama, 2004).

Moreover, cultures may be similar in some dimensions, but different in other characteristics. One study examined similarities in happiness and meaningfulness between seven countries (Brdar, 2010). Cluster analysis classified these countries into three groups based on their similarities, but the group composition for happiness and meaningfulness across life domains was different. Only Australia and South Africa were classified into same clusters for both criteria. According to happiness, Italy shared the same cluster with Portugal and Croatia, but for meaningfulness Italy was more like Spain. Germany and Spain showed resemblance in happiness, but when it comes to meaningfulness, Germany was much the same as Croatia. Although culturally diverse, Germany and Spain share the similar pattern of domain happiness. On the other hand, some differences were found for Portugal and Spain, which were not expected. These results show that assumed similarities and diversities between cultures need to be examined.

Another example could be found in the field of life aspirations. Western and non-Western dichotomization cannot explain some differences related to life goals and well-being. Past research in Western countries suggest that striving for extrinsic goals (mostly materialistic) is associated with lower well-being (Ryan et al., 1999). Nevertheless, the generalizability of this effect has yet to be tested in other cultures. Some studies suggest that people living in non-Western countries may attach different meaning to extrinsic goals and that negative effects of extrinsic aspirations may apply only to affluent countries (for a review see Brdar, Rijavec, & Miljković, 2009). However, affluence is associated with individualism (Hofstede, 1980), so future research needs to find whether these differences occur because of economic factors or because of individualism-collectivism (or possibly both).

Methodological Issues

Taking all cultural differences into account, how can we compare psychological phenomena in different cultures? Researchers need to consider all relevant sources that could produce between-country differences. Not all observed differences between countries can be attributed to culture. Countries may differ on one dimension, but they often differ on other dimensions too. Additional source of variability are the cultural heterogeneity of nations and the complexity of culture. Future research needs to exclude the possibility that non-cultural sources contribute to observed group differences (Matsumoto & Yoo, 2006).

There is still no generally accepted methodology to separate intracultural variations (within-cultural differences) from intercultural variations (culture-level differences), although this field has significantly developed in the last decade. Advanced multivariate methods are used, like multiple group confirmatory analysis (MGCFA) and multigroup structural equation modeling (MGSEM), multilevel analysis, latent class analysis and item response theory.

Measurement equivalence and bias are important issues in cultural and cross-cultural research. Researchers often assume that measurement instruments have exact the same meaning within different culture and that it measures the same construct. Equivalence concerns the level of comparability of measurement outcomes. One of the major problems refers to equivalence between languages, and the other concerns the response scales in questionnaires. Use of the same measurement instruments in different cultures does not guarantee comparability of obtained results between the groups. Two instruments are equivalent if they measure the same construct in the original and the target cultures, although the item contents of the two instruments may be different.

Cultural and cross-cultural research methodologies have developed in the last two decades. But it is time for cross-cultural research methods to go further. Matsumoto and Yoo (2006) argue that the next phase will be characterized by linkage studies, which will empirically link the observed differences among variables with the specific cultural sources that might account for those differences.

Cultural and Cross-cultural Approach

Cross-cultural psychology is focused on differences between cultures and establishes psychological universals. It consists mostly of comparative research aimed at studying the influence of various cultural factors on human development and behavior. Cultural psychology offers another approach, which views culture and psychology as "mutually constitutive phenomena" (Miller, 1997, p. 88), focusing on culture as integral to all psychological processes. It assumes that human behavior is meaningful within the specific cultural context in which it occurs (Segall, Loner, & Berry, 1998). Some authors distinguish between etic and emic approach. Etic studies refer to comparative studies across cultures, while emic research focuses on specific psychological phenomenon within local culture.

Cultural studies provide valuable descriptions of life in diverse countries and explain the possible mechanisms that account for the cultural differences. They also describe social and historical context which broaden our understanding of psychological phenomena. Cross-cultural research must start with examination of the meaningfulness of a given construct and the way it is used in a specific cultural context. This will ensure that non-cultural sources do not account for observed group differences

Betancourt and Lopez (1993) propose two approaches to enhance the study of culture. The first is a bottom-up approach, which begins with a phenomenon observed in the study of culture, and continues with cross-cultural comparisons to test theories of human behavior. The second is a top-down approach, beginning with a theory (usually one that ignores culture) and incorporating cultural elements to broaden the theoretical domain.

In conclusion, future research in positive psychology should take into account a wide variety of cultural influences in order to better understand the very nature of the good life.

References

Betancourt, H., & Lopez, S. R. (1993). The study of culture, ethnicity, and race in American psychology. *American Psychologist, 48*, 629–637.

Brenner, P. S. (2011). Identity importance and the over reporting of religious service attendance: Multiple imputation of religious attendance using American time use study and the General Social Survey. *Journal for the Scientific Study of Religion, 50*, 103–115.

Brdar, I. (2010). *A cross-country study of happiness across life domains*. Paper presented at the 5th European Conference on Positive psychology, Copenhagen, Denmark, 23–26 June 2010.

Brdar, I., Rijavec, M., & Miljković, D. (2009). Life goals and well-being: Are extrinsic aspirations always detrimental to well-being? *Psychological Topics, 18*(2), 303–316.

Csikszentmihalyi, M. (2009). The promise of positive psychology. *Psychological Topics, 18*(2), 203–211.

Gable, S. L., & Haidt, J. (2005). What (and why) is positive psychology? *Review of General Psychology, 9*(2), 103–110.

Hofstede, G. H. (1980). *Culture's consequences: International differences in work-related values*. Beverly Hills, CA: Sage Publications.
Matsumoto, D. (2007). Culture, context, and behavior. *Journal of Personality, 75*(6), 1285–1319.
Matsumoto, D., & Yoo, S. H. (2006). Toward a new generation of cross-cultural research. *Perspectives on Psychological Science, 1*, 234–250.
Miller, J. G. (1997). Theoretical issues in cultural psychology. In J. W. Berry, Y. H. Poortinga, & J. Pandey (Eds), *Handbook of Cross-Cultural Psychology: Theory and Method* (Vol. 1, pp. 85–128). Boston: Allyn & Bacon.
Park, N., Peterson, C., & Seligman, M. E. P. (2006). Character strengths in fifty-four nations and the fifty US states. *The Journal of Positive Psychology, 1*(3), 118–129.
Segall, M. H., Lonner, W. J., & Berry, J. W. (1998). Cross-cultural psychology as a scholarly discipline: On the flowering of culture in behavioral research. *American Psychologist, 53*, 1101–1110.
Ryan, R. M., Chirkov, V. I., Little, T. D., Sheldon, K. M., Timoshina, E., & Deci, E. L. (1999). The American dream in Russia: Extrinsic aspirations and well-being in two cultures. *Personality and Social Psychology Bulletin, 25*, 1509–1524.
Seligman, M. E. P. (2002). Positive psychology, positive prevention, and positive therapy. In C. R. Snyder & S. J. Lopez (Eds.), *Handbook of positive psychology* (pp. 3–9). New York: Oxford University Press.
Snyder, C. R., & Lopez, S. J. (2007). *Positive psychology: The scientific and practical explorations of human strengths*. Thousand Oaks, CA: Sage.
Suh, E. M., Diener, E., Oishi, S., & Triandis, H. (1998). The shifting basis of life satisfaction judgments across cultures: Emotions versus norms. *Journal of Personality and Social Psychology, 74*, 482–493.
Uchida, Y., Norasakkunkit, V., & Kitayama, S. (2004). Cultural constructions of happiness: Theory and empirical evidence. *Journal of Happiness Studies, 5*, 223–239.

Part I
Happiness and Well-Being

Chapter 1
Can We Get Happier Than We Are?

Ruut Veenhoven

What Is the Final Goal of Public Policy?

Jeremy Bentham (1789/1970) would say: *greater happiness for a greater number.* He thought of happiness as subjective enjoyment of life; in his words, it is "the sum of pleasures and pains." In his time, the happiness could not be measured. It was, therefore, difficult to assess how happiness could be furthered and to determine whether attempts to do so were successful or not. Hence, happiness remained a subject of philosophical speculation.

Today, we can do better. Social scientists have found that happiness can be measured using questions about life-satisfaction, and they have gone on to apply such questions in large-scale surveys of general population worldwide.

How Happy Are We?

Most inhabitants of modern society are happy. This is seen from their responses to the question: "*All things considered, how satisfied are you with your life as a whole nowadays?* Please indicate using a number from 0 to 10, where 0 is 'extremely dissatisfied' and 10 'extremely satisfied'." The responses to this question in Germany are depicted in Fig. 1.1. More than 50% of the Germans rate their life at seven or higher and fewer than 15% of Germans rate their lives at five or below five. Studies that use slightly different questions have yielded similar results. The average "school mark" that Germans give for their quality of life is currently 7.2[1].

[1] Average of several surveys. Reported in World Database of Happiness, Happiness in Nations, Rank Report 2007-1.

R. Veenhoven (✉)
Faculty of Social Sciences, Erasmus University, Rotterdam,
The Netherlands
e-mail: veenhoven@fsw.eur.nl

I. Brdar (ed.), *The Human Pursuit of Well-Being: A Cultural Approach*,
DOI 10.1007/978-94-007-1375-8_1, © Springer Science+Business Media B.V. 2011

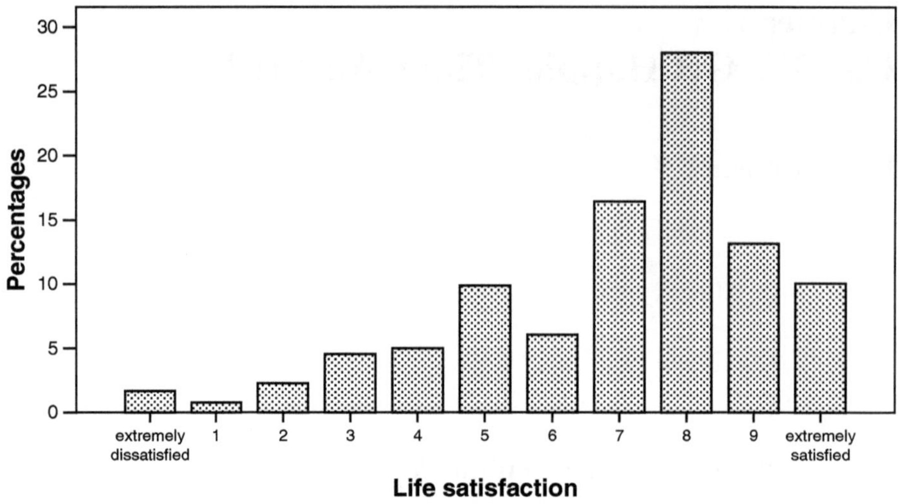

Fig. 1.1 Happiness in Germany (Data: European Social Survey 2003)

Table 1.1 Happiness in nations around 2000

Nation	Happiness
Denmark	8.2
Switzerland	8.1
Sweden	7.7
USA	7.4
Germany	7.2
France	6.5
Japan	6.2
Poland	5.9
Russia	4.4
Zimbabwe	3.3

Source: World Database of Happiness, Happiness in Nations, Rank Report 2007-1
Note: Average on scale 0–10

Rank of Happiness in Nations

How does German happiness rank in comparison to other nations? Some illustrative findings are presented in Table 1.1, and although Germany falls in the middle of this list, it is actually in the top range for the world. As one can see, average happiness varies between 8.2 (Denmark) and 3.3 (Zimbabwe), and with 7.2, Germany ranks high in the five-point interval between the highest and lowest average happiness.

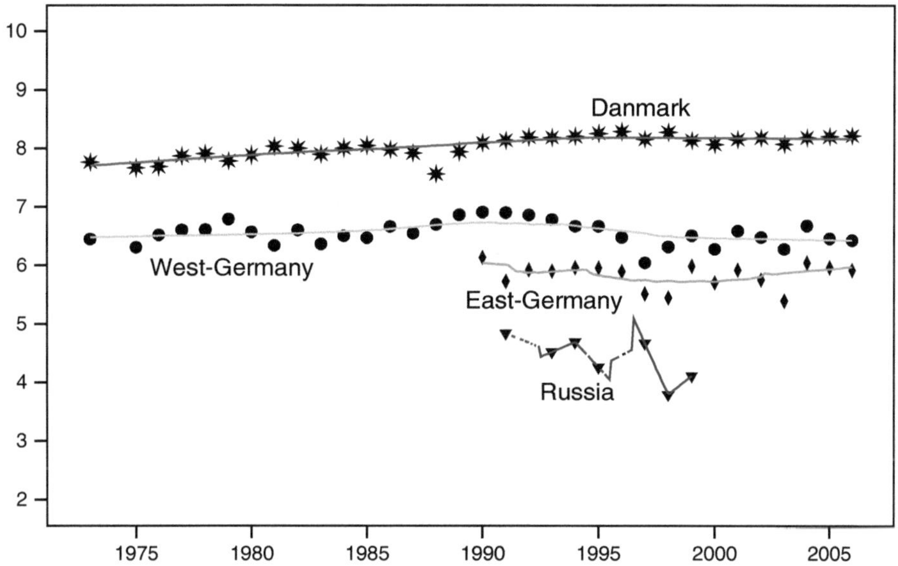

Fig. 1.2 Trend average happiness in three nations (Source: World Database of Happiness, data file TrendsInNations 2007)

Trend of Happiness in Nations

Survey research on happiness started in the late 1940s and took off in the early 1970s. Until recently, it was difficult to discern a pattern in the data; changes over time tend to be small and our view of the trend is often blurred by minor variations in sampling and questioning. Now that we have more and better data, a pattern of rising happiness has begun to emerge (Veenhoven & Hagerty, 2006). Some illustrative cases are presented in Fig. 1.2.

Greater Happiness Possible?

Can public policy create greater happiness? Several scientists think not. Some psychologists maintain that happiness is largely inborn or at least embedded in stable personality. Hence, a better society will not yield happier citizens. This view is known as the "set point" theory (Lykken, 1999). Some sociologists draw the same conclusion, because they think happiness depends on social comparison and that one is not better off than the neighbors if conditions for everybody improve. In this vein, the case of the USA is often mentioned as an example; material wealth would have doubled there since the 1950s, while average happiness seems to have

Table 1.2 Societal correlates of happiness

		Correlation with average happiness		
	Condition in nation	Zero-order	Wealth controlled	*N*
Wealth	Purchasing power per head	.65	–	88
Freedom	Economic	.60	.26	88
	Political	.48	.17	90
	Personal[a]	.35	–.13	83
Equality	Inequality of incomes	.05	.42	82
	Discrimination of women	–.52	–.25	58
Brotherhood	Tolerance	.52	.40	76
	Trust in compatriots	.39	.17	79
	Social security	.35	–.16	66
Justice	Rule of law	.64	.20	90
	Respect of civil rights	.47	.09	90
	Corruption	–.56	–.03	62
Explained variance		83%		60

[a]Not included in regression due to limited number of cases
Data: World Database of Happiness, data file 'States of Nations'

remained at the same level (Easterlin, 1995). These scientists are wrong, both empirically and theoretically.

Empirical Indications

There is a clear relation between average happiness and societal quality. Think of the case of Zimbabwe in Fig. 1.1, where this country is at the bottom with an average of 3.3. Apparently, people cannot live happily in a failed state, even if their neighbors suffer in a similar way. The correlations in Table 1.2 show that this is no exception; differences in quality of society explain about 80% of the variation in average happiness in the present day world.

Average happiness *has* changed in most nations and typically for the better (Veenhoven & Hagerty, 2006). Figure 1.2 depicts a gradual rise of happiness in Denmark over the last 30 years and a dramatic fall in average happiness in Russia, following the Ruble Crisis of 1995. Clearly, happiness is not fixed to a set point!

Figure 1.2 also shows that greater happiness is possible in most nations of the world. Average happiness is currently highest in Denmark, with an average of 8.2. What is possible in Denmark should also be possible in other countries. We cannot object that Danish happiness is a matter of genetic endowment or national character, because Fig. 1.2 shows that happiness has improved in Denmark since 1973.

Present-day happiness in Denmark may be close to the maximally possible level. If so, there is still a long way to go for most nations of this world, since the world's average happiness is now about 5.5. If we ever reached the maximum of average happiness, there is still the possibility to extend the duration of our happiness and create more happy life years for a greater number (Veenhoven, 2005).

Theoretical Underpinning

The erroneous idea that greater happiness is not possible has its roots in erroneous theories about the nature of happiness. One of these mistaken theories is that happiness is merely a matter of outlook on life and that this outlook is set in fixed dispositions, which are part of an individuals' personality as well as of their national character. Another faulty theory is that happiness results from cognitive comparison, in particular from social comparison. Elsewhere, I have shown that these theories are wrong (Veenhoven, 1991, 1995).

My alternative theory of happiness holds that we appraise life on the basis of affective information in the first place. We experience positivc as well as negative affects, and in appraising how much we like the life we live, we assess to what extent the former outbalances the latter. This theory fits Bentham's concept of happiness as "the sum of pleasures and pains." In my view, positive and negative affects signal the gratification of basic human needs, so in the end, happiness is determined by need gratification. Elsewhere, I have discussed this theory in more detail (Veenhoven, 2009).

How Can Happiness Be Raised?

Apparently, greater happiness for a greater number is possible. How can this be achieved? I see possibilities at three levels: (1) at the macro-level of society, (2) at the meso-level of organizations, (3) at the micro-level of individual citizens.

Macro-level: Improving the Livability of Society

Happiness also depends on the quality of the wider society. As we have seen in Table 1.1, there are wide differences in happiness across nations, and these differences are clearly linked to societal qualities, some of which are presented in Table 1.2.

Will further economic growth make us happier? Table 1.2 suggests so, because happiness is strongly correlated with the wealth of the nation. Yet, material affluence appears to be subject to the law of diminishing return, and economic growth yields more happiness in poor nations than in rich nations. This is not to say that economic development does not add to happiness at all in rich nations. Happiness is still on the rise in affluent nations, and it is well possible that this rise is linked to economic growth, directly or indirectly. We simply do not know what the underlying links are, as yet.

Still another reason to keep the economy going is that the "playing" may be as important as the prizes. Happiness is not only found in consumption, it is also found in productive activity. Like most animals, we have an innate need to use our potentials. The biological function of this need is to keep us sharp, in the human case, in particular, to keep the brain in shape. The human species evolved under the conditions of a hunter-gatherer existence that involved a lot of challenge. In today's conditions, as an industrial society, we still need some challenges and most of us find them mainly in our work life. In this perspective, we better not follow Layard's (2005) advice to discourage economic competition, though there is a point in keeping the competition nice and leaving room for other arenas in society.

The data in Table 1.2 do not suggest that a reduction of income differences will add to happiness; the zero-order correlation is close to zero, and when the wealth of the nation is taken into account, we even see a positive effect of income inequality. Though income inequality may be unfair, we can apparently live with it. Likewise, the data do not suggest that happiness can be advanced by increasing the offerings of a welfare state. At first sight, there is some correlation between expenditures for social security and happiness in nations, but the statistical relationship disappears when we take into account that big spending nations tend to be richer. For instance, happiness is fairly high in Sweden, and Sweden is known for its extended welfare state; yet, it is equally high in Iceland, which scores equally high and spends much less on social security (Veenhoven, 2000; Ouweneel, 2002).

The greatest gains seem to be possible in the realms of freedom and justice. Good governance also appears to contribute much to average happiness in nations, irrespective of the political color of the parties in the saddle.

Meso-level: Improving the Livability of Institutions

Another source of happiness is the institutional settings in which we spend most of our time, such as at work or at school. Systematic improvements in those realms will probably add to the average happiness of a nation.

This requires that we know which settings produce the most happiness, for example, determine the kind of schools where pupils enjoy their school years the most. Curiously, little investigation has been done in this field as yet, not even for old age homes. The prime product of such a research would be the number of happy life years. There is a lot of talk about quality of life in institutions, but little research. This is probably because there is little incentive to bother about the happiness of pupils and residents of care homes.

Governments can create an incentive by investigating the happiness output of institutions. Once differences are visible, the market will do its work. For instance, most parents will prefer a school where most children are happy over a school where the majority is not, even if the latter school produces higher grades.

Micro-level: Helping Individuals to Live Happier

Happiness can be furthered at the individual level in three ways by: (1) training art-of-living skills, (2) informing people about the probable outcomes of choices, and (3) improving professional guidance in self-development and life choice. Below, I will expand on these options, since they are particularly relevant for positive psychology.

Training Art-of-Living Skills

Many people think that they would be happier if they had more money or a higher position on the social ladder. However, research shows that these things do not matter very much, at least not in affluent and egalitarian societies. Differences in income and social status explain only some 5% of the differences in Fig. 1.1. Current images about condition for happiness are misleading.

What then does matter for happiness? About 10% of the differences can be attributed to social relations, in particular to a good marriage. Another 10% is due to good or bad luck, probably more so in countries where life is less predictable. Most of the difference appears to be due to personal characteristics; about 30% can be attributed to variation in life ability (Headey & Wearing, 1992). The relative importance of inner strengths should not be surprising if we realize that living conditions are typically very good in modern nations; the better the external conditions, the less they account for differences in happiness. In Paradise, all the difference in happiness will be due to inner competence, neurotics will quarrel with Angels. In Hell, the differences in happiness (if any) will largely be determined by closeness to the fire, because nobody can stand that environment. So the most evident way to advance happiness in modern society is to strengthen life abilities.

Part of these abilities is genetically determined or little alterable for other reasons. Still, there are also capabilities that can be improved through therapy and training. Psychotherapy is now well established in modern nations but still underutilized. There is also an emerging field of training in art of living in line with the new "positive psychology." "Art of living" is the knack of leading a satisfying life, and in particular, the ability to develop a rewarding life style (Veenhoven, 2003). This involves various aptitudes, some of which seems to be susceptible to improvement using training techniques. Four of these aptitudes are: (1) the ability to enjoy, (2) the ability to choose, (3) the ability to keep developing, and (4) the ability to see meaning.

Learning to Enjoy

The ability to take pleasure from life is partly in-born (trait negativity-positivity), but can to some extent be cultivated. Learning to take pleasure from life was part of traditional leisure-class education, which emphasized prestigious pleasures, such as the tasting of exquisite wines and the appreciation of difficult music. Yet, it is also possible to develop an enjoyment of the common things in life, such as eating breakfast or watching the sunset. Training in savoring simple pleasures is part of some religious practices.

Hedonistic enjoyment is valued in present day modern society and figures prominently in advertisements. Yet, techniques that help us to gain the ability to enjoy are underdeveloped. There are no professional enjoyment trainers, at least no trainers aiming at improving our general level of enjoyment. There is professional guidance for specific types of pleasures, such as how to appreciate fine arts, and often the main goal is to sell a particular product.

Still, it would seem possible to develop wider enjoyment training techniques. One way could be to provide training in "attentiveness," possibly using meditation techniques. Another option could be the broadening of one's repertoire of leisure activities, which could link up with expertise in various stimulation programs. A third way could be looking at ways to remove inner barriers to enjoy, which could be linked to clinical treatment of a-hedonie.

Learning to Choose

Happiness depends on also the choices one makes in life and hence also on one's ability to choose. The art of choosing involves several skills.

One such skill is getting to know what the options are. This aptitude can be improved by learning, and this is one of the things we do in consumer education. Expertise in this field can be used for training in the charting of wider life options. Another requirement is an ability to estimate how well the various options would fit one's nature. This requires self-knowledge and that is also something that can be improved, self-insight being a common aim in training and psychotherapy. Once one knows what to choose, there is often a problem of carrying through. This phase requires aptitudes such as perseverance, assertiveness, and creativity, all of which can be strengthened and are, in fact, common objectives in vocational trainings. The next step in the choice process is assessing the outcomes, in terms of the above-mentioned distinction, whether "expected utility" fits "experienced utility." This phase calls for openness to one's feelings and a realistic view on one's overall mood pattern. Training in mood monitoring is a common practice in psychotherapy and could possibly be improved using computer-based techniques of experience sampling.

The problem is not so much to develop such training techniques, but to separate the chaff from the corn. That will require independent effect studies. Once such techniques have been proven to be effective, a market culture will develop.

Learning to Grow

Happiness depends largely on the gratification of basic needs, and an important class of such needs is "growth needs" (Maslow, 1954), also referred to as "functioning needs" or "mastery needs." These needs are not restricted to higher mental functions; they also concern the use and development of the body and senses. In animals, gratification of these needs is largely guided by instinct, but in humans, it requires conscious action. Cultures typically provide standard action patterns for this purpose, such as providing for vocational career scripts or artistic interests, but people must also make choices of their own, in particular in multiple-choice societies. Failure to involve oneself in challenging activities may lead one to diffused discontent or even depression, this, for example, happens regularly after retirement from work. Thus, another art of living is to keep oneself going and developing.

Intervention would also seem possible in this case. Mere information will probably be useful and one can also think of various ways to get people going. Once again training techniques can build on available experience, and in this case, experience in various activation programs. There is already an ample supply of "growth trainings" on the peripheries of psychology, but, as yet, little evidence is available for the effectiveness of such interventions and certainly no proof of long-term effects on happiness.

Helping to See Meaning

Probably, but not certainly, happiness also depends on one seeing meaning in one's life. Though it is not sure that we have an innate need for meaningfulness as such, the idea of it provides at least a sense of coherence. Seeing a meaning in one's life requires that one develops a view of one's life and that one can see worth in it. These mental knacks can also be strengthened, and it is possible that one can also learn to live with the philosophical uncertainties that surround this issue. There is experience on this matter in existential counseling and in practices such as "life reviewing" (Holahan, Holahan, & Wonacott, 1999) and "logo therapy" (Frankl, 1946). As far as I know, the impact of such interventions on happiness has yet to be investigated.

Information: Enabling More Informed Choice

Another way of improving happiness at the individual level is to inform people about the consequences of major choices in life. We have to realize that we live in a "multiple-choice society," in which about 40% of the differences in happiness seems to be due to "intentional activity" (Sheldon & Lyubomirsky, 2004, p. 131). Better informed choices will give rise to greater happiness.

Life choices are for the most part based on expected happiness, for instance, we typically choose a profession we think we will like. Economists call this "expected utility," or "decision utility" and acknowledge that this may differ from later "experienced utility," because decisions are mostly made on the basis of incomplete information. An example of a malinformed choice is the decision to accept a higher paying job that requires more commuting. People typically accept such jobs in the expectation that the extra money will compensate for the travel time, but follow-up research has shown that they are mostly wrong and that happiness tends to go down in such cases (Frey & Stutzer, 2004).

Research of this kind can help people to make more informed choices. Though there is no guarantee that things will work out in the same way for you, it is still useful to know how it has worked out for other people in the recent past. Such research is particularly useful if it concerns similar people. This policy does not involve paternalism; it does not push people into a particular way of life, but it provides them with information for making a well-informed autonomous decision. Paternalism would only be involved if research is manipulated or its results communicated selectively, for instance, if the observed negative effect of parenthood on happiness is disguised (Veenhoven, 2007, World Database of Happiness: Correlational Findings on Happiness and Having Children).

This approach to the furthering of happiness is similar to the current evidence-based health education. As in the case of happiness, we are often not sure about the consequences of life style choices on our health. How much drinking is too much? Is eating raw vegetables really good for your health? We cannot answer such questions on the basis of our own experience, and common wisdom is often wrong. Hence, we increasingly look to the results of scientific studies that provide us with more information, the results of which are disseminated systematically.

As yet, the information basis for such a way of furthering happiness is still small. Although there is a considerable body of research on happiness, this research is typically cross-sectional and does not inform us about cause and effect. What we need is panel data that allows us to follow the effects of life choices over time. Still another problem is that current happiness research deals mainly with things over which we have little control, such as personality and social background. What we need is research into things we can choose, for example, working part time or full time or raising a family or not.

Once such information becomes available, it will quickly be disseminated to the public, through the life style press and the self-help literature. It can also be included in organized health education, broadened to become education for "living well" – happiness education. The problem is not in the dissemination of knowledge but in the production of it.

Professional Life Counseling

If we feel unhealthy, we go to a medical general practitioner, who makes a diagnosis and either prescribes a treatment or refers us to a medical specialist. If we feel unhappy, there is no such generalist. We have to guess about the possible causes ourselves, and on that basis, consult a specialist who may be a psychologist, a marriage counselor, or a lawyer. Professional guidance for a happier life is unavailable as yet. This is a remarkable market failure, given the large number of people who feel they could be happier. The size of the demand is reflected in the booming sales of self-help books and the willingness to pay for things that promise greater happiness, such as cosmetic surgery and second homes. The main reason is probably that the knowledge basis for such a profession is still small and that trust in happiness counseling is undermined by the many snake oil merchants operating in this area.

Still there seems to be a future for professional counseling for a happier life and for related life coaching and trainings. There is demand for such services, but as yet no proper supply. Much can be gained by developing that supply. One of the ways forward is to stimulate the professionalization of current activities in that area, among other things, by following people who use such services to establish what interventions added to happiness or did not. The development of professional life counseling could also profit from the above-advised research into long-term changes in happiness following major life choices.

Do We Need Greater Happiness?

If we *can* create greater happiness for a greater number, *should* we? Several voices say "no." Part of the objections comes from preachers of penitence, who like to see us suffer to clean our sinful souls. Yet, there are also objections from scientists who believe that the pursuit of happiness involves negative effects. One of their qualms is that mass happiness will be achieved at the cost of freedom, and another misgiving is that happy people tend to be passive and uncreative. These notions figure in Huxley's (1932) science fiction novel *Brave New World*, in which happiness for everybody is achieved using genetic manipulations and mind control and where the happy citizens are short-sighted consumer slaves.

Yet, research into the consequences of happiness shows another picture. It appears that happiness fosters activity, creativity, and an open mind. Happy people do better as a spouse and parent. They are also better citizens; they are typically better informed than unhappy compatriots; they involve themselves more in social action, while being more moderate in their political views (Lyubomirsky, King, & Diener, 2005). Still another thing is that happiness lengthens life, the effect of happiness being comparable to smoking or not (Veenhoven, 2008). This evidence on positive effects of happiness fits well with the theory that feeling good works as a "go-signal"; it tells the organism that the situation is OK and it can go ahead. Consequently, happy people "broaden" their behavioral scope and "build" more resources (Fredrickson, 2004).

So, happiness is worth pursuing for its own sake, and for its positive side effects.

References

Bentham, J. (1970). In: J. H. Burns & H. L. A. Hart (Ed.), *An introduction to the principles of morals and legislation*. London: Althone Press (original work published 1789 by London: Payne).

Easterlin, R. A. (1995). Will raising the incomes of all increase the happiness of all? *Journal of Economic Behavior and Organization, 27*, 35–47.

Frankl, V. E. (1946). *De zin van het bestaan, een inleiding tot de logotherapie [The meaning of life, an introduction to logotherapy]* (Nederlandse vertaling 2002). Rotterdam: Donker.

Fredrickson, B. L. (2004). The broaden-and-build theory of positive emotions. *Philosophical Transactions of the Royal Society of London. Series B, Biological Sciences, 359*, 1367–1377.

Frey, B., & Stutzer, A. (2004). *Economic consequences of mispredicting utility*. Working paper, Institute for Empirical Research in Economics, Zürich, Switzerland. Available at: www.crema-research.ch/papers

Headey, B., & Wearing, A. (1992). *Understanding happiness: A theory of subjective well-being*. Melbourne: Longman Cheshire.

Holahan, C. K., Holahan, C. J., & Wonacott, N. L. (1999). Self appraisal, life satisfaction and retrospective life choices across one and three decades. *Psychology and Aging, 14*, 238–244.

Huxley, A. (1932). *Brave new world*. London: Shatto & Windus.

Layard, R. (2005). *Happiness: Lessons of a new science*. New York: Penguin.

Lykken, D. T. (1999). *Happiness: What studies on twins show us about nature, nurture and the happiness set-point*. New York: Golden Books.

Lyubomirsky, S., King, L. A., & Diener, E. (2005). The benefits of frequent positive affect: Does happiness lead to success? *Psychological Bulletin, 131*, 803–855.

Maslow, A. H. (1954). *Motivation and personality*. New York: Harper.

Ouweneel, P. (2002). Social Security and well-being of the unemployed in 42 nations. *Journal of Happiness Studies, 3*, 167–192.

Sheldon, K., & Lyubomirsky, S. (2004). Achieving sustainable new happiness: Prospects, practices and prescriptions. In P. A. Linley & S. Joseph (Eds.), *Positive psychology in practice* (pp. 127–145). Hoboken: Wiley.

Veenhoven, R. (1991). Is happiness relative? *Social Indicators Research, 24*, 1–34.

Veenhoven, R. (1995). The cross national pattern of happiness: Tests of predictions implied in three theories of happiness. *Social Indicators Research, 34*, 33–68.

Veenhoven, R. (2000). Well-being in the welfare state: Level not higher, distribution not more equitable. *Journal of Comparative Policy Analysis, 2*, 91–125.

Veenhoven, R. (2003). Arts of living. *Journal of Happiness Studies, 4*, 373–384.

Veenhoven, R. (2005). Apparent quality of life: How long and happy people live. *Social Indicators Research, 71*, 61–86.

Veenhoven, R. (2007). World Database of Happiness, continuous register of scientific research on subjective enjoyment of life. Erasmus Universiteit Rotterdam: http://worlddatabaseofhappiness.eur.nl.

Veenhoven, R. (2008). Healthy happiness: Effects of happiness on physical health and the consequences for preventive health care. *Journal of Happiness Studies, 9*(3), 449–469.

Veenhoven, R. (2009). How do we assess how happy we are? In A. Dutt & B. Radcliff (Eds.), *Happiness, economics and politics* (pp. 45–69). Northampton: Edward Elger.

Veenhoven, R., & Hagerty, M. (2006). Rising Happiness in nations 1946–2004: A reply to Easterlin. *Social Indicators Research, 77*, 1–16.

Chapter 2
Self-serving Attributional Bias and Hedonic and Eudaimonic Aspects of Well-Being

Pilar Sanjuán, Alejandro Magallares, and Rodolfo Gordillo

The self-enhancement motive is defined as the tendency to see oneself in a positive way (Baumeister, 1998; Taylor & Brown, 1988). Different phenomena can be viewed as ways of self-enhancement. Thus, people recall information about their successes better than their failures; they rate themselves as above average on positive personality traits and abilities and more favorably than they rate their peers based on identical behavioral evidence (Sedikides, Horton, & Gregg, 2007). One of these phenomena is labeled "self-serving attributional bias" (SSAB), which is defined as the tendency of individuals to explain positive situations with *internal* (the cause of positive situations come s from within them), *stable* (the cause of positive situations will continue in the future), and *global* (the cause of positive situations will arise in lots of different areas) causes, and negative situations with *external* (the cause of negative situations comes from someone or something else), *unstable* (the cause of negative situations will not repeat in the future), and *specific* (the cause of the negative situations only arises in that specific situation) causes.

Research has shown that the different ways of self-enhancement, including SSAB, have as goal the protection or enhancement of self-esteem (Campbell & Sedikides, 1999). Due to this fact, some authors consider that this phenomenon would be a universal human motive (Sedikides, Gaertner, & Toguchi, 2003; Sedikides, Gaertner, & Vevea, 2005, 2007). However, research has shown that different ways of self-enhancement depend on cultural aspects and that are only displayed in societies where self-esteem is the best predictor of well-being, that is,

P. Sanjuán (✉) • R. Gordillo
Department of Personality Psychology, School of Psychology,
Universidad Nacional de Educación a Distancia (UNED), Madrid, Spain
e-mail: psanjuan@psi.uned.es

A. Magallares
Department of Social Psychology, School of Psychology,
Universidad Nacional de Educación a Distancia (UNED), Madrid, Spain

I. Brdar (ed.), *The Human Pursuit of Well-Being: A Cultural Approach*,
DOI 10.1007/978-94-007-1375-8_2, © Springer Science+Business Media B.V. 2011

in individualistic cultures like the United States, Canada, or Western Europe (Hamamura & Heine, 2008; Heine, Kitayama, & Hamamura, 2007; Heine, Lehman, Markus, & Kitayama, 1999; Kitayama, Takagi, & Matsumoto, 1995; Markus & Kitayama, 1991). Specifically, SSAB has been found in samples from the United States and other Western countries, such as Canada or Australia (Heine, 2005; Heine & Hamamura, 2007; Mezulis, Abramson, Hyde, & Hankin, 2004), while this bias is reversed, absent, or strongly attenuated in samples from Asian societies like Japan (Heine et al., 1999; Kitayama, et al., 1995; Mezulis et al., 2004), China (Anderson, 1999), or India (Pal, 2007).

Cultural psychologists have suggested that the protection of self-esteem would be only an important goal in individualistic cultures since these cultures fundamentally value competent and successful people, and individualistic people define themselves by the internal traits that they perceive as changeless. Thus, perceiving one's self in a positive way is an important motivation, since one would consider these characteristics impossible to change (Heine et al., 2001). The self-perceptions of individualistic people would tend to be biased toward a positive view of self, and they would view themselves in a manner consistent with their culture (Heine & Hamamura, 2007; Heine et al., 1999; Markus & Kitayama, 1991).

Some studies have also found that SSAB is associated with psychological well-being (Koenig, 1997; Wallbridge, 1997), while the absence of SSAB or even a reversed SSAB has been associated with psychological distress (Sweeney, Anderson, & Bailey, 1986) and psychopathologies, such as depression (Alloy, Just, & Panzarella, 1997; Mezulis et al., 2004; Morris, 2007), anxiety (Fresco, Alloy, & Reilly-Harrington, 2006; Mezulis et al., 2004) or schizophrenia (Moore et al., 2006; Sanjuán, Fraguas, Magallares, & Merchán-Naranjo, 2009).

Actually, the studies that have associated SSAB and well-being, summarized above, have focused on negative aspects of well-being. Thus, what these studies have revealed is an inverse relationship between SSAB and negative symptoms, such as depressive symptoms. However, well-being is not the absence of mental illness or negative symptoms. In fact, it has been shown that positive and negative aspects of psychological well-being are two related but also independent constructs (Huppert & Whittington, 2003; Karademas, 2007).

In this way, if only negative aspects of well-being are evaluated, the conclusions would probably be biased, since a person not being depressed (or anxious) does not mean that this person is satisfied or happy. Focusing on the study of the positive aspects of human functioning, and not only in the absence of negative ones, is in line with the principles of positive psychology. From positive psychology approach arises the understanding of the positive aspects of human functioning interests by themselves, since it is considered that an effective psychological functioning is more than not malfunction (Seligman & Csikszentmihalyi, 2000; Seligman, Steen, Park, & Peterson, 2005).

Indeed, the well-being is a complex construct which includes different aspects. According to Ryan and Deci (2001, 2002), there are two perspectives in the study of well-being, which can be labeled as hedonism and eudaimonism, and which reflect different aspects of well-being. Hedonistic approach defines well-being as happiness, which would be attained by the maximization of pleasure and minimization of displeasure. Most of hedonic psychologists have used measures of subjective well-being, which have two components: a cognitive evaluation of the satisfaction with one's life as a whole and an affective component that refers to predominance of positive over negative affect (or affect balance; Diener, 2000).

On the eudaimonic view, well-being is not simply the attainment of pleasure, but also the realization of one's true potential or the congruence between the goals that the person pursues and his/her true self (or daimon). The measures used by eudaimonic psychologists, sometimes labeled psychological well-being, include subjective evaluations of effective psychological functioning. Ryff's (1989) model of psychological well-being, which has an eudaimonic perspective, conceives well-being as a multidimensional construct made up of life attitudes such as self-acceptance, positive relation with others, autonomy, environmental mastery, purpose in life, and personal growth.

Research has revealed that hedonic and eudaimonic aspects of well-being are strongly interrelated; however, they are also distinguishable, since they are differentially related to various criteria (Waterman, Schwartz, & Conti, 2008). Thus, it would be advisable to consider well-being as a multidimensional construct which includes both hedonic and eudaimonic aspects (Ryan & Deci, 2001).

The main goal of the current research was to study the relationships between SSAB and positive aspects of well-being, something which has not been studied up till now. Specifically, we studied SSAB by examining individuals' explanatory styles for positive and negative situations, and we assessed positive hedonic and eudaimonic aspects of well-being in a Spanish sample.

In the past, Spain has been considered a collectivist culture. However, over the past decades, there have been different cultural and economic changes in Spain, and the current characteristics of the Spanish society do not fit those of collectivist cultures (Triandis, 2000, 2001). Thus, the economy is no longer based on agriculture, work distribution is not interdependent, and the exposure to mass media of other individualistic societies is very high. Likewise, Spanish society fundamentally values competent and successful people.

These observations were supported by a recent study (Kuppens, Realo, & Diener, 2008) that has assessed the individualism-collectivism cultural dimension, and has revealed that Spain is an individualistic society.

According to these arguments, we expected that the current sample of Spanish people would display SSAB. Moreover, we also expected to find positive or direct relationships between SSAB and positive aspects of well-being.

On the other hand, the average value of SSAB may be positive, which would show that, overall, people have displayed this bias. But, since SSAB is also a dimensional variable, the intensity with which each individual displays the bias may vary. The cultural psychology has also reported this fact, pointing out that individuals vary in the degree to which they conform to the prevailing values of their culture (Triandis & Suh, 2002). Therefore, we also expected that the individuals that displayed SSAB would show higher scores on different measures of well-being than individuals that did not display SSAB.

Method

Participants

Two hundred and fifty-five individuals (114 male and 141 female, mean age 36.46 years, SD 10.83, and range from 18 to 60) participated in the study. Participants were recruited from different workplaces in various urban areas of the Spanish territory. They were included if they had no past or current history of psychological disorders. On average, the participants had completed 14 years of education. Twenty (7.84%) had finished elementary school, 108 (42.35%) had finished high school, and 127 (49.80%) were holders of a university degree.

Measures

All the subjects who agreed to participate in the study were asked to complete the following four questionnaires:

Attributional Style Questionnaire (ASQ; Peterson et al., 1982; Spanish version: Sanjuán & Magallares, 2006). The ASQ is a self-report instrument containing 12 hypothetical events: six negative and six positive. For each situation, subjects decide what they believe would be the major cause of the event, and they indicate on three seven-point scales the extent to which they would attribute these events to internal, stable, and global causes. A rating of "1" on the scales indicates an external (totally due to other people or circumstances), unstable (the cause will never again be present), and specific (the cause influences just this particular situation) attribution, while, on the other extreme, a "7" reflects an internal (totally due to me), stable (the cause will always be present), and global (the cause influences all situations in my life) attribution.

Two composite scores for positive and negative events were calculated, which respectively correspond to attributional style for positive and negative situations. These scores were computed by averaging items of positive or negative situations, respectively. Alpha coefficients of current sample for composite positive and negative were .83 and .80, respectively.

A self-serving attributional score is calculated by subtracting attributions for negative outcomes from attributions for positive outcomes. This score provides an index of the direction or valence (negative or positive) of bias as well as its magnitude. A positive score reflects a SSAB (or stronger attributions for positive than for negative outcomes), a negative score reflects a self-derogating bias (or weaker attributions for positive than for negative outcomes), and a score of 0 reflects even-handedness.

Positive and Negative Affect Schedule (PANAS; Watson, Clark, & Tellegen, 1988; Spanish version: Sandin et al., 1999). The PANAS is a 20-item measure that evaluates two dimensions: positive affect (10 items) and negative affect (10 items). The response scale was a five-point Likert-type. Respondents were asked to report how they usually felt. Positive and negative affect scores were computed by averaging items of positive or negative affect scales, respectively. In our study, alpha coefficient was .85 for the positive affect subscale and .89 for the negative affect subscale. The negative affect score was subtracted from the positive affect score to obtain a measure of affect balance. Thus, a positive score reflects predominance of positive over negative affect, while a negative score reflects predominance of negative over positive affect.

Satisfaction with Life Scale (SWLS; Pavot & Diener, 1993; Spanish version: Cabañero et al., 2004). The SWLS is a five-item measure of global life satisfaction, or a person's satisfaction with life as a whole, rather than any specific domain. Respondents are asked to rate the extent of their agreement to these items across a seven-point Likert-type scale ranging from 0 (strongly disagree) to 6 (strongly agree). The score was computed by averaging the five items of scale. Higher scores on the SWLS reflect greater life satisfaction. In the current sample, the alpha coefficient was .88.

Scales of Psychological Well-Being (SPWB; Ryff, 1989; Spanish version: Díaz et al. 2006). The SPWB is a 29-item self-report instrument which is based on six dimensions that point to different aspects of positive psychological functioning: self-acceptance (four items), positive relations with others (five items), autonomy (six items), environmental mastery (five items), purpose in life (five items), and personal growth (four items). Items are scored on a seven-point scale ranging from 0 (strongly disagree) to 6 (strongly agree).

Six scores were computed, one for each dimension, by averaging the corresponding items for each of these dimensions. Higher scores on different dimensions or subscales reflect greater positive psychological functioning. Alpha coefficients obtained for the present study were: .81 for self-acceptance, .79 for positive relations with others, .68 for autonomy, .71 for environmental mastery, .73 for purpose in life, and .73 for personal growth.

Results

Since no differences were found on the analyzed variables (SSAB, affect balance, satisfaction with life, self-acceptance, positive relations with others, autonomy, environmental mastery, purpose in life, and personal growth) either in terms of gender or age, all data were analyzed together. Table 2.1 shows descriptive statistics of the analyzed variables.

The positive valence of the mean on SSAB shows that, overall, the current sample of Spanish individuals displayed the self-serving bias.

In order to analyze the relationships between SSAB and different aspects of well-being, Pearson's correlations were calculated. As can be seen in Table 2.1, these correlations show that SSAB is directly and significantly associated with all the positive hedonic and eudaimonic aspects of well-being.

Table 2.1 Descriptive data for hedonic and eudaimonic measures of well-being and their correlations with self-serving attributional bias (SSAB)

	Mean	SD	*r*
SSAB	1.08	0.96	–
Affect balance	1.39	1.03	.41***
Satisfaction with life	3.88	1.16	.29***
Self-acceptance	4.19	0.99	.38***
Positive relation with others	4.28	1.12	.23***
Autonomy	4.01	0.92	.32***
Environmental mastery	4.06	0.99	.38***
Purpose in life	4.19	1.04	.22***
Personal growth	4.69	0.94	.25***

***$p<.001$

Group Differences

In order to further analyze the relationships between SSAB and well-being, we also wanted to know whether there were differences in well-being variables among individuals who displayed or did not display SSAB. Only 27 individuals had scores less than or equal to zero on SSAB, that is, only 10.59% of people did not display this bias.

Since the groups with and without SSAB had no equivalent sizes, we decided to select individuals with more extreme scores. Thus, the groups of participants were formed by categorizing those individuals with the higher and lower scores on SSAB (25% above and 25% below) as groups with and without SSAB, respectively. Comparisons between these two groups on all the well-being variables were made by means of the Student's *t*-test. Cohen's *ds* (Cohen, 1988) were also calculated as indices of effect size. The effect sizes are indices that measure the magnitude of an effect. These indices assess the strength of the difference between two means. Cohen (1988) defined *d* as the difference between means divided by standard deviation of either group. Unlike significance test, these indices are standardized and are independent of sample size ($d \geq .2$ is considered medium effect size and $d \geq .8$ large effect size; Cohen, 1988).

According to previous criterion, 125 individuals were selected (with-SSAB group $n=63$; and without-SSAB group $n=62$). These groups were correctly formed, given that the mean scores on classification variable (SSAB score) were significantly different between groups, with-SSAB group = 2.41, ranging from 1.67 to 4.11, *vs.* without-SSAB group = 0, ranging from –0.89 to 0.33 ($t_{123}=28.18$, $p<.001$; $d=5.08$).

Table 2.2 shows means and standard deviations by groups, as well as summarized results of analyses (*t* values) and effect sizes (d values). As can be seen, these analyses revealed statistically significant differences for all dependent variables, indicating that with-SSAB group scored on all the well-being variables higher than without-SSAB group.

Table 2.2 Differences between SSAB groups on hedonic and eudaimonic measures of well-being

		Self-serving attributional bias			
		With-SSAB	Without-SSAB		
Well-being measure		$N=63$	$N=62$	t_{123}	d
Satisfaction with life	M	4.33	3.59	3.90***	.69
	SD	1.02	1.11		
Affect balance	M	1.88	0.85	5.57***	1.00
	SD	0.95	1.1		
Self-acceptance	M	4.68	3.77	5.22***	.99
	SD	0.80	1.03		
Positive relation with others	M	4.55	3.94	3.18**	.58
	SD	1.03	1.08		
Autonomy	M	4.38	3.65	4.73***	.86
	SD	0.80	0.90		
Environmental mastery	M	4.51	3.64	5.01***	.93
	SD	0.81	1.04		
Purpose in life	M	4.43	3.9	3.09**	.55
	SD	0.88	1.04		
Personal growth	M	5.06	4.42	3.37***	.69
	SD	0.87	0.98		

Note: *SSAB* Self-serving attributional bias, *d* effect size
$^{**}p<.01$; $^{***}p<.001$

Discussion

The main goal of the present study was to analyze the relationships between SSAB and positive hedonic and eudaimonic aspects of well-being in a Spanish sample. Current results allow us to confirm that most Spanish people display SSAB and also allow us to show that this bias is related to positive aspects of well-being. Specifically, on one hand, we have found positive correlations between SSAB and hedonic and eudaimonic aspects of well-being, and the other hand, we have found that people that display SSAB score on all the positive aspects of well-being higher than people that do not display SSAB.

The most relevant contribution of this study is to show, for the first time, that SSAB is not only associated with an absence of negative symptoms, but also with satisfaction with life, predominance of positive affect and positive life attitudes such as self-acceptance, positive relation with others, autonomy, environmental mastery, purpose in life and personal growth. Although it is required that these findings be confirmed in subsequent studies, these results seem to suggest that SSAB is an adaptive feature of human cognition which would have a protective role for mental health. Since SSAB is a relevant predictor of positive aspects of well-being, it should be included in any program that seeks promotion of psychological well-being.

It could be said that different ways of self-enhancement motive, including SSAB, serve to protect the individual against emotional distress. However, further research is needed to deepen the understanding of the relationship between this motive and well-being. We think this relationship depends on the magnitude of the self-enhancement displayed. When self-enhancement biases are not too extreme, it would be normally associated with adaptation. However, an excessive self-enhancement bias would be associated with different experiences that produce long-term emotional distress. Thus, since modesty is generally valued, people with inflated self-view could be socially rejected. In the same way, people who excessively self-enhance can be prone to feelings of invulnerability that can lead to the realization of risk behaviors. Moreover, people with excessive self-enhancement could also be prone to aggression when their feelings of self-worth are threatened.

Up till now, little attention has been paid to SSAB. However, we think that is a relevant issue, which needs to be investigated in depth. The possible complex relationship that this bias could have with psychological well-being has already been mentioned above. In addition, the study of this bias provides also an alternative approach to analyze the combined effects of attributional styles for negative and positive situations. Both styles have been studied separately, and it has been shown that each of them is a powerful predictor of well-being.

On one hand, attributional style research has revealed that positive attributional style, or tendency to explain negative situations through external, unstable, and specific causes, is associated with a variety of wellness-relevant outcomes, from different aspects of psychological well-being (Abramson et al., 2002; Alloy et al., 2006; Sanjuán, 2007; Sweeney et al., 1986) to physical health (Buchanan, 1995; Peterson, 1995; Peterson & Bossio, 2001).

On the other hand, with respect to attributional style for positive situations, although less studies have been conducted than for the attributional style for negative situations, these have also shown that the tendency to explain good results with internal, stable, and global causes, which has begun to be labeled as *enhancing explanatory style*, is related to work success, psychological well-being, and high self-esteem (Cheng & Furnham, 2001, 2003; Corr & Gray, 1996).

However, attributional style research has not paid enough attention to the study of the interactive or synergic effects between attributional styles for negative and positive situations. We believe that studying the two attributional styles together can be a very fruitful line of research. In fact, in a recent study, we have found that the interaction between attributional style for negative and positive situations can predict psychological well-being better than each of attributional styles separately (Sanjuán, Pérez, Rueda, & Ruiz, 2008). It is necessary that these results can be corroborated, and, as we indicated above, through the study of SSAB, it is possible to analyze the combined effect of both attributional styles.

This study was subject to some limitations that deserve mention. First, we use self-reports, which are likely to be distorted. It would be necessary for future studies to analyze the relationships between the different manifestations of self-enhancement and well-being, using not only self-reports, but also more objective criteria. The measure of self-enhancement is, in fact, the measure of a bias, given that it reflects that people report more internal, stable, and global attributions for positive situations than for negative ones. However, to better understand the links between

SSAB and well-being, it would be advisable to use accurate measures of well-being which reflect its actual level. A recent study has shown that when well-being is evaluated by alternative measures to self-reports, the relationships between self-enhancement and well-being remain (Colvin & Griffo, 2008), but it would be necessary to corroborate these results.

Second, we analyze the relationships between SSAB and well-being with a cross-sectional study. However, only longitudinal studies can provide insight into how SSAB interacts with different stressful experiences and whether SSAB is a relevant predictor of well-being.

Third, although the sample is heterogeneous at educational level, the sample size has not allowed us to analyze possible differences in SSAB and well-being in relation to that variable. However, it is possible that educational level and other related variables like income level and socio-economic status can affect well-being variables (Deaton, 2008).

Despite these limitations, the study provides new data with potential applications in relation to the promotion of well-being and the prevention of psychological distress.

References

Abramson, L. Y., Alloy, L., Hogan, M., Whitehouse, W., Donovan, P., Rose, D., et al. (2002). Cognitive vulnerability to depression: Theory and evidence. In R. L. Leahy & E. T. Dowd (Eds.), *Clinical advances in cognitive psychotherapy: Theory and applications* (pp. 75–92). New York: Springer.

Alloy, L. B., Abramson, L. Y., Whitehouse, W. G., Hogan, M. E., Panzarella, C., & Rose, D. T. (2006). Prospective incidence of first onsets and recurrences of depression in individuals at high and low cognitive risk for depression. *Journal of Abnormal Psychology, 115*(1), 145–156.

Alloy, L. B., Just, N., & Panzarella, C. (1997). Attributional style, daily life events, and hopelessness depression: Subtype validation by prospective variability and specificity of symptoms. *Cognitive Therapy and Research, 21*, 321–344.

Anderson, C. (1999). Attributional style, depression, and loneliness: A cross-cultural comparison of American and Chinese students. *Personality and Social Psychology Bulletin, 25*, 482–499.

Baumeister, R. F. (1998). The self. In D. T. Gilbert, S. T. Fiske, & G. Lindzey (Eds.), *The handbook of social psychology* (pp. 680–740). New York: McGraw-Hill.

Buchanan, G. M. (1995). Explanatory style and coronary heart disease. In G. M. Buchanan & M. E. P. Seligman (Eds.), *Explanatory style* (pp. 225–232). Hillsdale, NJ: Lawrence Erlbaum Associates.

Cabañero, M. J., Richart, M., Cabrero, J., Orts, M. I., Reig, A., & Tosal, B. (2004). Reliability and validity of satisfaction with life scale in a sample of pregnant women. *Psicothema, 16*, 448–455.

Campbell, K., & Sedikides, C. (1999). Self-threat magnifies the self-serving bias: A meta-analytic integration. *Review of General Psychology, 3*, 23–43.

Cheng, H., & Furnham, A. (2001). Attributional style and personality as predictors of happiness and mental health. *Journal of Happiness Studies, 2*, 307–327.

Cheng, H., & Furnham, A. (2003). Attributional style and self-esteem as predictors of psychological well-being. *Counselling Psychology Quarterly, 16*, 121–130.

Cohen, J. (1988). *Statistical power analysis for the behavioral sciences*. Hillsdale, NY: Lawrence Erlbaum Associates.
Colvin, C., & Griffo, R. (2008). On the psychological costs of self-enhancement. In E. Chang (Ed.), *Self-criticism and self-enhancement: Theory, research, and clinical implications* (pp. 123–140). Washington: American Psychological Association.
Corr, P. J., & Gray, J. A. (1996). Attributional style as a personality factor in insurance sales performance in the UK. *Journal of Occupational and Organizational Psychology, 69*, 83–87.
Deaton, A. (2008). Income, health, and well-being around the world: Evidence from the Gallup World Poll. *The Journal of Economic Perspectives, 22*, 53–72.
Díaz, D., Rodríguez-Carvajal, R., Blanco, A., Moreno-Jiménez, B., Gallardo, I., Valle, C., et al. (2006). Spanish adaptation of Ryff's scales of psychological well-being. *Psicothema, 18*, 572–577.
Diener, E. (2000). Subjective well-being: The science of happiness and proposal for a national index. *American Psychologist, 55*, 34–43.
Fresco, D. M., Alloy, L. B., & Reilly-Harrington, N. (2006). Association of attributional style for negative and positive events and the occurrence of life events with depression and anxiety. *Journal of Social and Clinical Psychology, 25*, 1140–1159.
Hamamura, T., & Heine, S. (2008). The role of self-criticism in self-improvement and face maintenance among Japanese. In E. Chang (Ed.), *Self-criticism and self-enhancement: Theory, research, and clinical implications* (pp. 105–122). Washington: American Psychological Association.
Heine, S. (2005). Where is the evidence for pancultural self-enhancement? A reply to Sedikides, Gaertner, and Toguchi (2003). *Journal of Personality and Social Psychology, 89*, 531–538.
Heine, S., & Hamamura, T. (2007). In search of East Asian self-enhancement. *Personality and Social Psychology Review, 11*, 4–27.
Heine, S., Kitayama, S., & Hamamura, T. (2007). Which studies test whether self-enhancement is pancultural? Reply to Sedikides, Gaertner, and Vevea, 2007. *Asian Journal of Social Psychology, 10*, 198–200.
Heine, S. J., Kitayama, S., Lehman, D. R., Takata, T., Ide, E., Leung, C., et al. (2001). Divergent consequences of success and failure in Japan and North America: An investigation of self-improving motivations and malleable selves. *Journal of Personality and Social Psychology, 81*, 599–615.
Heine, S., Lehman, D., Markus, H., & Kitayama, S. (1999). Is there a universal need for positive self-regard? *Psychological Review, 106*, 766–794.
Huppert, F., & Whittington, J. (2003). Evidence for the independence of positive and negative well-being: Implications for quality of life assessment. *British Journal of Health Psychology, 8*, 107–122.
Karademas, E. (2007). Positive and negative aspects of well-being: Common and specific predictors. *Personality and Individual Differences, 43*, 277–287.
Kitayama, S., Takagi, H., & Matsumoto, H. (1995). Causal attribution of success and failure: Cultural psychology of the Japanese self. *Japanese Psychological Review, 38*, 247–280.
Koenig, L. (1997). Depression and the cultural context of the self-serving bias. In U. Neisser & D. Jopling (Eds.), *The conceptual self in context: Culture, experience, self-understanding* (pp. 62–74). New York: Cambridge University Press.
Kuppens, P., Realo, A., & Diener, E. (2008). The role of positive and negative emotions in life satisfaction judgment across nations. *Journal of Personality and Social Psychology, 95*, 66–75.
Markus, H., & Kitayama, S. (1991). Culture and self: Implications for cognition, emotion, and motivation. *Psychological Review, 98*, 224–253.
Mezulis, A., Abramson, L. Y., Hyde, J., & Hankin, B. (2004). Is there a universal positivity bias in attributions? A meta-analytic review of individual, developmental, and cultural differences in the self-serving attributional bias. *Psychological Bulletin, 130*, 711747.
Moore, R., Blackwood, N., Corcoran, R., Rowse, G., Kinderman, P., Bentall, R., et al. (2006). Misunderstanding the intentions of others: An exploratory study of the cognitive etiology of

persecutory delusions in very late-onset schizophrenia-like psychosis. *The American Journal of Geriatric Psychiatry, 14*(5), 410–418.
Morris, S. (2007). Attributional biases in subclinical depression: A schema-based account. *Clinical Psychology & Psychotherapy, 14*, 32–47.
Pal, G. (2007). Is there a universal self-serving attribution bias? *Psychological Studies, 52*, 85–89.
Pavot, W., & Diener, E. (1993). Review of the satisfaction with life scale. *Psychological Assessment, 5*, 164–172.
Peterson, C. (1995). Explanatory style and health. In G. M. Buchanan & M. E. P. Seligman (Eds.), *Explanatory style* (pp. 233–2246). Hillsdale, NJ: Lawrence Erlbaum Associates.
Peterson, C., & Bossio, L. M. (2001). Optimism and physical well-being. In E. C. Chang (Ed.), *Optimism and pessimism: Implications for theory, research, and practice* (pp. 127–145). Washington, DC: American Psychological Association.
Peterson, C., Semmel, A., Baeyer, C., Abramson, L. Y., Metalsky, G. I., & Seligman, M. E. P. (1982). The attributional style questionnaire. *Cognitive Therapy and Research, 6*, 287–300.
Ryan, R., & Deci, E. (2001). On happiness and human potentials: A review of research on hedonic and eudaimonic well-being. *Annual Review of Psychology, 52*, 141–166.
Ryan, R., & Deci, E. (2002). An overview of self-determination theory: An organismic-dialectical perspective. In E. Deci & R. Ryan (Eds.), *Handbook of self-determination research* (pp. 3–33). Rochester, NY: The University of Rochester Press.
Ryff, C. (1989). Beyond Ponce de León and life satisfaction: New directions in quest of successful aging. *International Journal of Behavioral Development, 12*, 35–55.
Sandin, B., Chorot, P., Lostao, L., Joiner, T. E., Santed, M. A., & Valiente, R. M. (1999). Positive and Negative Affect Scales (PANAS): Factorial validity and cross-cultural convergence. *Psicothema, 11*, 37–51.
Sanjuán, P. (2007). Explanatory styles, psychological well-being and health. *Ansiedad y Estrés, 13*, 203–214.
Sanjuán, P., Fraguas, D., Magallares, A., & Merchán-Naranjo, J. (2009). Depressive symptomatology and attributional style in patients with schizophrenia. *Clinical Schizophrenia and Related Psychoses, 3*, 31–38.
Sanjuán, P., & Magallares, A. (2006). The relationship between dispositional optimism and attributional style and their predictive power in a longitudinal study. *Revista de Psicología General y Aplicada, 59*, 71–89.
Sanjuán, P., Pérez, A., Rueda, B., & Ruiz, M. A. (2008). Interactive effects of attributional styles for positive and negative events on psychological distress. *Personality and Individual Differences, 45*, 187–190.
Sedikides, C., Gaertner, L., & Toguchi, Y. (2003). Pancultural self-enhancement. *Journal of Personality and Social Psychology, 84*, 60–79.
Sedikides, C., Gaertner, L., & Vevea, J. (2005). Pancultural self-enhancement reloaded: A meta-analytic reply to Heine (2005). *Journal of Personality and Social Psychology, 89*, 539–551.
Sedikides, C., Gaertner, L., & Vevea, J. (2007). Evaluating the evidence for pancultural self-enhancement. *Asian Journal of Social Psychology, 10*, 201–203.
Sedikides, C., Horton, R., & Gregg, A. (2007). The way's the limit: Curtailing self-enhancement with explanatory introspection. *Journal of Personality, 75*, 783–824.
Seligman, M. E. P., & Csikszentmihalyi, M. (2000). Positive psychology: An introduction. *American Psychologist, 55*, 5–14.
Seligman, M. E. P., Steen, T. A., Park, N., & Peterson, C. (2005). Positive psychology progress: Empirical validation of interventions. *American Psychologist, 60*, 410–421.
Sweeney, P. D., Anderson, K., & Bailey, S. (1986). Attributional style in depression: A meta-analytic review. *Journal of Personality and Social Psychology, 50*, 974–991.
Taylor, S. E., & Brown, J. D. (1988). Illusions and well-being: A social psychological perspective on mental health. *Psychological Bulletin, 103*, 193–210.
Triandis, H. C. (2000). Culture and conflict. *International Journal of Psychology, 35*, 145–152.

Triandis, H. C. (2001). Individualism-Collectivism and personality. *Journal of Personality, 69*, 907–924.
Triandis, H. C., & Suh, E. M. (2002). Cultural influences on personality. *Annual Review of Psychology, 53*, 133–160.
Wallbridge, H. (1997). Self-enhancing illusion and mental health: A longitudinal panel latent-variable structural equation model. *Dissertation Abstract International, 57*(10-B), 6638.
Waterman, A. S., Schwartz, S. J., & Conti, R. (2008). The implications of two conceptions of happiness (hedonic enjoyment and eudaimonia) for the understanding of intrinsic motivation. *Journal of Happiness Studies, 9*, 41–79.
Watson, D., Clark, L. A., & Tellegen, A. (1988). Development and validation of brief measures of positive and negative affect. *Journal of Personality and Social Psychology, 54*, 1063–1070.

Chapter 3
Affect Specificity as Indicators of National Well-Being: Representative Sample of Croatia*

Zvjezdana Prizmić-Larsen, Ljiljana Kaliterna Lipovčan, and Tihana Brkljačić

Growing evidence suggests that besides the economic indicators, subjective well-being should also be taken into account when measuring national welfare (Deaton, 2008; Diener, Kesebir, & Lucas, 2008; Diener & Seligman, 2004; Kahneman, Krueger, Schkade, Schwarz, & Stone, 2004). Evaluating national well-being can help policy makers by giving them information about domains where quality of life needs to be improved and about possible side effects of implemented measures (Diener et al., 2008; Lyubomirsky, King, & Diener, 2005). As such, they can complement existing economic indicators of national welfare in determining the developmental progress of the nation.

Measuring population well-being and examining the impact of individual well-being on the wealth of society are increasing in countries around the world and in some instances become a standard follow-up procedure (Bonini, 2008; Deaton, 2008; Selim, 2008). For example, Gallup started gathering, systematically, data on many aspects of respondents' well-being and their behaviors from 132 countries worldwide, where the samples are nationally representative (Deaton, 2008). This makes opportunity for cross-country comparisons. Many national and international surveys are using measures that allow the comparison of well-being across different nations, subpopulations, regions, and other groups of interest (Bonini, 2008; Kaliterna Lipovčan & Prizmić-Larsen, 2006a, 2006b; 2007; Selim, 2008).

Researchers distinguish between cognitive and affective components of well-being (Diener, 2006; Kuppens, Realo, & Diener, 2008). The cognitive component

*This research was conducted as a part of a project "Development of National Indicators of Quality of Life" funded by the grant from the Ministry of Science, Education and Sport of the Republic of Croatia.

Z. Prizmić-Larsen (✉)
Washington University in St. Louis, St. Louis, USA
e-mail: zprizmic@artsci.wustl.edu

L.K. Lipovčan • T. Brkljačić
Institute of Social Sciences Ivo Pilar, Zagreb, Croatia

I. Brdar (ed.), *The Human Pursuit of Well-Being: A Cultural Approach*,
DOI 10.1007/978-94-007-1375-8_3, © Springer Science+Business Media B.V. 2011

refers to people's subjective evaluation of their life circumstances, while the affective component refers to the balance of positive and negative affective states experienced over time. Researches show that positive and negative affect should be measured separately since they are relatively independent constructs displaying different relationships with predictor variables (Huppert & Whittington, 2003; Lucas, Diener, & Suh, 1996). For example, Huppert and Whittington (2003) found that unemployment was strongly related to lack of positive affect and weakly to negative affect, while social support was strongly related to negative affect and weakly to positive affect.

Regarding the ways of measuring well-being, Kahneman and Krueger (2006) support the distinction between "experienced utility," which is the way people feel about an experience in real time, and "remembered utility," which refers to the way people remember their experience after it is over. They pointed out the differences between the measures which elicit a global evaluation of one's life and the measures of experienced affect or happiness reported in real time (Kahneman, Krueger, Schkade, Schwarz, & Stone, 2006). Depending on the purpose of the research, well-being indicators vary from evaluative assessments of global life satisfaction and specific life domains satisfaction to momentary or time-related assessments of subjective experience (Diener, 2006; Kahneman & Krueger, 2006; Kahneman et al., 2006; Kuppens et al., 2008).

The predictors of well-being have been researched widely, as well as the factors associated with it (Diener and Seligman, 2004; Oishi, Diener, Lucas, & Suh, 1999). The links between well-being measures and factors such as income, health, marital status, age, sex, job moral, and education have been demonstrated (for review see Diener and Seligman, 2004; Diener, Suh, Lucas, & Smith, 1999; Dolan, Peasgood, & White, 2008). In recent years, the research questions about how human behavior shapes and influences positive growth in society are also of interest to other disciplines. For instance, behavioral economics, which incorporates well-being indicators with existing economic ones, connect two discipline, psychology and economics, to investigate psychological aspects of different economic activity (Hobcraft, 2006; Kahneman & Krueger, 2006).

Besides the widely used well-being measures, such as happiness and life satisfaction, which represent hedonic well-being, the importance of eudaimonic well-being, which refers to positive psychological and social functioning in life and human potential, is also emphasized (Diener et al., 1999; Keyes, Shmotkin, & Ryff, 2002). Psychological well-being is tapping into areas of personal growth and development, feelings of respect and reward, while social well-being is concerned with quality of a person's relationship with other people, the community, and feeling of social trust (Deci & Ryan, 2008; Keyes et al., 2002; Ryan & Deci, 2001).

The main goal of our study was to examine different life domains as predictors of evaluative and experiential measures of well-being on the nationally representative sample. The evaluative assessments of life satisfaction and assessment of six emotions (two positive and four negative) experienced over the past month were used as well-being measures. We examined their correlates with different variables covering the physical, social, and psychological domains.

Method

Subjects

Subjects were a representative sample of 1,129 Croatian citizens recruited as a part of a public opinion research project (November 2007). Median age was 49 years (range 18–95 years). Women made up 56% of the sample and men 44%.

In terms of household monthly income, 17% reported to have less than 137 Euros[1] per family member, 33% had between 137 and 273 Euros, 34% had between 273 and 546 Euros, and 16% reported to have more than 546 Euros per family member.

Procedure

The data were obtained from the national survey on public opinion conducted in November 2007 in Croatia. The survey was carried out by in-person interviews in the respondents' home. Interviews were done by trained persons who attended training sessions on the use of the questionnaire and procedures. The Troldahl–Carter method of selecting adult respondents within households was used to achieve a balance of males and females, younger and older adults in the sample. The respondents were told that their responses were anonymous.

Measures

Well-Being Variables

As evaluative assessment measures of well-being, we used measures of life satisfaction. As experiential measures of well-being, we measured specific emotions experienced over the past month.

Life satisfaction. As a measure of global life satisfaction, one-item life satisfaction measure was used. Subjects rated how much they were satisfied with their life as a whole using an 11-point scale, where 0 was "totally unsatisfied" and 10 was "totally satisfied."

Specific emotions. The ratings of specific emotions were obtained by asking subjects about their emotions over the past month. They reported how often they experienced two positive (i.e., happy and satisfied) and four negative emotions

[1]The income was calculated in Euro based on currency rate of November 2007 (1 Euro = 7.32 Croatian Kuna).

(i.e., sad, angry, depressed, and stressed) over the past month using the seven-point scale where 1 was "almost never" and 7 was "almost always."

Life Domains Variables

As predictors of well-being, various measures representing different domains such as physical domain (i.e., health), social domain (i.e., social and family support, trust and fairness) and psychological domain (i.e., learning, respect, recognition and spirituality) were included.

Physical domain. Perceived health was measured with one item "In general, how would you describe your health?" on the scale of 1 as "very poor"and 5 as "excellent."

Social domain. Social and family support questions covered aspects such as the frequency of seeing friends, receiving support from the community, and family support. Question concerning *seeing friends* asked about the frequency of meeting friends or work colleagues socially and rated it on a seven-point scale from 1 as "never" to 7 as "everyday." *Receiving support* was assessed by asking subjects if they thought that people in a community help one another and rated it on a seven-point scale, from 1 as "never" to 7 as "always." *Family support* question asked subjects if they can ask their family for help and rated it on a five-point scale, from 1 as "never" to 5 as "always." Higher results on each question reflected better social and family support.

Trust. Perception of trust in society was examined by the question "Would you say that most people could be trusted?" and the subject had to rate it on an 11-point scale, from 0 as "cannot be trusted" to 10 as "could be completely trusted."

Fairness. Perception of fairness in society was examined by the question "Do you think that most people would try to take advantage of you?" and the subject rated it on an 11-point scale, from 0 as "most people would take advantage" to 10 as "most people would be fair to me."

Psychological domain. Questions in this domain covered aspects of personal growth such as learning, respect, recognition and spirituality. *Learning* was covered by asking subjects to report if they get a chance to learn new things. *Respect* was examined by asking subjects if people respect them, while *recognition* by asking them if they feel that they get the recognition they deserve for what they do. All three questions were rated on a seven-point scale, from 1 as "never" to 7 as "almost always." *Spirituality* was assessed by questioning how much religion was important in their life, which was rated on a five-point scale, from 1 as "completely unimportant" to 5 as "extremely important."

Results

Descriptive statistics for the well-being and life domains variables are presented in Table 3.1.

Table 3.1 Descriptive statistics for the sample

		Theoretical range	Mean	SD
Well-being	Life satisfaction	0–10	6.8	2.04
	Specific emotions			
	Happy	1–7	4.9	1.19
	Satisfied	1–7	4.9	1.21
	Sad	1–7	3.4	1.34
	Angry	1–7	3.5	1.25
	Depressed	1–7	2.5	1.43
	Stressed	1–7	3.2	1.70
Life domains variables	*Physical domain*			
	Health	1–5	3.0	1.10
	Social domain			
	Seeing friends	1–7	5.4	1.46
	Receiving help	1–7	4.4	1.14
	Family support	1–5	4.4	0.94
	Trust	0–10	5.2	1.98
	Fairness	0–10	5.0	2.25
	Psychological domain			
	Learning	1–7	4.4	1.44
	Respect	1–7	5.2	1.06
	Recognition	1–7	4.4	1.38
	Spirituality	1–5	3.9	1.08

While evaluating their life from 0 as the "most unsatisfied" to 10 as "totally satisfied," 61% of Croatian citizens reported 7 and higher satisfaction. On the low spectrum of the scale, 8% of Croatian citizens rated satisfaction with their life from 0 to 4, and the rest of Croatians, i.e., 31%, were between 5 and 6 on life satisfaction scores.

Among the various emotions experienced over the last month, the average person experienced the "most often" feelings of being happy and satisfied and the "least often" feeling of being depressed.

Well-Being and Predictors – the Regression Analyses

The correlations between well-being and predictors (socio-demographic and life domains variables) are shown in Table 3.2 and the inter-correlations between predictors' variables in Appendix. Because of the very large sample size, most of the correlations are significantly different from zero.

The strongest correlation with well-being among the socio-demographic variables showed income, which was positively associated with life satisfaction and positive emotions and negatively associated with negative emotions except with feeling of being stressed.

Table 3.2 Zero-order correlations between well-being variables and predictors

	Life satisfaction	Happy	Satisfied	Sad	Angry	Depressed	Stressed
Age	−.20**	−.26**	−.16**	.09**	−.21**	.05	−.21**
Gender	−.03	−.02	−.03	.22**	.08*	.12**	.14**
Income	.29**	.18**	.23**	−.15**	−.13**	−.08*	.02
Health	.32**	.35**	.31**	−.24**	.02	−.24**	−.01
Seeing friends	.14**	.25**	.20**	−.07*	−.03	−.10**	.01
Receiving help	.10**	.14**	.17**	−.08*	−.03	−.14**	−.08*
Family support	.23**	.22**	.23**	−.10**	−.07*	−.15**	−.04
Trust	.28**	.16**	.22**	−.20**	−.16**	−.21**	−.16**
Fairness	.22**	.15**	.21**	−.19**	−.16**	−.21**	−.15**
Learning	.23**	.30**	.26**	−.15**	−.01	−.13**	.04
Respect	.13**	.13**	.22**	−.14**	−.08*	−.22**	−.14**
Recognition	.17**	.12**	.20**	−.13**	−.13**	−.20**	−.18**
Spirituality	.04	−.02	.03	.01	.00	−.02	−.06*

*$p<.05$; **$p<.01$

Among the life domains predictors, health showed the highest correlations with well-being variables followed by variables of trust, fairness and learning. The lowest correlations were found between spirituality and well-being variables.

To explore the associations more systematically, hierarchical regression analyses were conducted separately on each of the well-being variables (life satisfaction, six emotions). Also, age, gender and family income were entered at the first step as covariates. Results are shown in Table 3.3.

The strongest predictor of life satisfaction was health, i.e., better health predicted better life satisfaction. Even after controlling it, income stayed as significant predictor of life satisfaction. Other significant predictors were variables from social domains, such as trust and family support, while spirituality barely reached significance. People, who reported higher trust in community and more family support, as well as importance of religion in their life, reported better life satisfaction. Together, the measured variables accounted for 22% of life satisfaction variance.

Concerning the positive emotion, better health, more family support, more chance to learn new thing and more often meeting friends predicted being happier and more satisfied over the past month. Respect and fairness appeared to be significant but not too strong in predicting satisfaction. People who perceived more fairness in society and more respect from others also reported to be more satisfied. Total explained variance for feeling happy over the past month was 20%, while for feeling satisfied was 21%.

In predicting the experience of negative emotions over the past month, health again showed significant negative betas for all emotions expect for angry feelings. Lower trust in society and feeling that people take advantage of you repeatedly predicted experiencing more negative emotions. Also, less family support and help was related to the experience of feeling depressed and angry. The feeling not being respected was associated with being sad, depressive, and stressed, while perception of not getting the deserved recognition was associated with feeling stressful.

Table 3.3 Summary of hierarchical regression analyses (beta weights) for life domains variables predicting life satisfaction and specific emotions

	Life satisfaction	Emotions					
		Happy	Satisfied	Sad	Angry	Depressive	Stressed
Step 1							
Age	−.14**	−.24**	−.11**	.06*	−.24**	.04	−.21**
Gender[a]	−.01	−.02	−.02	.22**	.07*	.12**	.13**
Income	.26**	.13**	.20**	−.12**	−.17**	−.04*	−.01
R	.32**	.29**	.26**	.27**	.28**	.15**	.25**
Step 2							
Age	−.01	−.05	.05	−.05	−.29**	−.09*	−.25**
Gender	−.02	−.02	−.03	.23**	.07*	.13**	.14**
Income	.18**	.04	.12**	−.05	−.13**	.01	.03
Health	.20**	.21**	.20**	−.21**	−.05	−.23**	−.12**
Seeing friends	−.01	.11**	.07*	.03	−.05	−.01	.01
Receiving help	−.01	.05	.04	.02	.04	−.01	.02
Family support	.12**	.09**	.12**	−.04	−.07*	−.08*	−.04
Trust	.16**	.03	.06	−.10**	−.07*	−.08*	−.09*
Fairness	.04	.04	.07*	−.09*	−.10**	−.10**	−.08*
Learning	.05	.13**	.08*	−.04	.02	−.01	.05
Respect	.00	.02	.10**	−.09*	−.02	−.13**	−.08*
Recognition	.05	.00	.02	−.01	−.06	−.05	−.10**
Spirituality	.06*	−.02	.03	−.02	.01	−.01	−.04
R	.47**	.45**	.46**	.40**	.35**	.39**	.36**

Note: [a]Gender is coded into *1* male and *2* female
$*p<.05$; $**p<.01$

Total explained variances of being sad, depressive, stressed, and angry over the past month, by measured variables, were 16%, 15%, 13%, and 12%, respectively.

Discussion

The study explored evaluative and experiential measures of well-being and their correlates with different life domains variables. We examined those research questions on a large, nationally representative sample. Examining people's well-being at the national-level groups can provide important information to government and policy making organizations in guiding and improving the quality of life in society and specific groups.

Widely used life satisfaction was examined as evaluative measure of well-being as it elicits global evaluation of one's life. Also, we employed time-based measure of well-being, measuring experience of two positive and four negative emotions[2]

[2]In the experience sampling studies, it was shown that positive emotions are highly intercorrelated, while the correlations among the negative emotions, still positive, are lower; thus we used more negative than positive emotions (Kahneman & Krueger, 2006).

over the past month. Usually, experienced well-being is concerned with momentary emotions and their experiences in the real time (Kahneman & Krueger, 2006). Due to the nature of our survey, which was conducted at only one time period, respondents were asked to report the experience of certain emotions in the last month. The given time frame reduced the extent of memory bias, as reports are more likely to be anchored in actual experiences than are reports of emotions in general.

Predictors were number of specific items which covered physical (i.e., health), social (i.e., seeing friends, family support, receiving help, trust, fairness), and psychological (i.e., learning, respect, recognition, spirituality) domains, and thus provided insight on respondents' view of society, relationships, and personal growth.

Concerning the life satisfaction, 61% respondents reported to be very satisfied (ratings of 7 and higher), while on the lower end of spectrum, there were only 8% of them (ratings of satisfaction less than 4). If we borrow the terminology from the Gallup organization (Harter, Arora, & Neftzger, 2008), which they use for the cross-country comparisons, first group (61%) could be considered as "thriving," which means that they have their basic needs, such as food and shelter, met. Second group (8%) could be considered as "suffering" residents and they are less likely to have their basic needs met. The middle group (31% respondents in our sample) refers to "struggling" residents who tend to have lower income and are much more likely to worry about money on a daily basis (Harter & Gurley, 2008). Asked about their emotions, Croatian citizens reported experiencing significantly more positive emotions, i.e., to be happy and satisfied, than negative ones, i.e., to be depressed, angry, sad, and stressed, over the past month.

Further, we examined what are the predictors of evaluative and experienced measures of well-being, while controlling for possible effects of age, gender, and income. Even after controlling for income, higher income was still significant predictor of better life satisfaction, and in less extent of being more satisfied and less angry over the past month. This is in accordance with previous findings that the country's income level is positively correlated with ratings of citizens' global judgments of life satisfaction, while more weakly correlated with experienced feelings over time (Diener, Ng, Harter, & Arora, 2010; Diener & Seligman, 2004; Kahneman et al., 2006). Also, being female was a significant predictor of being sad and depressive over the past month, which is in the line of research that women appear more likely to develop cognitive strategies that are associated with increased susceptibility to depressive states (Nolen-Hoeksema, 2006).

Life satisfaction was best predicted by health variable, i.e., better health was associated with higher ratings of life satisfaction. Health consistently shows a strong relationship with well-being measures, which is reported in many studies and literature reviews (Dolan et al., 2008; Diener & Seligman, 2004; Lelkes, 2006). Following are the variables from social domain such as trust and family support. Trusting others more and getting more help from family predicted better life satisfaction. Social trust, which is trust in other people, was found in previous research to be associated with higher life satisfaction (Helliwell, 2006). To maintain good well-being, people need supportive and positive family and social relationships (Diener & Seligman, 2004; Lelkes, 2006).

As for positive emotions, better health and more family support predicted happiness and satisfaction over the past month. Kaliterna Lipovčan and Prizmić-Larsen (2006a) found that health is a strong predictor of happiness in the Croatian society. Another two strong predictors were learning new things and seeing friends. In terms of eudaimonic well-being, learning could be seen as variable of self-realization and personal growth (Ryan & Deci, 2001). In the research of Park, Peterson and Seligman (2004), love for learning, defined as one of the character strengths, added little bit to life satisfaction, while it added almost nothing to life satisfaction in our research. However, we found that opportunity to learn new things was associated with positive emotions. People who had more of it felt happier and more satisfied over the past month than ones who did not.

Numerous other studies provide evidence for the positive relationship between social support and well-being (Diener & Seligman, 2004; Dolan et al., 2008; Lelkes, 2006). Some authors emphasized the importance of social relationships in the maintenance of health and well-being, pointing out that social support promotes well-being by influencing cognition and behaviors in the way that promotes positive emotions (Cohen, Gottlieb, & Underwood, 2001).

In predicting the experience of negative emotions, only two predictors, health and family support, were similar to those of positive emotions, both showing negative associations with negative emotions. It confirms again that health and family support are very important predictors for both evaluative and experienced well-being (Diener and Seligman, 2004; Dolan et al., 2008). Additional strong predictors were fairness and social trust, followed by respect and recognition. Perceived quality of society, like trusting one another and being mutually helpful, described in literature as social capital, are usually examined in connection with life satisfaction (Böhnke, 2008; Helliwell, 2006). Having high social capital indicates higher well-being (Diener & Seligman, 2004). In our data, lower perceived social capital was particularly associated with citizens' experience of negative emotions, i.e., of being more sad, depressed, angry and stressed over the past month. Not being respected was associated with being sad, depressed, and stressed, while not having recognition was associated with more stress. Those variables, which in some ways reflect position of individual in social context and relationships in society, like perceived social actualization and contribution, were also related to experiencing negative emotions.

This study showed that different components of well-being were predicted by similar variables, on one hand, but also has distinct variables predicting it, on the other. Positive and negative emotions demonstrated different relationships to predictors, and again confirmed their independence found in the literature (Lucas et al., 1996). In some way, those experiential responses were strongly related to variables from social and personal domains, than evaluative measure. Positive emotions showed association with personal growth variables and aspects of life more related to individual and his or her growth (i.e., psychological well-being), while negative emotions were related to social domain, like aspects of life related to other people, relationships, and community (i.e., social well-being).

However, there are several limitations of the study, which should be mentioned. The cross-sectional design and the correlative nature of the study do not allow any casual interpretation of relationships between well-being measures and various life domains variables. Since only self-report measures were used, in future research, it would be important to utilize a multimethod approach by including peer reports. Although the life domains variables used were quite diverse, there are still areas of life that we might overlook such as personal safety, leisure, etc. Finally, specific emotions were assessed over the last month, so retrospective component in measuring the affect exists to some extent. If the mood was assessed momentarily or in reference to the previous day, it would reduce the extent of bias in recalling past experiences.

In summary, the most important predictors of life satisfaction were income, health and family support. Distinctive predictors of positive emotions were learning and seeing friends, while for negative emotions, significant predictors were trust, fairness, and recognition. Those results could be valuable tools for government and policy makers in improving well-being of the nation not only through economic changes but also by improving health care, supporting family values, promoting trust and fairness in social climate, and expanding opportunities for learning.

The national accounts of well-being can have broad benefits for society. Targeting specific groups within society can give more detailed answers for applying specific intervention and programs too. As many researchers now point out, governments that effectively promote well-being can produce engaged citizens who influence growth and prosperity of the country and build a happy society (Diener & Seligman, 2004; Diener et al., 2008; Kahneman et al., 2006).

Appendix: Zero-Order Correlations Between Predictors' Variables

	1	2	3	4	5	6	7	8	9	10	11	12
1. Age	–											
2. Gender	−.03	–										
3. Income	−.22**	−.07*	–									
4. Health	−.52**	.02	.27**	–								
5. Seeing friends	−.26**	−.02	.09**	.25**	–							
6. Receiving help	−.01	−.04	−.05	.07*	.13**	–						
7. Family support	−.17**	.05	.10**	.15**	.25**	.14**	–					
8. Trust	−.08*	−.03	.14**	.14**	.17**	.24**	.17**	–				
9. Fairness	−.05	.01	.12**	.15**	.07*	.20**	.09**	.57**	–			
10. Learning	−.31**	−.02	.28**	.32**	.22**	.23**	.25**	.13**	.12**	–		
11. Respect	.23**	.07	.07	.11**	.09**	.33**	.20**	.15**	.15**	.20**	–	
12. Recognition	.04	−.05	.10**	.09**	.11**	.36**	.15**	.21**	.19**	.23**	.51**	–
13. Spirituality	.06*	.13**	−.16**	.01	.02	.03	.05	.04	.04	−.05	.05	.05

*$p < .05$; **$p < .01$

References

Böhnke, P. (2008). Does society matter? Life satisfaction in the enlarged Europe. *Social Indicators Research, 87*, 189–210.

Bonini, A. (2008). Cross-national variation in individual life satisfaction: Effects of national wealth, human development, and environmental conditions. *Social Indicators Research, 87*, 223–236.

Cohen, S., Gottlieb, B., & Underwood, L. (2001). Social relationships and health: Challenges for measurement and intervention. *Advances in Mind-Body Medicine, 17*, 129–141.

Deaton, A. (2008). Income, health, and well-being around the world: Evidence from the Gallup world poll. *The Journal of Economic Perspectives, 22*, 53–72.

Deci, E., & Ryan, R. (2008). Hedonia, eudaimonia, and well-being: An introduction. *Journal of Happiness Studies, 9*, 1–11.

Diener, E. (2006). Guidelines for national indicators of subjective well-being and ill-being. *Journal of Happiness Studies, 7*, 397–404.

Diener, E., Kesebir, P., & Lucas, R. (2008). Benefits of accounts of well-being— for societies and for psychological science. *Applied Psychology: An International Review, 57*, 37–53.

Diener, E., Ng, W., Harter, J., & Arora, R. (2010). Wealth and happiness across the world: Material prosperity predicts life evaluation, whereas psychosocial prosperity predicts positive feeling. *Journal of Personality and Social Psychology, 99*(1), 52–61.

Diener, E., & Seligman, M. (2004). Beyond money: Toward an economy of well-being. *Psychological Science in the Public Interest, 5*, 1–31.

Diener, E., Suh, E., Lucas, R., & Smith, H. (1999). Subjective well-being: Three decades of progress. *Psychological Bulletin, 125*, 276–302.

Dolan, P., Peasgood, T., & White, M. (2008). Do we really know what makes us happy? A review of the economic literature on the factors associated with subjective well-being. *Journal of Economic Psychology, 29*, 94–122.

Harter, J. K., Arora, R., & Neftzger, A. (2008). More Americans struggling than six months ago, those struggling outnumber those thriving for fourth consecutive month. *The Gallup Organization.* Retrieved from www.gallup.com/poll/109501/More-Americans-Struggling-Than-Six-Months-Ago.aspx

Harter, J. K., & Gurley, V. F. (2008). Measuring well-being in the United States. *Observer, 21*, 17–20.

Helliwell, J. (2006). Well-being, social capital and public policy: What's new? *The Economic Journal, 116*, 34–45.

Hobcraft, J. (2006). The ABC of demographic behaviour: How the interplays of alleles, brains, and contexts over the life course should shape research aimed at understanding population processes. *Population Studies, 60*, 153–187.

Huppert, F., & Whittington, J. (2003). Evidence for the independence of positive and negative well-being: Implications for quality of life assessment. *British Journal of Health Psychology, 8*, 107–122.

Kahneman, D., & Krueger, A. (2006). Developments in the measurement of subjective well-being. *The Journal of Economic Perspectives, 20*, 3–24.

Kahneman, D., Krueger, A., Schkade, D., Schwarz, N., & Stone, A. (2004). Toward national well-being accounts. *The American Economic Review, 94*, 429–434.

Kahneman, D., Krueger, A., Schkade, D., Schwarz, N., & Stone, A. (2006). Would you be happier if you were richer? A focusing illusion. *Science, 312*, 1908–1910.

Kaliterna Lipovčan, L., & Prizmić-Larsen, Z. (2006a). What makes Croats happy? Predictors of happiness in representative sample. In A. Delle Fave (Ed.), *Dimensions of well-being: Research and intervention* (pp. 53–59). Milano: Franco Angeli.

Kaliterna Lipovčan, L., & Prizmić-Larsen, Z. (2006b). Quality of life, life satisfaction and happiness in Croatia in comparison to European countries. In K. Otti (Ed.), *Croatia's accession to the European Union: The challenges of Participation* (pp. 189–208). Zagreb, Croatia: Institute for Public Finances.

Kaliterna Lipovčan, L., & Prizmić-Larsen, Z. (2007). Importance and satisfaction with life domains in Croatia: Representative sample. In R. J. Estes (Ed.), *Advancing quality of life in a turbulent world* (pp. 41–51). Dordrecht, The Netherlands: Springer.

Keyes, C., Shmotkin, D., & Ryff, C. (2002). Optimizing well-being: The empirical encounter of two traditions. *Journal of Personality and Social Psychology, 82*, 1007–1022.

Kuppens, P., Realo, A., & Diener, E. (2008). The role of positive and negative emotions in life satisfaction judgment across nations. *Journal of Personality and Social Psychology, 95*, 66–75.

Lelkes, O. (2006). Knowing what is good for you: Empirical analysis of personal preferences and the 'objective good'. *Journal of Socio-Economics, 35*, 285–307.

Lucas, R., Diener, E., & Suh, E. (1996). Discriminant validity of well-being measures. *Journal of Personality and Social Psychology, 71*, 616–628.

Lyubomirsky, S., King, L., & Diener, E. (2005). The benefits of frequent positive affect: Does happiness lead to success? *Psychological Bulletin, 131*, 803–855.

Nolen-Hoeksema, S. (2006). The etiology of gender differences in depression. In C. M. Mazure & G. P. Keita (Eds.), *Understanding depression in women: Applying empirical research to practice and policy* (pp. 9–43). Washington, DC: American Psychological Association.

Oishi, S., Diener, E., Lucas, R., & Suh, E. (1999). Cross-cultural variations in predictors of life satisfaction: Perspectives from needs and values. *Personality and Social Psychology Bulletin, 25*, 980–990.

Park, N., Peterson, C., & Seligman, M. (2004). Strengths of character and well-being. *Journal of Social and Clinical Psychology, 23*, 603–619.

Ryan, R., & Deci, E. (2001). On happiness and human potentials: A review of research on hedonic and eudaimonic well-being. *Annual Review of Psychology, 52*, 141–166.

Selim, S. (2008). Life satisfaction and happiness in Turkey. *Social Indicators Research, 88*, 531–562.

Chapter 4
The Effect of Leisure Activities on Life Satisfaction: The Importance of Holiday Trips

Jeroen Nawijn and Ruut Veenhoven

In recent years, the phenomenon of happiness has been receiving increased interest. People want to know what can possibly make them happier. Generally speaking, there are two ways to improve happiness, one is to change one's *view* on life and the other is to change one's *way* of life. The latter way is promising since approximately 40% of variance in happiness is attributable to intentional activity (Lyubomirksy, Sheldon, & Schkade, 2005). Still, there is a lack of knowledge of what ways of life are the most satisfying and, in particular, about the happiness revenues of different leisure activities.

Research into Happiness and Leisure

Happiness researchers are quite knowledgeable on the subject of work but less so on leisure. The World Database of Happiness currently lists 585 correlations between work and happiness and only 91 correlations between leisure activities and happiness (Veenhoven, 2008). Thus, the effect of work on happiness is a well-explored area of research, but far less is known about how participating in leisure activities affects happiness. Work, leisure, and happiness are interrelated (Haworth, 1997). For example, the number of working hours has a strong negative effect on leisure satisfaction, whereas the effect of the number of hours spent on leisure has only a small positive effect on leisure satisfaction (Van Praag, Frijters, & Ferrer-i-Carbonell, 2003).

J. Nawijn (✉)
NHTV Breda University of Applied Sciences & Faculty of Social Sciences, Erasmus University, Rotterdam, The Netherlands
e-mail: nawijn@fsw.eur.nl

R. Veenhoven
Faculty of Social Sciences, Erasmus University, Rotterdam, The Netherlands
e-mail: veenhoven@fsw.eur.nl

I. Brdar (ed.), *The Human Pursuit of Well-Being: A Cultural Approach*,
DOI 10.1007/978-94-007-1375-8_4, © Springer Science+Business Media B.V. 2011

Happiness and Leisure Satisfaction

The subjective evaluation of different aspects of life is known to correlate fairly strongly with life satisfaction (Ateca-Amestoy, Serrano-del-Rosal, & Vera-Toscano, 2008; Lloyd & Auld, 2002; Van Praag & Ferrer-i-Carbonell, 2004; Van Praag et al., 2003). Evaluations of finance, health, and job satisfaction, together with leisure satisfaction are the four most important correlates (Van Praag et al., 2003). Ateca-Amestoy et al. (2008) and Spiers and Walker (2009) find positive associations between leisure satisfaction and life satisfaction. Neal et al. (1999) constructed a model based on the assumption that "life satisfaction is functionally related to satisfaction with all of life's domains and subdomains" (Neal, Sirgy, & Uysal, 1999, p. 154). In 2004, Neal and Sirgy (2004) further validated this model by demonstrating that there is a correlation between satisfaction with leisure life and satisfaction with life in general. A similar model was developed by Sirgy, Rahtz, Cicic, and Underwood (2000), whose model includes leisure as part of the "global satisfaction with other life domains" (Sirgy & Cornwell, 2001; Sirgy et al., 2000).

Happiness and Leisure Activities

Increased satisfaction with leisure and higher frequency of participation in leisure activities positively correlate with life satisfaction (Lloyd & Auld, 2002). Others also find that participating in leisure activities has a positive correlation with life satisfaction (Baldwin & Tinsley, 1988; Dowall, Bolter, Flett, & Kammann, 1988; Wankel & Berger, 1990). Research efforts to date tend to focus on the total frequency of a group of leisure activities on either happiness or leisure satisfaction. However, not enough attention has been paid to the effect of specific leisure activities on happiness. Whenever a happiness study does address leisure activities, it usually involves one specific leisure activity, such as listening to music (Laukka, 2007) or watching television (Bruni & Stanca, 2006, 2008; Delle Fave & Bassi, 2003; Frey, Benesch, & Strutzer, 2005).

The majority of leisure studies are cross-sectional; therefore, it is difficult to determine cause and effect.

Happiness and Tourism

Specifically addressing the component of holiday trips, several studies have examined its correlation with happiness (Gilbert & Abdullah, 2002, 2004; Milman, 1998; Neal, 2000; Neal & Sirgy, 2004; Neal et al., 1999). Milman's study, based on a sample of senior citizens, shows that holiday trippers are not happier after their holiday (Milman, 1998). Nawijn (2007) finds a low, but positive, correlation between holiday trips and happiness. His findings confirm those of Gilbert and Abdullah (2004) and Neal and Sirgy (2004), who conclude that holiday trips positively influence the sense of well-being of tourists. On the other hand, not every study finds only positive consequences of holiday tripping. High job stress, caused by work not being done during the vacation, for instance, is associated with poorer well-being (Strauss-Blasche, Ekmekcioglu, & Marktl, 2002). Returning to work where one finds more work piled up compared to the prevacation period results in higher levels of stress.

None of the aforementioned studies measured both happiness and tourism over a long period of time. Thus, cause and effect are not always clear.

Aim of This Chapter

In this chapter, we try to disentangle cause and effect in the relationship between happiness and leisure activity and seek an answer to the following questions: What is the effect of leisure activities on happiness? Do holiday trips have a bigger impact than other leisure activities? And finally, does everyone benefit from these activities?

The purpose of this chapter is to determine the effect of leisure activities on happiness in terms of strength and cause and effect. This study clarifies which leisure activities increase happiness. Over-time correlations were calculated, to be certain that happy people did not participate more in leisure activities in general. Additionally, to further determine the cause–effect relationship, all effects were controlled for by demographic variables and personality.

Method

These questions are answered by means of data of the German Socio-Economic Panel Study (SOEP), which were made available to us by SOEP at the German Institute for Economic Research (DIW Berlin). Four waves of that study involved questions about leisure activities. The longitudinal design allows the separation of cause and effect and rich background variables allow a check for possible spurious correlation.

Data

SOEP is a large-scale representative panel of private households, which exists since 1984. Participants are interviewed once a year. Leisure activities are not automatically included in the questionnaires but were included in the waves of 1990, 1995,

1998, and 2003. The wave of 1990 consists of ~9,500 West Germans and 4,300 East Germans. The 1995 wave holds ~13,600 people, the 1998 wave ~14,500 people, and the 2003 wave ~20,400. The panel consists of Germans living in the former eastern and western part, foreigners and recent immigrants to Germany. SOEP contains 18 main topics including "health," "education and qualification," "job market and occupation," and "socialization." The topic "Basic orientation, participation, and integration" includes measures of subjective well-being.

Variables the Following Variables are Used

Dependent Variable: Life Satisfaction

The dependent variable of the present study is *life satisfaction*, which we define as "the overall appreciation of one's life as a whole." This concept is delineated in more detail in Veenhoven (1984) and is also labeled as "happiness." The focus of this chapter is on *present* satisfaction with life.

Life satisfaction is measured using a self-report on a single question: "And finally, we would like to ask you about your satisfaction with your life in general. Please answer by using the following scale, in which 0 means totally unhappy, and 10 means totally happy." The exact question was phrased as: "How satisfied are you at present with your life as a whole?" This question is in SOEP's core questionnaire and responses are, therefore, available for all respondents in all years.

Independent Variable: Leisure Activities

The 1990 wave of the SOEP study included the following leisure activities: *go out to eat or drink, visit neighbors, visit family member, play card and board games, participate in local politics, perform volunteer work, attend church or other religious events, watch television, video, read nonfiction and fiction, engage in artistic and musical activities, perform handicraft and home repairs, participate in sports, attend sports event, attend cinema, pop, jazz concerts* and *attend cultural events*. The East German data did not contain the variable of *holiday trips*, but included two different activities: *attend community events* and *attend social gatherings*. The 1990 data for East Germany contain only a small range of leisure activities (6 out of the 15), which were used in the West German sample. For this reason, the East German data were excluded from analysis. The 1995 wave included the same leisure activities as the 1990 West German wave. The 1998 wave omits *play card and board games, engage in artistic and musical activities, perform handicraft and home repairs* and *read nonfiction and fiction*. The 1998 wave contained some new activities, namely, *private personal computer use, tinkering and garden work, car repairs* and *attend opera/classical concerts and theater*. The 2003 activities were almost the same as those of 1998, with just one addition: *private internet usage*.

Holiday Trips

The focus of this chapter is on "holiday trips," i.e., daytrips and short holidays. This independent variable was part of the SOEP study in 1990 (West Germany), 1995, 1998, and 2003. The wording of the questions and answers slightly varies over the years. In 1990 and 1995, the following phrasing was used: "Now some questions about your free time. How frequently do you undertake the following activities?" Then several items were listed, among which were outings or short trips. This variable contained the following choices: "daily, once a week, once a month, less than once a month, never." In 1995, instead of asking how frequently one participated in the activities, the question was as follows: "Please indicate how often you engage in the following activities: daily, at least once a week, at least once a month, less often or never?" The responses were equal to the ones pointed out in the question itself. The name of the variable had "excursions" added to it: outings, excursions, short trips. Again, in 2003, some minor changes were made. The question was rephrased as: "Please indicate how often you take part in each activity: daily, at least once a week, at least once a month, seldom, or never." with corresponding answers. Finally, the variable was renamed: go on a trip or short holiday.

Control Variables

To ensure that correlations between leisure activities and happiness are not driven by a common third variable, personality, health and socio-demographic variables are used as control variables.

Personality

The "big five" most important personality traits are: extraversion, agreeableness, conscientiousness, neuroticism and openness to experience (McCrae & John, 1992, p. 175). The SOEP study includes measures of these five dimensions (Dehne & Schupp, 2007). As personality traits are deemed fairly stable (Costa & McCrae, 1994; Gustavsson, Weinryb, Göransson, Pedersen, & Åsberg, 1997; Hampson & Goldberg, 2006; McCrae & Costa, 2003; Terraciano, Costa, & McCrae, 2006), the 2005 measurement is used for each year of analysis.

Health

Health is measured as the total number of doctor visits in the past 3 months.

Socio-demographic Variables

Age, sex, marriage, education, work and income are the socio-demographic variables used in this study. Income is defined as the average gross amount of salary.

Analytic Approach

We started with a same-time analysis to see whether happiness and leisure activities are related. Next, we did an over-time comparison to get an idea about cause and effect.

The same-time analysis was done using Pearson correlations. First, we computed simple zero-order correlations for assessing to what extent happiness goes together with leisure activities. To check whether these same-time correlations are spurious, we also computed partial correlations. Over-time correlations were used to gain an insight into cause and effect and to determine the duration of effects. Again, we computed both zero-order and partial correlations. Missing values were deleted list-wise. Each wave contained ~500 cases with missing values, the final wave ($n=22{,}400$) had more missing values, namely ~2,000 cases.

Results

Correlations for each of the four waves are presented in the appendices to this chapter. Table 4.1 presents the average correlation across all four waves. These averages were computed as a weighted mean, whereby the weights were equal to the inverse variance of each wave's effect estimator.

Same-Time Zero-Order Correlations

Just five leisure activities (LAs) have significant correlations with life satisfaction (LS). The LAs with significant correlations are *holiday trips*, *attending church*, *handicrafts*, *home repairs* and *attending cultural events*.

The leisure activity with the largest correlation each year is *holiday trips* (shown in Appendix 1). The waves of 1990, 1995, 1998 and 2003 have effect sizes of .15 ($p<.01$), .15 ($p<.01$), .18 ($p<.01$) and .19 ($p<.01$), respectively. Thus, the effect sizes are rather similar for each wave. On top of that, *holiday trips* is the only leisure activity which has a significant effect each year. Three of the other activities do not have a significant effect each year, but their mean effects are significant. The leisure activities that have significant mean zero-order correlations are *holiday trips*, *attending church*, *handicraft*, *home repairs* and *attend cultural events*.

Same-Time Partial Correlations

When examining the mean partial correlations (shown in Table 4.1, Column 3), it is immediately obvious that, out of the four significant mean zero-order effects, just

Table 4.1 Correlations between leisure activities and life satisfaction

	Same-time correlations		Over-time correlations	
Leisure activities	*r*	Partial *r*[a]	LS→LA	LA→LS
Holiday trips	.18**	.14**	–.01	.01
Eating and drinking	.05	–.01	.02	.01
Visiting neighbors	.06	.01	.01	–.01
Visiting family	.04	.01	.00	.00
Card and board games	.03	.02	–.03	–.01
Local politics	–.19	–.01	–.02	.00
Volunteer work	.02	–.01	.03	.00
Attend church	.03*	.01	.01	.00
Watch television, video	.00	.01	.01	.00
Private computer use	.00	–.01	.00	–.01
Private internet use	.00	–.01	–.01	–.01
Reading	.03	.00	–.01	–.02
Artistic, musical activities	.02	.01	.01	–.02
Tinkering and garden work	–.02	–.01	.02	.00
Car repairs	–.01	–.01	.01	.01
Handicraft, home repairs	.03**	.01	–.02	–.02
Participate in sports	.03	.00	–.01	–.02
Attend sports events	.02	–.01	.01	–.01
Attend cinema, concerts	.02	.00	.01	–.02
Attend opera, theater	.01	– .02	.01	.00
Attend cultural events	.02*	.00	– .00	– .03

LS Life satisfaction ; *LA* Leisure activities
*$p<.05$; ** $p<.01$
[a]Partial correlation is controlled for age, sex, marriage, education, work, income, personality and health

one remains significant. Beyond any doubt, *holiday trips* is the most important leisure activity with mean partial effect sizes of .11 ($p<.01$), .09 ($p<.01$), .19 ($p<.01$) and .16 ($p<.01$). *Holiday trips* is the only leisure activity that has an independent effect on happiness; all the other mean zero-order correlations are no longer significant after controlling for *age*, *sex*, *marriage*, *education*, *work*, *income*, *personality* and *health*. The size of the correlation is small but considerable; *holiday trips* accounts for ~2% of the variance in life satisfaction.

Over-Time Correlations

This leaves us with the question of cause and effect: do holiday trips make us happier? Or, does happiness make us take holiday trips? To answer these questions, we did an across-time comparison. Since the SOEP study involves annual interviews, the minimal period we can use is 1 year.

Does Life Satisfaction Predict Leisure Activity 1 Year Later?

Could it be that happiness is the cause, happy people being more open to fun? This does not seem to be the case, as life satisfaction scores do not predict leisure activity scores 1 year later. The correlation is in fact negative, suggesting that it is unhappiness that predisposes people to take a holiday trip (see Column 4 in Table 4.1 and the detail in Appendix 2). No leisure activity has a consistent significant over-time correlation with the preceding life satisfaction score.

Does Leisure Activity Predict Life Satisfaction 1 Year Later?

Is the same-time correlation due to an effect of holiday trips on happiness? The over-time correlation is positive (.01) but does not reach statistical significance. So if there is an effect of holiday trips on happiness, it is apparently short lived and hardly visible anymore after a year. None of the leisure activities have consistent significant correlations with life satisfaction in the following year (see Column 5 in Table 4.1 and the detail in Appendix 3).

Discussion

Do Holiday Trips Boost Happiness?

Probably, but not certainly. People who did a trip a year appear to be somewhat happier in that year, and this applies to all kinds of people: working or not, an extrovert or an introvert, healthy or sick, rich or poor, married or single, and old or young. Still, it is not established that this correlation is due to an effect of holiday trips on happiness or an effect of happiness on holiday taking. None of these effects is reflected in significant correlations after 1 year, but these correlations of earlier trips on later happiness are positive, while the correlation of earlier happiness on later trip tends to the negative.

Suppose that the effect of holiday trips on happiness is the main driver of the same-year correlation. Holiday trips then have a short-lived effect on happiness. Is this effect big enough to be important? The answer to that question should be "yes." A 2% increase in happiness may not seem like a lot as such, but it is, when compared to other methods to increase happiness (Seligman, Steen, Park, & Peterson, 2005). Unlike this study, Seligman et al.'s study included people who were eager to improve their happiness. Even so, some of their techniques were less successful. Their positive intervention of gratitude visits had an effect size of .06 after 1 month (Seligman et al., 2005, p. 417), which is lower than the .14 effect size of holiday trips. Otake, Shimai, Tanaka-Matsumi, Otsui and Fredrickson (2006) conducted a study on counting kindness, among women. Their counting kindness intervention increased happiness by .44 on a seven-point scale (Otake et al., 2006), which is equal to a .06 effect size, much lower than the .14 of holiday trips. Apart from the smaller effect, women are also more attuned to kindness (Baskersville et al., 2000). The "identifying signature strengths" intervention technique (Seligman et al., 2005) has an effect size of .25 at the immediate post-test, which is higher than the effect size of holiday trips, but its effect is short lived as there is only immediate gratification (1 week post-tests were not significantly different from the control group).

These positive interventions were intentional activities. What if we compare the importance of holiday trips to an unintentional event? According to Lyubomirksy et al. (2005), unintentional activity makes up about 10% of happiness. One unintentional event may be a "medium-sized" lottery win of £50,000. Such a financial windfall increases happiness by ~3% (Gardner & Oswald, 2001, p. 7). (When dividing Gardner and Oswald's 1.09-point increase on their 36-point scale.) We should compare this to the uncontrolled effect of holiday trips, as Gardner and Oswald did not control their effect either. When doing so, we discover that winning £50,000 is less beneficial than going on a few holiday trips in a year. Additionally, the effect of the lottery win does not even have immediate gratification; it takes 2 years to take full effect. It seems that going on a holiday trip several times a year has a much bigger effect than winning £50,000 in the lottery, with the additional benefit of getting an immediate reward instead of having to wait for 2 years.

We argue that going on holiday trips is more beneficial for one's happiness in terms of intensity and duration compared to techniques such as "identifying signature strengths," "counting kindness," and "gratitude visits," especially as these studies involved people more attuned to the measurement (Otake et al., 2006) or more eager to increase their happiness (Seligman et al., 2005). Going on a holiday is just as beneficial, or even more so, than some positive intervention techniques (Seligman et al., 2005) and financial windfalls (Gardner & Oswald, 2001).

Why No Effect of Other Leisure Activities?

This study finds that out of all leisure activities, only *holiday trips* boost happiness. None of the other leisure activities have a significant effect on happiness. This finding partly contradicts previous findings by others (Brown, Frankel, & Fennell, 1991; Hills & Argyle, 1998; Suh & Diener, 1996). The cause of this probably lies in that fact that the leisure activities all seem to fall into the category of casual leisure (Stebbins, 2007). Two other categories, project-based leisure and serious leisure (Stebbins, 2007), which may be more beneficial to one's happiness, particularly if used purposefully (Winefield, Tigermann, & Winefield, 1992) and in congruence to their personality (Melamed, Meir, & Samson, 1995), are not included in the data. Additionally, the measurement level is likely to be the cause of some of the nonsignificant correlations, for instance, with watching TV. Other studies (Bruni & Stanca, 2006, 2008; Delle Fave & Bassi, 2003; Frey et al., 2005) found that watching TV negatively influences happiness. As most people watch TV daily, no distinction could be made between heavy users and regular viewers. This most likely explains the absence of significant correlations regarding watching TV in this study.

Limitations

The SOEP data have some limitations. The biggest limitation is that leisure activities are not measured every year. When measured, they are measured just once a year. Furthermore, the measurement level of the leisure activities is ordinal, and the categories are not very well chosen. This may have caused inaccurate reports as certain answers are not possible (e.g., twice a month). Future studies should incorporate more accurate methods of measuring leisure behavior. Another point of criticism is the choice of leisure activities. Some activities seem illogically combined into one variable (*attend cinema, pop, jazz concerts*) whereas others appear to have been excluded completely (*playing computer games* or *visiting museums*).

Further Research

Short-Term Follow-up

If holiday trips have a causal effect on happiness, that effect is apparently shorter than 1 year. To capture the short-lived effect, we need follow-up studies at shorter intervals, preferably every month. It is in the interest of the travel industry to fund such research.

Further Analysis of SOEP Data

Two facets of the SOEP data have not been analyzed yet. One is the total frequency and diversity of leisure activities. Do people with a wide range of leisure activities benefit more, in terms of happiness, than people with a small range of activities? The same applies to the total frequency of leisure activities; does a high frequency of leisure activities boost happiness? The other facet is the moderating effect of demographic criteria. We now know that everyone benefits, but do certain people benefit more than others from going on holiday?

Optimal Tourist Lifestyle

The interesting thing about holiday trips is that you start enjoying the experience before it actually starts. There is clearly an anticipation effect (Ryan, 1991). In that sense, it is quite a different experience from some of the aforementioned intervention techniques.

Also, the findings presented in this study are based on current behavior. Further work needs to be done to establish whether this current behavior is optimal, in the sense that it maximizes the potential happiness boost it generates. Future research should, therefore, focus on finding out what an optimal tourist lifestyle could be. Taking short holiday trips may be particularly favorable when more evenly spread over the year. Further analysis of different tourist lifestyles is a must. Finally, future research needs to determine the exact duration of the effect of holiday trips.

Conclusion

Happy people report more holiday trips in the past year, probably because holiday trips boost happiness. Though the effect is short lived, it is substantial, accounting for about 2% of the variance in happiness. Holiday trips affect happiness more than other leisure activities.

Acknowledgments The authors thank associate professor Paul Peeters and Nina Delbressine for their valuable comments and help.

Appendix 1. Same-Time Correlations of Leisure Activities and Life Satisfaction

	r				Partial *r*[a]			
Leisure activities	1990	1995	1998	2003	1990	1995	1998	2003
Holiday trips	.15**	.15**	.18**	.19**	.11**	.09**	.19**	.16**
Eating and drinking	.08**	.00	.04**	.05**	.01	.00	–.03	–.02
Visiting neighbors	.07**	.02	.03**	.02**	.06**	.01	–.01	–.02
Visiting family	.05**	.01	–.01	.00	.03	.00	.01	–.03
Card and board games	.06**	–.01	–	–	.05**	–.02	–	–
Local politics	.03**	.00	–.01	.01	.01	.00	–.02	–.02
Volunteer work	.06**	–.02**	.02*	.02**	.01	–.03	.01	–.02
Attend church	.05**	–.02	.06**	.04**	.06**	–.04**	.00	.02
Watch television, video	.02**	.01	–.02*	–.01*	.04*	.01	–.01	.01
Private computer use	–	–	.00	.03**	–	–	–.01	–.01
Private internet use	–	–	–	.03**	–	–	–	–.01
Reading	.07**	–.01	–	–	.02	–.02	–	–
Artistic, musical activities	.07**	–.02*	–	.03**	.05**	–.02	–	.01

(continued)

Appendix 1 (continued)

	r				Partial *r*[a]			
Leisure activities	1990	1995	1998	2003	1990	1995	1998	2003
Tinkering and garden work	–	–	–.02*	–.01	–	–	–.02	–.01
Car repairs	–	–	–.01	–.01*	–	–	.00	–.02
Handicraft, home repairs	.07**	–.03**	–	–	.04*	–.02	–	–
Participate in sports	.12**	–.01	.00	.03**	.05**	–.02	.00	–.03
Attend sports events	.07**	–.01	.01	.02*	.02	.00	–.01	–.03
Attend cinema, concerts	.07**	.00	–.01	.01	.01	.02	.00	–.02
Attend opera, theater	–	–	.00	.04**	–	–	–.03	–.01
Attend cultural events	.07**	–.02*	.00	–	.02	–.01	.00	–

'–' = No measurement *p<.05; **p<.01 [a]Partial correlations are controlled for age, sex, marriage, education, work, income, personality and health

Appendix 2. Over-Time Partial Correlations of Earlier Life Satisfaction and Later Leisure Activities

Leisure activities	1989–1990	1994–1995	1997–1998	2002–2003
Holiday trips	.02	–.01	.00	–.01
Eating and drinking	–.03*	–.01	.01	.01
Visiting neighbors	–.02	.002	.00	–.01
Visiting family	.02	–.02	.01	.00
Card and board games	–.01	–.02	–	–
Local politics	.00	–.01	.01	.01
Volunteer work	–.01	.01	.01	–.01
Attend church	.01	.00	–.01	.00
Watch television, video	.00	.01	–.02	.02
Private computer use	–	–	.00	–.01
Private internet use	–	–	–	–.01
Reading	.00	–.04**	–	–
Artistic, musical activities	–.03	–.05**	–	–.01
Tinkering and garden work	–	–	.00	.01
Car repairs	–	–	.01	.01
Handicraft, home repairs	–.03	.00	–	–
Participate in sports	–.05**	–.03*	.00	–.01
Attend sports events	–.03	–.01	.00	–.01
Attend cinema, concerts	–.03	–.04**	–.01	.00
Attend opera, theater	–	–	–.01	.00
Attend cultural events	–.02	–.04	.01	–

'–' No measurement; Partial correlations are controlled for age, sex, marriage, education, work, income, personality and health *p<.05; **p<.01

Appendix 3. Over-Time Partial Correlations of Earlier Leisure Activities and Later Life Satisfaction

Leisure activities	1990–1991	1995–1996	1998–1999	2003–2004
Holiday trips	.00	.04*	–.01	.00
Eating and drinking	.00	.04*	.02	.00
Visiting neighbors	–.01	.05*	–.02	.00
Visiting family	–.01	.02	.00	.00
Card and board games	–.03	–.03	–	–
Local politics	–.03	.00	–.04*	–.02
Volunteer work	–.01	.02	–.01	.01
Attend church	–.01	.03	.01	.01
Watch television, video	.01	.00	.00	.02
Private computer use	–	–	.00	.00
Private internet use	–	–	–	–.01
Reading	–.01	.00	–	–
Artistic, musical activities	.00	.03	–	.01
Tinkering and garden work	–	–	.02	.02
Car repairs	–	–	.03	.01
Handicraft, home repairs	–.01	–.04*	–	–
Participate in sports	.00	–.03	.01	–.02
Attend sports events	–.01	.02	.01	.01
Attend cinema, concerts	.01	.00	.02	.00
Attend opera, theater	–	–	.01	.02
Attend cultural events	.00	–.01	.00	–

'–' No measurement; Partial correlations are controlled for age, sex, marriage, education, work, income, personality and health *p<.05; **p<.01

References

Ateca-Amestoy, V., Serrano-del-Rosal, R., & Vera-Toscano, E. (2008). The leisure experience. *The Journal of Socio-Economics, 37*(1), 64–78.

Baldwin, K., & Tinsley, H. (1988). An investigation of the validity of Tinsley and Tinsley's (1986) Theory of leisure experience. *Journal of Counseling Psychology, 35*(3), 263–267.

Baskersville, K., Johnson, K., Monk-Turner, E., Slone, Q., Standley, H., Stansbury, S., et al. (2000). Reactions to random acts of kindness. *The Social Science Journal, 37*(2), 293–298.

Brown, B. A., Frankel, G. B., & Fennell, M. (1991). Happiness through leisure: The impact of type of leisure activity, age, gender and leisure satisfaction on psychological well-being. *Journal of Applied Recreation Research, 16*(4), 368–392.

Bruni, L., & Stanca, L. (2006). Income aspirations, television and happiness: Evidence from the world values survey. *Kyklos: internationale Zeitschrift für Sozialwissenschaften, 59*(2), 209–226.

Bruni, L., & Stanca, L. (2008). Watching alone: Relational goods, television and happiness. *Journal of Economic Behavior & Organization, 65*(3), 506–528.

Costa, P. T., & McCrae, R. R. (1994). Set like plaster? Evidence for the stability of adult personality. In T. F. Heatherton & J. L. Weinberger (Eds.), *Can personality change?* (pp. 21–40). Washington, DC: American Psychological Association Books.

Dehne, M., & Schupp, J. (2007). *Persönlichkeitsmerkmale im sozio-oekonomischen panel (Soep) – Konzept, umsetzung und empirische eigenschaften*. Berlin: DIW.
Delle Fave, A., & Bassi, M. (2003). Italian adolescents and leisure: The role of engagement and optimal experience. *New Directions for Child and Adolescent Development, 99*, 79–94.
Dowall, J., Bolter, C., Flett, R., & Kammann, R. (1988). Psychological well-being and its relationship to fitness and activity levels. *Journal of Human Movement Studies, 14*(1), 39–45.
Frey, B. S., Benesch, C., & Strutzer, A. (2005). *Does watching TV make us happy?* Zurich, Switzerland: University of Zurich, Institute for Empirical Research in Economics.
Gardner, J., & Oswald, A. J. (2001). *Does money buy happiness? A longitudinal study using data on windfalls*. Mimeo: Warwick University.
Gilbert, D., & Abdullah, J. (2002). A study on the impact of the expectation of a holiday on an individual's sense of well-being. *Journal of Vacation Marketing, 8*(4), 352–361.
Gilbert, D., & Abdullah, J. (2004). Holidaytaking and the sense of well-being. *Annals of Tourism Research, 31*(1), 103–121.
Gustavsson, J. P., Weinryb, R. M., Göransson, S., Pedersen, N. L., & Åsberg, M. (1997). Stability and predictive ability of personality traits across 9 years. *Personality and Individual Differences, 22*(6), 783–792.
Hampson, S. E., & Goldberg, L. R. (2006). A first large cohort study of personality trait stability over the 40 years between elementary school and midlife. *Journal of Personality and Social Psychology, 91*(4), 763–779.
Haworth, J. T. (1997). *Work, leisure and well-being*. London and New York: Routledge.
Hills, P., & Argyle, M. (1998). Positive moods derived from leisure and their relationship to happiness and personality. *Personality and Individual Differences, 25*(3), 523–535.
Laukka, P. (2007). Uses of music and psychological well-being among the elderly. *Journal of Happiness Studies, 8*(2), 215–241.
Lloyd, K., & Auld, C. J. (2002). The role of leisure in determining quality of life: Issues of Content and measurement. *Social Indicators Research, 57*(1), 43–71.
Lyubomirksy, S., Sheldon, K. M., & Schkade, D. (2005). Pursuing happiness: The architecture of sustainable change. *Review of General Psychology, 9*(2), 111–131.
McCrae, R. R., & Costa, P. T. (2003). *Personality in adulthood: A five-factor theory perspective*. New York: Guilford.
McCrae, R. R., & John, O. P. (1992). An introduction to the five-factor model and its applications. *Journal of Personality, 60*(2), 175–215.
Melamed, S., Meir, E. I., & Samson, A. (1995). The benefits of personality-leisure congruence: Evidence and implications. *Journal of Leisure Research, 27*(1), 25–40.
Milman, A. (1998). The Impact of tourism and travel experience on senior travelers' psychological well-being. *Journal of Travel Research, 37*(2), 166–170.
Nawijn, J. (2007, April 23–25). *Happiness and long haul leisure trips*. Paper presented at the tourism, mobility and technology, Nice, France.
Neal, J. D. (2000). *The effects of different aspects of tourism services on travelers' quality of life: Model validation, refinement, and extension*. Blacksburg, Virginia: Virginia Polytechnic Institute And State University.
Neal, J. D., & Sirgy, M. J. (2004). Measuring the effect of tourism services on travelers' quality of life: Further validation. *Social Indicators Research, 69*(3), 243.
Neal, J. D., Sirgy, M. J., & Uysal, M. (1999). The role of satisfaction with leisure travel- tourism services and experience in satisfaction with leisure life and overall life. *Journal of Business Research, 44*(3), 153–164.
Otake, K., Shimai, S., Tanaka-Matsumi, J., Otsui, K., & Fredrickson, B. L. (2006). Happy people become happier through kindness: A counting kindness intervention. *Journal of Happiness Studies, 7*(3), 361–375.
Ryan, C. (1991). *Recreational tourism: A Social science approach*. London: Routledge.
Seligman, M., Steen, T. A., Park, N., & Peterson, C. (2005). Positive psychology progress. *The American Psychologist, 60*(5), 410–421.

Sirgy, M. J., & Cornwell, T. (2001). Further validation of the Sirgy et al.'s Measure of Community Quality of Life. *Social Indicators Research, 56*(2), 125–143.

Sirgy, M. J., Rahtz, D., Cicic, M., & Underwood, M. (2000). A method for assessing residents' satisfaction with community-based services: A quality-of-life perspective. *Social Indicators Research, 49*(3), 279–316.

Spiers, A., & Walker, G. J. (2009). The effects of ethnicity and leisure satisfaction on happiness, peacefulness, and quality of life. *Leisure Sciences, 31*(1), 84–99.

Stebbins, R. A. (2007). *Serious leisure: A perspective for our time*. New Brunswick and London: Transaction Publishers.

Strauss-Blasche, G., Ekmekcioglu, C., & Marktl, W. (2002). Moderating effects of vacation on reactions to work and domestic stress. *Leisure Sciences, 24*(2), 237–249.

Suh, E. M., & Diener, E. (1996). Events and subjective well-being: Only recent events matter. *Journal of Personality and Social Psychology, 70*(5), 1091–1102.

Terraciano, A., Costa, P. T., & McCrae, R. R. (2006). Personality plasticity after age 30. *Personality and Social Psychology Bulletin, 32*(8), 999–1009.

Van Praag, B. M. S., & Ferrer-i-Carbonell, A. (2004). *Happiness quantified: A satisfaction calculus approach*. Oxford: Oxford University Press.

Van Praag, B. M. S., Frijters, P., & Ferrer-i-Carbonell, A. (2003). The anatomy of subjective well-being. *Journal of Economic Behavior & Organization, 51*(1), 29–49.

Veenhoven, R. (1984). *Conditions of happiness*. Dordrecht, Netherlands: Reidel.

Veenhoven, R. (2008). World database of happiness. Correlational findings: http://worlddatabaseofhappiness.eur.nl.

Wankel, L., & Berger, B. (1990). The psychological and social benefits of sport and physical activity. *Journal of Leisure Research, 22*(2), 167–182.

Winefield, A. H., Tigermann, M., & Winefield, H. R. (1992). Spare time use and psychological well-being in employed and unemployed young people. *Journal of Occupational and Organizational Psychology, 65*(1), 307–313.

Chapter 5
From Flow to Optimal Experience: (Re)Searching the Quality of Subjective Experience Throughout Daily Life

Teresa Freire

A great amount of research and theoretical considerations have been updated for several years about flow and optimal experience in the domain of psychology. Since the 1970s, with the work of Csikszentmihalyi, flow theory has been a main conceptual framework for the understanding of daily life and subjective experience of human beings. Several studies have been focused on knowing more about optimal functioning and its consequences and impact on all kinds of psychological and social domains (Csikszentmihalyi, 1997; Massimini & Delle Fave, 2000; Nakamura & Csikszentmihalyi, 2005).

This chapter is aimed at showing the investigation of a Portuguese research group focused on the study of optimal functioning (*Grupo de Investigação para o funciomento óptimo* – GIFOp), from the Department of Psychology, University of Minho. Several research lines integrate this group, with several studies about optimal experience, aimed to discuss empirical results but also to present new guidelines for future studies and research goals about this psychological issue. According to this, several on-going studies are being conducted, defining specific research lines focused on five main life contexts (school, family, leisure, therapy, and physiology) with participants from four main populations (adolescents, young adults, adults and the elderly) in order to study the quality of the subjective experience, mainly the optimal experience. Each research line is aimed to contribute to the study of the role or relation of optimal experience with specific contexts and populations, and psycho-social-physiological issues. All together they are aimed to contribute to, on one hand, the study of the concept of optimal experience, such as its conceptual characteristics, conditions for emergence and maintenance, and its impact on individual and social development. On the other hand, and at the same time, they also contribute to the study of its evaluation and measurement methods, in order to answer the methodological concerns.

T. Freire (✉)
School of Psychology, University of Minho, Portugal
e-mail: tfreire@psi.uminho.pt

I. Brdar (ed.), *The Human Pursuit of Well-Being: A Cultural Approach*,
DOI 10.1007/978-94-007-1375-8_5,

Conceptual Framework and Empirical Methodology

Some researchers have defined optimal experience as a state of consciousness characterized by clear goals and feedback from the situation, intrinsic motivation, personal satisfaction, involvement, control of the situation, perception of a balance between high environmental challenges and high personal skills and also concentration and engagement (Csikszentmihalyi, 1997; Csikszentmihalyi & Csikszentmihalyi, 1988; Massimini & Delle Fave, 2000). Although it is clear what flow and optimal experience are, concerning their characteristics, different perspectives are still present in the empirical literature concerning the clarification of the core of such subjective experiences.

The main conceptual framework underlying all the presented ongoing studies is based on the Experience Fluctuation Model (EFM, Csikszentmihalyi & Massimini, 1985; Massimini, Csikszentmihalyi, & Delle Fave, 1988; Massimini & Delle Fave, 2000). Although they focus on specific topics and issues about the study of subjective experience and optimal experience, results have been discussed in order to validate the model as theoretical explanation for the understanding and knowledge of subjective experience in daily life. This model states that the perceived level of environmental challenges and the personal skills in facing them is crucial in shaping the global individuals' quality of daily experience. Considering these two variables (challenges and skills), this model is set on a Cartesian plan, in which the skills are reported on the *x* axis and the challenges on the *y* axis. This plan has been divided into eight sectors, denominated channels that correspond to experiential states and are defined as a function of challenges/skills ratios. According to this, perceived high challenges, matched with the perceived adequate skills to face them, characterize Channel 2, which is associated with optimal experience. All the other channels, such as relaxation, apathy, anxiety, arousal, control, boredom, and worry express different balances and experiential states of subjective experience. Each one of these channels, besides its perceived balance between challenges and skills, integrates different characteristics of emotional, motivational, and cognitive dimensions that are interdependent throughout the ongoing experience of the subject in relation with the context (Delle Fave & Bassi, 2000; Delle Fave & Massimini, 2005; Nakamura & Csikszentmihalyi, 2005).

Apart from the same theoretical framework, all the presented research lines use the same methodological approach, integrating online and retrospective measures. As for the first, the Experience Sampling Method (ESM) has been used, in accordance to the perspective that it is the most adequate to the study of people's daily life and the associated quality of experience (Csikszentmihalyi & Larson, 1987). It is a signal-contingent sampling method, in which participants respond to repeated self-report assessments across a time period while functioning within their natural settings, reducing recall and estimation errors inherent to surveys and retrospective interviews and avoiding any expectancy effects (Scollon, Kim-Prieto, & Diener, 2003). This method is associated with high levels of ecological, internal, and situational validity, as well as reliability of measurement (Hektner, Schmidt, & Csikszentmihalyi, 2007). The ESM permits the identification and analysis of how patterns in people's subjective experience relate to the wider conditions of their lives, without compromising the essential personal meaning of the experience. Concerning retrospective measures, self-report instruments have been used, in order to evaluate some concepts related to the model, such as the Flow questionnaire (Delle Fave & Massimini, 1988) and the Life Theme questionnaire (Csikszentmihalyi & Beattie, 1979), as well as other specific psychological instruments related to the specific topics of each one of the research lines.

Main Research Lines

At the present moment, our studies about optimal experience are structured in six topics, as the result of crossing the different life contexts and specific populations being studied, and are defined as the following:

1. *Optimal experience, school and learning processes in adolescence* (Freire, 2004; Freire, Lima, & Fonte, 2009; Lima & Freire, 2006, 2007, 2008, 2009). The main aim of this research line with Portuguese adolescents in school contexts is to identify and characterize specific experiential patterns associated with different learning activities. This has been studied considering, on one hand, the eight channels of the *Experience Fluctuation Model,* articulating the cognitive, emotional, and motivational dimensions of experience, which are considered critical for understanding students' educational experiences. On the other hand, the analysis of which conditions foster the experience of *flow* in classroom settings contribute to optimize the role of teachers in providing adolescents with opportunities for optimal learning and positive growth, with important implications for the promotion of academic success and adolescents' development.
2. *Optimal experience, leisure and substance abuse in adolescence* (Fonte & Freire, 2006, 2007, 2008; Freire, 2006a, 2006b; Freire & Fonte, 2007; Freire, Fonte, & Lima, 2007b). The main aim of this research line is to analyze the daily life of Portuguese adolescents in terms of the leisure's quality of experience, focusing on the emergence and impact of optimal experience in their lifestyles and developmental processes. According to this, the analysis of specific experiential patterns associated with leisure activities and leisure experience, differentiating among drug users and nonusers is a main focus of these studies. The role of leisure experience in terms of intervention for preventing health risk behaviours is highlighted, in order to understand how to promote proactive and engaged healthy individuals in adolescence.
3. *Optimal experience, family and parental influence on adolescence* (Freire, 2009; Freire, Fonte, & Lima, 2007a). The aim of this research line is to analyze the quality of subjective experience inside the context of family relations, mainly to know how this context and associated social relations between parents and adolescents can contribute to the emergence and maintenance of specific experiential states concerning daily life, such as the optimal experience and, in an opposite way, apathy and boredom. In particular, these studies are aimed to

analyze how the relations between adolescents and their parents shape their subjective experience and what the consequent implications are for identity building and autonomy improvement in adolescence.

4. *Optimal experiences and well-being in older age* (Ferreira & Freire, 2008a, 2008b, 2009a, 2009b, 2010). The main aim of this research line is to study the quality of subjective experience in later life, and its association with the psychological well-being as well as the life satisfaction and the feelings of loneliness. More specifically, the focus is to understand the daily life structure of the elderly; the interactions they establish with others and with places; their resources and opportunities for action; and the associated cognitions, emotions, and motivations. The comparison of these results with other age groups and life patterns is a main research goal, contributing to a better understanding of the subjective experiential processes through the lens of the life span perspective.
5. *Optimal experience, physiological and psychological experience patterns in young adults* (Matias, Nicolson, & Freire, 2008, 2009a, 2009b, 2011). The main aim of this research line is to understand the associations of the physiology of cortisol and the flow experience, focusing on the long-term consequences of flow and overall positive experiences, through the study of the autotelic personality and cortisol daily patterns. The knowledge of how positive events and characteristics influence and are influenced by physiological processes raise awareness of the importance of promoting these experiences in daily life, thus increasing the development of an optimal psychological and physical functioning.
6. *Optimal experience, psychotherapy and related daily life in adults* (Mourão, Freire, & Fernandes, 2008a, 2008b, 2008c; Mourão, Ribeiro, & Freire, 2009). The aim of this research line is to understand the interaction among intersession life factors, such as the events of clients' daily life outside the therapeutic context, and intrasession factors related to therapeutic alliance, analysing three different phases of the therapeutic process (initial, intermediate, and final phase). In addition, the study of the role of the optimal experience in this individual change process is a main goal in order to know about the conditions for its occurrence and the associated cognitive, motivational, and affective dimensions underlying the impact of the psychotherapy process in promoting more positive and healthy lives.

Main Research Issues for Theoretical and Empirical Discussion

Independent of the specific research topic, these studies with Portuguese subjects showed optimal experience as a balance between challenges and skills perceptions with opposite channels showing opposite experiential patterns. In relation to cognitive, affective and motivational dimensions, results showed different characteristics of flow experience according to different kinds of activities, showing that these dimensions may have different values in a precise moment or from one activity to another.

All these results underline the importance of the study of the quality of subjective experience, considering these two main features: the channels with the expressed balance between challenges and skills, and the psychological features concerning cognitive, affective and motivational dimensions. Only these two levels of analysis make possible a deep understanding about how and why specific patterns of experience emerge across different subjective experiential trajectories. At this point, our Portuguese results go in the same direction of different studies supported by the Experience Fluctuation Model. One of the main contributions of our investigation is the association of some physiological states and characteristics to the study of the subjective experience, trying to know where psychological and physiological patterns converge for the emergence of positive experiences and optimal functioning. In the perspective of person–environment interaction, as stated by the Experience Fluctuation model (cf. Massimini & Delle Fave, 2000), we are assuming that physiology has to be considered not only as an internal result of, but also as an intermediate state between environment and psychological features – being the influence or being influenced.

About methodological concerns related to this kind of daily life and real-time collecting data, all these studies are characterized by the use of both retrospective and online methods, with the aim of providing adequate methods in terms of validity and reliability. It is underlined that different methods make possible different information about individuals, contexts, and interactions. Besides this, we are guided by the perspective that, if there are different collected information, they need to be deeply analyzed in terms of "what does this mean" concerning knowledge about human functioning processes.

One of the most relevant results that require deep analysis and theoretical discussion is the motivational dimension of the quality of the experience, analyzed as short-term desirability (e.g., wanting to do the activity at present) versus long-term meaning (e.g., future goals) of the daily activities Concerning our results on adolescents, a paradox is clearly shown when results about school and leisure are compared, which is not new in literature (cf. Csikszentmihalyi & LeFevre, 1989; Delle Fave & Massimini, 2005). If in the school context, and in particular in school activities, short-term desirability shows low results and long-term meaning high ones, on the contrary, in the leisure context, results on short-term desirability are higher than those of long-term meaning. Apart from these opposite results, both contexts appeared as being related to developmental issues, action and awareness, socio-cognitive processes and meaning building. According to this, a main question emerges (Freire & Lima, 2009): Do these results contradict the model or, in turn, do they highlight the need for a conceptual discussion about the concept of flow and optimal experience?

In the same line, some of the most meaningful data about this issue is related to leisure and its association with optimal experience (Freire, 2006a, 2007). According to the Portuguese data, when using online measures, leisure experience appears to be the most positive optimal experience, showing high levels of activation and involvement. However, when using retrospective measures, requiring individuals' memories and associated meanings, results show that leisure experience is a main optimal activity, a source of optimal experiences and positive influences, but it is neither a present challenge nor a relevant future goal. As optimal experience, leisure appeared more frequently in retrospective than online measures which needs to be analyzed concerning psychological selection and life theme concepts (Freire & Matias, 2008).

From this point of view, some research questions are pointed out from a conceptual and methodological perspective, being a present research goal for the GIFOp group research. Conceptually, it is important to systematically analyze the process from action to awareness and meaningfulness and the role of attribution processes and life theme building, in order to know and characterize the core of optimal experience. Methodologically, the comparison between online and retrospective measures contributes for a deep knowledge about psychological processes, from action to awareness, which means, to analyze the socio-cognitive processes associated with physiological and social issues.

As a conclusion, a main research goal is highlighted that requires answering a main question about human functioning, which has to do with the definition of flow and optimal experience. At this stage of research, our research group is oriented to the hypothesis that flow and optimal experience are different and independent experiential states. This conclusion and emergent question is only possible to understand when several and different research studies are put together and a more supra-analysis is done. The presented studies are aimed to attain this research goal.

But, although different and independent, flow and optimal experience are related states, with the individuals' represented meanings about past experiences being the main issue that makes possible the relation, and at the same time, the differentiation of these two concepts. In this sense, and as it is shown in Fig. 5.1, we hypothesize that flow is an experiential state occurring during the course of the action, influenced and defined by the in-situation characteristics that lead to the emergent experience. Only when the individual becomes aware of this action and it is represented in his/her socio-cognitive map, it is possible to speak about optimal experience. This awareness process has to do with the meanings that individuals build along their life trajectory, being a consequence of the socialization process. These meanings are articulated both by internal physiological states as well as by social and cultural parameters about the external world, according to the process of psychological selection, as stated by the EFM.

In this awareness process, several patterns of the balance between challenges and skills can exist, integrating the cognitive, affective, and motivational dimensions of the experience. According to our own perspective, both flow and optimal experience deal with the balance between challenges and skills, but only when this balance is high and occurs simultaneously with high values of these three dimensions, we speak about the optimal experience (see Fig. 5.1). Otherwise, it could be a flow experience, but without this optimal level that characterizes the source for the continuing replication of the activity and the associated experience. This conceptual discussion does not ask for a new model. On the contrary, it expresses the great sensitivity of the Experience Fluctuation Model to analyze and explain the main

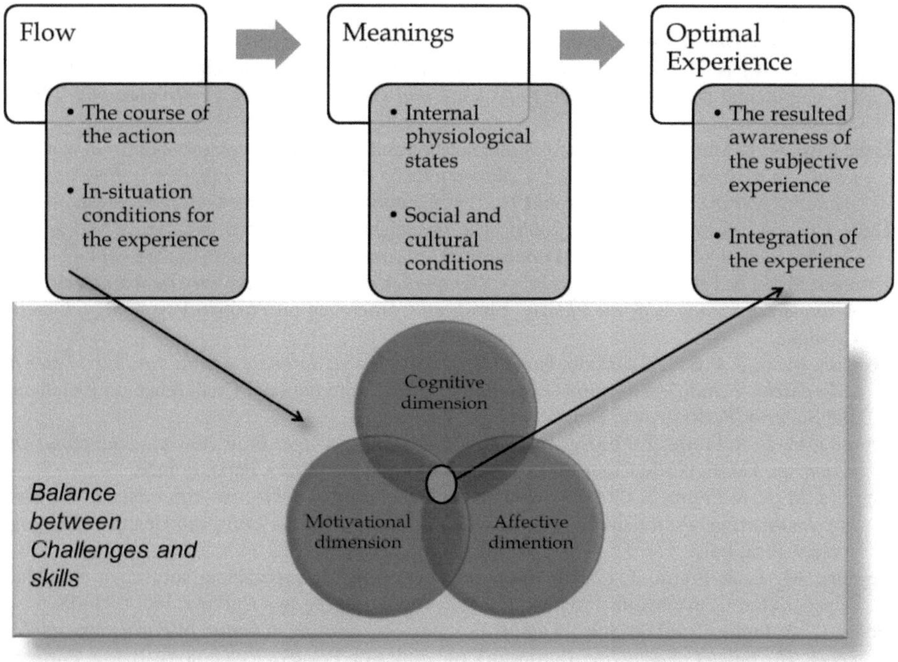

Fig. 5.1 A conceptual analysis of flow and optimal experiential states – a guide for future research (Source: Freire, 2008)

deep features of the quality of the subjective experience as it exists and is lived by individuals in their daily lives. This discussion and research can have a great impact on the study of human positive functioning, as well as on the way intervention is thought or defined and implemented in the various life contexts accross different populations and cultures, in order to promote individual and social development.

References

Csikszentmihalyi, M. (1997). *Finding flow: The psychology of engagement with everyday life*. New York: Basic Books.

Csikszentmihalyi, M., & Beattie, O. (1979). Life themes: A theoretical and empirical exploration of their origins and affects. *Journal of Humanistic Psychology, 19*, 45–63.

Csikszentmihalyi, M., & Csikszentmihalyi, I. (1988). *Optimal experience: Psychological studies of flow in consciousness*. Cambridge: Cambridge University Press.

Csikszentmihalyi, M., & Larson, R. W. (1987). Validity and reliability of the experience sampling method. *The Journal of Nervous and Mental Disease, 175*, 526–536.

Csikszentmihalyi, M., & LeFevre, J. (1989). Optimal experience in work and leisure. *Journal of Personality and Social Psychology, 56*(5), 815–822.

Csikszentmihalyi, M., & Massimini, F. (1985). On the psychological selection of bio-cultural information. *New Ideas in Psychology, 3*(2), 115–138.

Delle Fave, A., & Bassi, M. (2000). The quality of experience in adolescents' daily lives: Developmental perspectives. *Genetic, Social, and General Psychology Monographs, 126*(3), 347–367.

Delle Fave, A., & Massimini, F. (1988). Modernization and the changing contexts of flow in work and leisure. In M. Csikszentmihalyi & I. Csikszentmihalyi (Eds.), *Optimal experience: Psychological studies of flow in consciousness* (pp. 193–213). Cambridge: Cambridge University Press.

Delle Fave, A., & Massimini, F. (2005). The investigation of optimal experience and apathy: Developmental and psychosocial implications. *European Psychologist, 10*, 264–274.

Ferreira, M. J., & Freire, T. (2008a, July). *The quality of the subjective experience in daily life: A single case study with the elderly*. European Conference on Positive Psychology, Opatija, Croatia.

Ferreira, M. J., & Freire, T. (2008b, November). *Experiência óptima e Apatia nas actividades da vida diária: Estudo exploratório com idosos*. ICESP International Conference on Excellence and Superior Performance, Braga.

Ferreira, M. J., & Freire, T. (2009a, July). *Well-being in older age: From flow to eudaimonia and hedonism*. IAGG World Congress of Gerontology and Geriatrics, Paris, France.

Ferreira, M. J., & Freire, T. (2009b, September). *The quality of subjective experience in the daily life: Implications for a healthy aging*. Annual Conference of the European Health Psychology society, Pisa, Italy.

Ferreira, M. J., & Freire, T. (2010). Bemestar, qualidade da experiência subjectiva e solidão: relações com o envelhecimento humano. *Psicologia, Educação e Cultura, 14*(1), 41–58.

Fonte, C., & Freire, T. (2006, July). *Quality of experience in daily activities of Portuguese adolescents: The impact of drug use*. European Conference on Positive Psychology, Braga, Portugal.

Fonte, C., & Freire, T. (2007, April). *Quality of experience, future goals, and cannabis use in daily life: A study with Portuguese adolescents*. Applied Positive Psychology Conference – People at Their Best: Work, education and health, University of Warwick, Coventry, England.

Fonte, C., & Freire, T. (2008, July). *Leisure experience and alcohol consumption in adolescents' daily life: From boredom to optimal experience*. European Conference on Positive Psychology, Opatija, Croatia.

Freire, T. (2004, July). *Optimal experience in Portuguese adolescents: The role of the school context*. European Conference on Positive Psychology, Verbania, Itália.

Freire, T. (2006a). Leisure experience and positive development of adolescents: From theory to intervention. In A. Delle Fave (Ed.), *Dimensions of well-being: Research and intervention* (pp. 366–381). Milano: FrancoAngeli.

Freire, T. (2006b). Experiências óptimas e lazer: sobre a qualidade da experiência subjectiva na vida diária. *Psicologia: Teoria, investigação e Prática, 11*(2), 243–258.

Freire, T. (2007, April). *Optimal leisure experience of Portuguese adolescents: Implications for a positive development in daily life contexts*. Applied Positive Psychology Conference, Coventry, England.

Freire, T. (2008, July). *(Re)searching flow throughout daily life: From social contexts to internal states*. European Conference on Positive Psychology, 1–4 July, Opatija, Croatia. Invited Symposium, chaired by Jeanne Nakamura & Mihaly Csikszentmihalyi.

Freire, T. (2009). From vulnerability to skillfulness leisure and positive intervention in therapy with adolescents. In G. Burns (Ed.), *Happiness, healing, enhancement: Your casebook collection for applying positive psychology in therapy* (pp. 100–112). New York: John Wiley and Sons.

Freire, T., & Fonte, C. (2007, August). *Quality of experience in daily life, drug use and future goals in adolescents: Positive development and health implications*. International Congress European Society for Child and Adolescent Psyquiatry, Florence, Italy.

Freire, T., Fonte, C., & Lima, I. (2007a, July). *Quality of experience in social relations and interactions in daily life of Portuguese adolescents: With whom they feel better?* International Attachment Conference, University of Minho, Braga, Portugal.

Freire, T., Fonte, C., & Lima, I. (2007b). As experiências óptimas na vida diária de adolescentes: Implicações para um desenvolvimento positivo. *Psicologia, Educação e Cultura, XI*(2), 223–242.
Freire, T., & Matias, G. (2008, July). *Measurement of flow experience: An empirical comparison using on-line and retrospective measures*. Presented in the symposium: Varieties of optimal experiences: Conceptual and methodological issues, Convenor: Joar Viterso. European Conference on Positive Psychology. Opatija, Croatia.
Freire, T., & Lima, I. (2009, June). *Optimal experience of autotelic and non-autotelic adolescents in school and leisure: The role of motivation*. World Congress on Positive Psychology, Philadelphia, USA.
Freire, T., Lima, I., & Fonte, C. (2009). Life interests and optimal experiences in the school life of adolescents. In T. Freire (Ed.), *Understanding positive life: Perspectives on positive psychology* (pp. 131–151). Lisboa: Climepsi.
Hektner, J. M., Schmidt, J. A., & Csikszentmihalyi, M. (2007). *Experience sampling method: Measuring the quality of everyday life*. California: Sage Publications.
Lima, I., & Freire, T. (2006, July). *Adolescent's quality of experience in the school context: Optimal experiences and life interests*. European Conference on Positive Psychology, Braga, Portugal.
Lima, I., & Freire, T. (2007, April). *The quality of Portuguese students' classroom experiences: How they feel while they are learning*. Applied Positive Psychology Conference, University of Warwick, Coventry, England.
Lima, I., & Freire, T. (2008, July). *Meanings, challenges and future life goals related to adolescents' school experiences*. European Conference on Positive Psychology, Opatija, Croatia.
Lima, I., & Freire, T. (2009). Qualidade da experiência subjectiva no quotidiano escolar de adolescentes: Implicações desenvolvimentais e educacionais. *Análise Psicológica, 4*(XXVII), 523–534.
Massimini, F., Csikszentmihalyi, M., & Delle Fave, A. (1988). Flow and biocultural evolution. In M. Csikszentmihalyi & I. Csikszentmihalyi (Eds.), *Optimal experience: Psychological studies of flow in consciousness* (pp. 60–87). New York: Cambridge University Press.
Massimini, F., & Delle Fave, A. (2000). Individual development in a bio-cultural perspective. *The American Psychologist, 55*(1), 24–33.
Matias, G., Nicolson, N. A., & Freire, T. (2008, July). *Flow and cortisol: Where do subjective experience and physiology patterns converge? – An exploratory study*. European Conference on Positive Psychology, Opatija, Croatia.
Matias, G., Nicolson, N. A., & Freire, T. (2009a). Experiência óptima e cortisol: A psicofisiologia no quotidiano. *Psychologica, 50*.
Matias, G., Nicolson, N. A., & Freire, T. (2009b, September). *Cortisol awakening response and the autotelic personality: An exploratory study*. EHPS Annual Conference, Pisa, Italy.
Matias, G. P., Nicolson, N. A., & Freire, T. (2011). Solitude and cortisol: Associations with state and trait affect in daily life. *Biological Psychology, 86*(3), 314–319. doi: 10.1016/j.biopsycho.2010.12.011.
Mourão, J., Fernandes, E., & Freire, T. (2008a, June). *Relationships in psychotherapy and daily life*. International Annual Meeting of the Society for Psychotherapy Research, Barcelona, Spain.
Mourão, J., Fernandes, E. & Freire, T. (2008b, September). *Constructivist and cognitive-behavioural therapy through the lens of positive psychology*. EABCT Annual Congress, Helsinki, Finland.
Mourão, J., Freire, T., & Fernandes, E. (2008c, July). *Thoughts and emotions: the daily experience in clients undergoing psychotherapy*. European Conference on Positive Psychology, Opatija, Croatia.
Mourão, J., Ribeiro, E., & Freire, T. (2009). *Therapeutic alliance: From the client's security to the client's sense of challenge*. European Conference of the Society for Psychotherapy Research, Bolzano, Itália.
Nakamura, J., & Csikszentmihalyi, M. (2005). The concept of flow. In C. R. Snyder & S. Lopez (Eds.), *Handbook of positive psychology* (pp. 89–105). Oxford: Oxford University Press.
Scollon, C., Kim-Prieto, C., & Diener, E. (2003). Experience sampling: Promises and pitfalls, strengths and weaknesses. *Journal of Happiness Studies, 4*, 5–34.

Chapter 6
Gender Differences in Psychological Well-Being and Distress During Adolescence

Dalila Visani, Elisa Albieri, Emanuela Offidani, Fedra Ottolini, Elena Tomba, and Chiara Ruini

Several investigations report a greater prevalence of depressive symptoms in girls compared to boys during adolescence (Baron & Campbell, 1993; Cyranowski, Frank, Young, & Shear, 2000). Moreover, females show higher anxiety levels compared to males both in clinical sample and general population (Spence, 2001).

Nowadays, however, there still are a paucity of studies exploring levels of psychological well-being in youth and few psychometric instruments for measuring this concept in adolescence. One of these is VSP-A, a French health-related quality of life instrument, specific for adolescents, encompassing a six-dimensional psychological well-being: energy, friends, parents, leisure, school, and a total index to indicate the general health status. Validation results of VSP-A showed that females reported lower scores in the most of VSP-A scales and on the global health-related quality of life index (Simeoni, Auquier, Antoniotti, Sapin, & San Marco, 2000; Sapin, Simeoni, El Khammar, Antoniotti, & Auquier, 2005).

A complete model of psychological well-being in an eudemonic perspective (Ryan & Deci, 2001) has been proposed by Carol Ryff (1989), encompassing six key dimensions: autonomy, environmental mastery, personal growth, positive relations with others, purpose in life, and self-acceptance. Once defining these dimensions, Ryff (1989) created a self-rating questionnaire (PWB scales) for measuring these constructs. Research, using this instrument on adult and aging individuals, have been already published and have pointed out that females show lower psychological well-being levels compared to males (Ryff, 1989; Ryff & Keyes, 1995; Steca, Ryff, D'Alessandro, & Delle Fratte, 2002; Ruini, Ottolini, Rafanelli, Ryff, & Fava 2003a; Ruini et al.,2003b). In two studies on an Italian population (Steca et al., 2002;

D. Visani (✉) • E. Albieri • E. Offidani • F. Ottolini • E. Tomba • C. Ruini
Department of Psychology, University of Bologna, Bologna, Italy
e-mail: dalila.visani@gmail.com

I. Brdar (ed.), *The Human Pursuit of Well-Being: A Cultural Approach*,
DOI 10.1007/978-94-007-1375-8_6, © Springer Science+Business Media B.V. 2011

Ruini, Ottolini, Rafanelli, Ryff, & Fava, 2003a; Ruini et al., 2003b), females reported significant lower levels in all PWB scales compared to males except in positive relations. Women showed higher scores in this scale also in US investigation (Ryff, 1989; Ryff & Keyes, 1995), but no other significant differences were found for any other dimensions of well-being.

Since, in above-mentioned studies, participants were already out of adolescence, the aim of this investigation is to explore gender differences in the levels of psychological well-being and distress during one of the most controversial period of human life: adolescence. As adolescence is a period of life during which a lot of changes follow quickly one after another, we conducted a follow-up study in order to explore if results would be stable over time.

Method

Participants

Participants were 568 adolescents aged from 11 to 18 years (Mean age = 13.68 years, SD = 1.90); 312 were female (54.9%) and 256 were male (45.1%). Adolescents attended both middle schools (N=223; 39.3%) and high schools (N=345; 60.7%). They were recruited through advertisements from various schools in Northern Italy, which volunteered to participate in the study.

Measures

Participants were administered the following rating scales in their schools.

Psychological Well-Being Scales (PWB, Ryff, 1989). This is an 18-item, self-rating scale that covers 6 areas of well-being: autonomy, environmental mastery, personal growth, positive relations with others, purpose in life, and self-acceptance. Each scale is made up of three items and its score may range from 0 to 6.

Symptom Questionnaire (SQ, Kellner, 1987). This is a 92-item, self-rating scale that yields four scales of distress (anxiety, depression, somatization, and hostility-irritability) and four scales of well-being (relaxation, contentment, physical well-being, and friendliness). Each symptom scale score may range from 0 to 17; each well-being scale may score from 0 to 6. In the present study, SQ well-being subscales were computed to represent the lack of these well-being dimensions, so the higher the score, the higher the distress.

A previous study, not already published, has shown that adolescent PWB mean scores tend to be stable over a 3-month period. Pearson's coefficients ranged from .48 to .77 and were significant for all six scales at $p \leq .01$. Test-retest Pearson's coefficients were satisfactory for all SQ scales as well. They ranged from .44 to .61 and were significant for all scales at $p \leq .01$.

Procedure

A 3-month follow-up has been undertaken. At follow-up, 59 subjects were not present. Written, informed consent for collecting and analyzing these data was obtained from students' parents and teachers.

Results

Descriptive statistics were used to calculate mean scores and standard deviations for all scales. Student *t*-test was used to analyze gender differences in PWB and SQ scores. *t*-test on adolescent PWB scales (Tables 6.1 and 6.2) indicated that there were no significant gender differences between males and females. However, at the first test, females tended to score lower on self-acceptance scale than males (Table 6.1).

Girls reported also higher levels of distress than boys. *t*-Test indicated significant gender differences in all SQ scales, except in friendliness (Table 6.2). On retest, results were very similar (Table 6.2). Females scored significantly higher than males in all SQ scales, except in contentment and friendliness, where females reported better levels compared to males.

Table 6.1 Gender differences in PWB and SQ scales (test)

		Females $N=312$		Males $N=256$		
Questionnaire	Scales	Mean	SD	Mean	SD	t^a
Psychological well-being scale	Autonomy	12.08	4.00	11.54	3.91	1.62
	Environmental mastery	13.38	3.56	12.96	3.74	1.38
	Personal growth	11.77	3.47	11.84	3.64	0.22
	Positive relations	12.42	4.44	12.43	4.36	0.02
	Purpose in life	12.09	4.50	12.78	4.56	1.81
	Self-acceptance	11.96	3.84	12.56	3.50	1.94*
	Total	73.69	14.77	74.10	15.69	0.32
Symptom questionnaire	Anxiety	4.85	3.82	3.47	2.92	4.86**
	Depression	4.80	3.87	3.19	3.17	5.48**
	Somatization	4.33	3.70	2.91	3.20	4.90**
	Hostility	4.79	4.07	3.56	3.57	3.83**
	Relaxation	2.42	1.83	1.66	1.50	5.44**
	Contentment	1.15	1.67	0.85	1.30	2.41*
	Physical well-being	2.53	1.89	1.90	1.57	4.29**
	Friendliness	1.34	1.46	1.48	1.52	1.12

$*p \leq .05$, $**p \leq .01$ [a]Degrees of freedom: For Psychological Well-Being Scales df=566; for Symptom Questionnaire from 563 to 566

Table 6.2 Gender differences in PWB and SQ scales (retest)

		Females $N=277$		Males $N=232$		
Questionnaire	Scales	Mean	SD	Mean	SD	t^{a}
Psychological well-being scale	Autonomy	11.76	4.08	11.48	4.10	0.78
	Environmental mastery	13.28	3.35	12.75	3.63	1.69
	Personal growth	11.98	3.53	11.74	3.70	0.76
	Positive relations	12.18	4.43	12.33	4.20	0.39
	Purpose in life	11.90	4.68	12.61	4.79	1.69
	Self-acceptance	12.22	3.67	12.39	3.68	0.51
	Total	73.32	15.29	73.30	16.99	0.01
	Anxiety	4.37	3.93	3.32	3.33	3.26**
Symptom questionnaire	Depression	4.26	4.09	3.16	3.50	3.26 **
	Somatization	3.87	3.68	2.72	3.56	3.56 **
	Hostility	4.34	4.24	3.50	3.84	2.33 *
	Relaxation	2.19	1.80	1.68	1.50	3.49 **
	Contentment	1.01	1.55	1.04	1.49	0.24
	Physical well-being	2.43	2.00	1.77	1.62	4.13 **
	Friendliness	1.37	1.45	1.66	1.63	2.14 *

*$p \leq .05$, **$p \leq .01$ [a]Degrees of freedom: For Psychological Well-Being Scales df=566; for Symptom Questionnaire from 563 to 566

Discussion

According to recent findings (Galambos, Barker, & Krahn, 2006; Goldbeck, Schmitz, Besier, Herschbach, & Henrich, 2007), differences between boys and girls have been found both in terms of psychological well-being and distress. In this investigation, females tend to report lower levels of psychological well-being (except in environmental mastery) and higher levels of distress than males. Particularly, girls display an impaired self-acceptance and higher levels of anxiety and depression compared to boys. This is in line with the findings of Galambos et al. (2006), which showed impaired levels of self-esteem, more depression and more anger in a sample of Canadian young girls compared to boys. Girls also report in our study, as well as in Goldbeck et al. (2007), a generally impaired sense of well-being and life satisfaction compared to boys. These gender differences could be due to the fact that females tend to have more negative cognitive styles than males (Boggiano & Barret, 1991; Hankin & Abramson, 2001) even if data on this issue are still controversial and need further investigations (Nolen-Hoeksema, Girgus, & Seligman, 1992; Abel, 2001). In the present study, girls show, in fact, similar scores compared to boys in PWB scales such as environmental mastery, autonomy, and positive relations. These aspects may constitute important strengths or resources for adolescent girls which may act as protective factors against stress and future adversities and reduce their greater risk of experiencing depression.

These findings are not completely in line with studies using PWB scales on Italian adults and aging population (Steca et al., 2002; Ruini et al., 2003a, 2003b), where females reported significant lower levels in all PWB scales compared to males except positive relations. In fact, differences between boys and girls in PWB scales are not statistically significant in the present investigation, although females report higher levels of distress than males also during adolescence. These results suggest that adolescence is a period of the life with peculiar characteristics in boys and girls, and further investigations are needed.

The present study has several limitations: a naturalistic design, a small and self-selected sample, and the absence of observed-rated instruments. Further, in this study, we have not taken into consideration the personality factors which can account for individual differences in experiencing well-being and negative emotions (Hand, Archer, Handel, & Forbey, 2007; Hendriks, Kuyper, Offringa, & Van der Werf, 2008). However, it underlines the importance of studying psychological well-being in adolescents as a route to identify protective resources that may moderate the risks of developing future distress in young generations. The findings, in fact, provide new insight concerning psychological well-being and its relationship to distress during adolescence.

References

Abela, J. (2001). The hopelessness theory of depression: A test of the diathesis–stress and causal mediation components in third and seventh grade children. *Journal of Abnormal Child Psychology, 29*, 241–254.

Baron, B., & Campbell, T. L. (1993). Gender differences in the expression of depressive symptoms in middle adolescence: An extension of earlier findings. *Adolescence, 28*, 903–911.

Boggiano, A. K., & Barret, M. (1991). Gender differences in depression in college students. *Sex Roles, 25*, 595–609.

Cyranowski, J. M., Frank, E., Young, E., & Shear, M. K. (2000). Adolescent onset and the gender difference in lifetime rates of major depression. *Archives of General Psychiatry, 57*, 21–27.

Galambos, N. L., Barker, E. T., & Krahn, H. J. (2006). Depression, self-esteem and gender in emerging adulthood: seven-year trajectories. *Developmental Psyhchology, 42*, 350–365.

Goldbeck, L., Schmitz, T. G., Besier, T., Herschbach, P., & Henrich, G. (2007). Life satisfaction decreases during adolescence. *Quality of Life Research, 16*, 969–979.

Hand, C. G., Archer, R. P., Handel, R. W., & Forbey, J. D. (2007). The classification accuracy of the Minnesota multiphasic personality inventory–adolescent: Effects of modifying the normative sample. *Assessment, 14*, 80–85.

Hankin, B. L., & Abramson, L. Y. (2001). Development of gender differences in depression: An elaborated cognitive vulnerability-transactional stress theory. *Psychological Bulletin, 127*, 773–796.

Hendriks, A. A. J., Kuyper, H., Offringa, G. J., & Van der Werf, M. P. C. (2008). Assessing young adolescents' personality with the five-factor personality inventory. *Assessment, 15*, 304–316.

Kellner, R. (1987). Symptom questionnaire. *Journal of Clinical Psychiatry, 48*, 269–274.

Nolen-Hoeksema, S., Girgus, J., & Seligman, M. (1992). Predictors and consequences of childhood depressive symptoms: A 5-year longitudinal study. *Journal of Abnormal Psychology, 101*, 405–422.

Ruini, C., Ottolini, F., Rafanelli, C., Ryff, C. D., & Fava, G. A. (2003a). La validazione italiana delle Psychological Well-being Scale (PWB). *Rivista di Psichiatria, 38*(3), 117–130.

Ruini, C., Ottolini, F., Rafanelli, C., Tossani, E., Ryff, C. D., & Fava, G. A. (2003b). The relationship of psychological well-being to distress and personality. *Psychotherapy and Psychosomatics, 72*, 268–275.

Ryan, R. M., & Deci, E. L. (2001). On happiness and human potentials: A review of research on hedonic and eudaimonic well-being. *Annual Review of Psychology, 52*, 141–166.

Ryff, C. D. (1989). Happiness is everything, or is it? Exploration on the meaning of psychological well-being. *Journal of Personality and Social Psychology, 57*(6), 1069–1083.

Ryff, C. D., & Keyes, C. L. M. (1995). The structure of psychological well-being revisited. *Journal of Personality and Social Psychology, 69*, 719–727.

Sapin, C., Simeoni, M. C., El Khammar, M., Antoniotti, S., & Auquier, P. (2005). Reliability and validity of the VSP-A, a health-related quality of life instrument for ill and healthy adolescents. *Journal of Adolescents Health, 36*, 327–336.

Simeoni, M. C., Auquier, P., Antoniotti, S., Sapin, C., & San Marco, J. L. (2000). Validation of a French health-related quality of life instrument for adolescents: The VSP-A. *Quality of Life Research, 9*, 393–440.

Spence, S. H. (2001). Prevention strategies. In M. W. Vasey & M. R. Dadds (Eds.), *The developmental psychopathology of anxiety*. Oxford: Oxford University Press.

Steca, P., Ryff, C. D., D'Alessandro, S., & Delle Fratte, A. (2002). Il benessere psicologico: Differenze di genere e di età nel contesto italiano. *Psicologia della Salute, 2*, 121–138.

Chapter 7
The Impact of Positive Affect: Two Weekly Assessment Studies on Benefits of Positive Emotions in Patients with a Chronic Painful Disease

Elin Strand

Rheumatoid Arthritis, Chronic Pain and Negative Affect

Rheumatoid arthritis (RA) is a chronic autoimmune disease with fluctuations in illness activity and pain. Pain is reported as the most widespread and challenging symptom by patients (Katz, 1998), and in one study, pain was described as an area of priority in which they needed more help (Heiberg & Kvien, 2002). Pain in arthritis is a potential stressor not only because the pain may fluctuate relatively unpredictable but also because it is an aversive bodily experience that really may hurt. Subjective experiences of the pain seem to vary between individuals and across situations both in intensity, duration, and unpleasantness, and negative affect is an important mediating variable (Blumer & Heilbronn, 1982; Fernandez & Milburn, 1994; Smestad, Vaglum, Moum, & Kvien, 1997). Research has revealed that there is a well-established relationship between pain and negative affect in general and also in patients with arthritis. Negative psychological responses may exert an effect on the illness course, increase the frequency of painful flares, lower pain threshold, increase pain reports, intensify pain behaviors, increase pessimism, and deteriorate coping (Affleck, Tennen, Urrows, & Higgins, 1992; Banks & Kerns, 1996; Bradley & Alberts, 1999; Gaskin, Greene, Robinson, & Geisser, 1992; Janssen, 2002; Lefebvre et al. 1999; Manne & Zautra, 1989). Identifying factors that may diminish this established connection are of great value to the patient's health. In the first paper, it was hypothesized that positive psychological states such as positive affect would make a difference to the pain-negative affect relationship.

E. Strand (✉)
Oslo University Hospital, Oslo, Norway
e-mail: Elin.Strand@su.hio.no

I. Brdar (ed.), *The Human Pursuit of Well-Being: A Cultural Approach*,
DOI 10.1007/978-94-007-1375-8_7, © Springer Science+Business Media B.V. 2011

Self-management and Pain Readiness to Change

Treatment programs with multidimensional approaches are developed to help patients adjust to and cope with their chronic pain condition. Such programs are often based on cognitive and behavioral principles and have been shown to be efficacious in pain reduction and in altering psychological aspects, particularly the negative ones. More specifically, researchers have documented benefits in reducing pain and in coping more successfully through the application of self-management skills (Astin, Beckner, Soeken, Hochberg, & Berman, 2002; Lorig & Holman, 2003; Newman, Steed, & Mulligan, 2004). Self-management may be understood as the daily activities a person undertakes to keep illness under control, minimize its impact on physical health status and functioning, and cope with psychological consequences of the illness as well as symptoms (Clark et al., 1991). Also for arthritis, patient's self-management is an important part of pain coping, and often, it requires behavior changes by the patient such as taking medication, doing physical exercise or relaxing, undertaking preventive action, or changing other aspects of their lifestyle. Patients often vary in their motivation to adopt such strategies, which may account for their varying degrees of participation, and ultimately, improvement during rehabilitations and treatment programs for persistent pain (Turk & Rudy, 1991). One approach to understand and handle the patient's motivation may be through the "pain readiness to change" model and its methods for assessment (Kerns & Habib, 2004). This approach is based on the Transtheoretical Model (Prochaska, DiClemente, & Norcross, 1992; Prochaska, Norcross, & DiClemente, 1999) that originally postulated behavior change to be a process going through five specific stages. When applied to chronic pain the readiness to change model holds four stages: precontemplation, contemplation, action, and maintenance (Kerns, Bayer, & Findley, 1999). Patients low in readiness place responsibility for pain relief on providers, and their treatment of choice is most often pain medication and other medical interventions. An attitude such as this is characteristic of the precontemplation stage. Some patients are more ready to change their coping strategies, and even if ambivalent, they do contemplate other alternatives for coping. Such an attitude is characteristic for the contemplation stage. Other patients agree to actively take part in rehabilitation and self-management programs, practice and acquire new pain coping strategies, and integrate them into their daily living. These kinds of behaviors are characteristic of the action and maintenance stages of change (Kerns, Bayer, & Findley, 1999). In the second paper, associations between the readiness to change approach, pain reports, and positive affect were investigated.

Positive Affect

Positive affect may be defined as feelings or emotions that reflect pleasurable engagement with environment such as interest, excitement, contentment, joy, engagement, love, and enthusiasm (Watson, 2000).

Positive emotions are key factors for well-being and quality of life and have benefits beyond making people feel good at the moment and actually broaden thoughts and behaviors (Fredrickson, 2001; Fredrickson & Branigan, 2005). Results obtained in different settings, using diverse methods and assessments, have revealed that positive emotions are associated with cognitive strategies for reframing a situation, to see it in a more positive light such as optimism, hope, and finding meaning (Ashby, Isen, & Turken, 1999; Estrada, Isen, & Young, 1997; Fredrickson & Branigan, 2005; Isen, Daubman, & Nowicki, 1987; Isen, Rosenzweig, & Young, 1991). Positive emotions increase a person's ability to organize ideas in multiple ways, access alternative cognitive perspectives, lead to greater cognitive flexibility, facilitate creative problem solving across a broad range of settings, and enhance cognitive elaboration. Also, research has documented that the threshold for labeling and reporting physiological states as symptoms vary with affect (Cohen & Williamson, 1991), and that individuals with more positive emotions respond to illness by reporting fewer and less severe symptoms (Cohen, Doyle, Turner, Alper, & Skoner, 2003).

In terms of action, positive affect relates to approach and promotes a readiness to engage in different activities. For example, joy and happiness incline the individual to interact and play, whereas interest motivates exploration of the environment. Positive emotions relate to increased interest and engagement in social, leisure, and physical activities, as well as a higher tendency to initiate social conversations (Folkman & Moskowitz, 2000; Fredrickson & Losada, 2005; Isen, 1987).

Positive Affect, Stress and Pain

Empirical evidence also shows that not only negative but also positive affect occurs during chronic stress, which is quite common and has significant importance in the coping process (Taylor, Kemeny, Reed, Bower, & Gruenewald, 2002; Tugade, Fredrickson, & Barrett, 2004). Positive emotions may be important in serving as buffers, giving a psychological break, or as restorers during aversive states (Lazarus, 1999). Little empirical attention has been given to the role of buffering factors in the process of recovery from stress or pain for populations with chronic pain. Positive emotions may be critical to preservation of well-being during times of high pain. Results from Zautra and his research team revealed that both for patients with fibromyalgia and arthritis conditions, higher levels of positive affect resulted in reduced negative emotional responses at pain (Zautra, Johnson, & Davis, 2005; Zautra, Smith, Affleck, & Tennen, 2001).

The impact of positive affect at pain fluctuations has hardly been studied in arthritis patients and the relationship between positive emotions and readiness to change has neither been tested in this patient group before. Based on the above-mentioned research, there are good reasons to focus on and study the impact of positive affect. In general, positive emotions trigger resources in people that might be of importance to arthritis patients in preventing stress as well as in coping with chronic pain on an emotional, cognitive, and behavioral level. In both studies presented here, it was hypothesized that positive affect would make a difference and the following research questions were asked:

In the first paper, we asked whether there was an association between pain and negative affect, and then it was asked if positive affect would serve as a buffer in this relationship.

In the second paper, we investigate associations between positive affect, pain, and readiness to change, and whether positive affect would make a difference in the relationship.

Method

Subjects

The sample initially consisted of 43 participants (70% women), that were diagnosed 12–14 years ago, mean age was 57.5 years (range 33–80), 60% were married/living with a partner, 23% had full time, while 12% had a part-time job and 65% were on age/disability pension. The patients were hardly depressed; they also had normal levels of affect and pain compared to other pain samples as well as low levels of interpersonal stress.

The same data set was applied in both studies. In the second study, $N=40$ because three of them missed the Pain Stages of Change Questionnaire (PSOCQ) scores and were thus removed from the sample. The participants were interviewed weekly by telephone during 8 subsequent weeks on pain, affect, and interpersonal stress. In addition, they were asked to fill in some baseline questionnaires on depression and readiness to change.

Measures

Pain. An 11-point numerical rating scale from 0 to 10, with separate rates on three aspects of the pain: last week's average, lowest, and most intense pain level was applied to measure pain. We rely on the rating of the most intense pain in Study 1 because this most closely identifies weeks when the person's pain is most stressful. We rely on the average level in Study 2 because we were interested in the patients' overall pain.

Affect. Positive and negative affects were measured weekly with the 20-item Positive and Negative Affect Schedule (PANAS) which taps the two major dimensions of mood with "pure" markers for each scale. Watson's own scoring for the affects with ten items in each affect category was employed (Watson, Clark, & Tellegen, 1988). Participants were asked to indicate on a five-point scale "To what extent did you experience each of the adjectives for positive and for negative affect during the previous week." The five-point scale was labeled as (1) Very slightly/Not at all, (2) A little, (3) Moderately, (4) Quite a bit, and (5) Very much.

Interpersonal stress. In addition, interpersonal stress was measured by the Inventory of Small Life Events (ISLE) (Zautra, Guarnaccia, & Dohrenwend, 1986). The patients were asked to indicate on a four-point scale the extent of interpersonal stress over the past weeks in the areas of family, friends, and spouse/partner.

Depression and readiness to change. Depression assessed by Beck Depression Inventory (BDI) (Beck, Steer, & Garbin, 1988), and readiness to change were measured at baseline. The Pain Stages of Change Questionnaire (PSOCQ) (Kerns, Rosenberg, Jamison, Caudill, & Haythornthwaite, 1997) has been developed to assess a patient's readiness to adopt a self-management approach to their chronic pain condition. This is a multidimensional instrument based on The Transtheoretical Model as well as influenced by empirical work (Kerns et al., 1997). The PSOCQ has not previously been used to assess Norwegian pain patients or patients with rheumatoid arthritis.

Statistical Analyses

The dataset contains data on two levels, where Level 1 examines within-person variation in weekly pain, interpersonal stress, positive affect and negative affect, respectively. All the weekly predictor variables were person-centered and calculated by subtracting each person's weekly score from the person's average score across 8 weeks. These scores identify weekly fluctuations in each variable. Level 2 identifies individual differences which were included as predictors (independent variables) in the model. The variables reflected the average interpersonal stress and affect scores across the weeks as well as the depression and readiness to change measured only at one time point. For the readiness to change variables, a centered sum score of the items loading on the three factors (precontemplation, contemplation, and action/maintenance) were applied in the analyses.

To test the relationships between the variables, we used hierarchical linear regression multilevel modeling in SAS PROC MIXED. Multilevel models adjust for biases resulting from nonindependence of observations as there is when the same person is repeatedly studied. Also, this method gives the opportunity to study both within- and between-person variables at the same time.

Results

Initial analyses provided descriptive statistics as well as correlations among the study variables. Only descriptive statistics are reported here (Table 7.1).

Associations between positive affect, stress, pain and negative affect were examined in the first paper. Analyses revealed that both weekly scores of most intense

Table 7.1 Descriptives of the variables from study 1 and 2 used in multilevel regression analyses

Variables	*N*	Mean	SD
Negative affect	336	1.38	4.67
Positive affect	336	3.08	7.81
Most intense pain	336	4.72	2.74
Average pain	336	3.51	2.15
Lowest pain	336	1.85	1.67
Interpersonal stress	43	0.22	0.35
Depression	41	8.38	4.20
Precontemlation	40	2.58	0.87
Contemplation	40	3.53	0.73
Action/maintenance	40	3.11	0.72

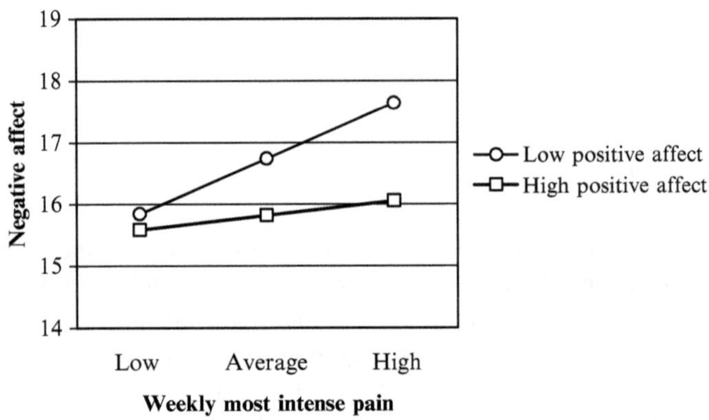

Fig. 7.1 Interaction of positive affect and weekly most intense pain on negative affect (*Note*: Weekly most intense pain: Low (Mean – 1 SD), High (Mean + 1 SD))

pain ($B = 0.37$, $p < .01$), interpersonal stress ($B = 2.42$, $p < .001$) as well as individual characteristics of depression ($B = 0.26$, $p < .02$) and stress ($B = 10.80$, $p < .001$) were related to weeks with more negative affect.

The main finding was an interaction between positive affect and pain, telling us that the relationship between pain and negative affect depended on the level of positive emotions ($B = -0.05$, $p < .02$). Graphing the interaction revealed that weeks of more intense pain and a higher level of positiv;e emotional states in that same week was related to less negative emotions. This finding is illustrated in Fig. 7.1. More specifically, the stressful impact of more intense pain was lessened by the presence of positive affect.

In the second paper, associations between positive affect, readiness to change and pain were investigated. The main finding from this study was a significant interaction effect between higher level of pain readiness to change and positive affect on weekly reports of pain ($B = -0.004$, $p < .01$). This is illustrated in Fig. 7.2. The findings

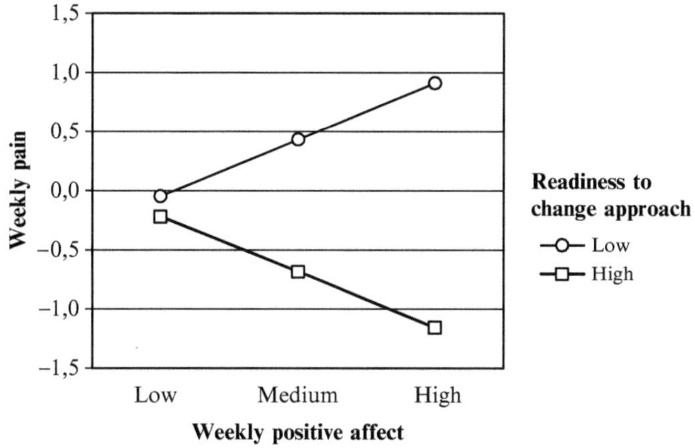

Fig. 7.2 Interaction of high readiness to change approach and positive affect on weekly reports of pain

imply that for those patients with higher level of readiness to change, higher scores on action was associated with less weekly pain reports but only in weeks when positive affect were higher than usual.

Analysis further revealed that in weeks with more positive affect, patients also reported significantly less pain ($B=-0.05$, $p<.01$), while individual differences in positive affect did not make any difference. Both weekly ($B=0.08$, $p<.01$) and average level ($B=0.20$, $p<.01$) of negative affect were associated with more weekly pain. There were no significant associations between the three readiness to change variables and pain.

Discussion

Positive affect such as being engaged, interested, enthusiastic, inspired, lively, etc. has greatest influence and is a buffer in the pain–negative affect relationship in weeks when pain is at a higher level; then, it relates to lower negative emotions. This finding is in accordance with a former research by Zautra et al. (2001, 2005) on arthritis patients as well as research showing benefits of positive emotions at different aversive states (Lazarus, 1999; Taylor et al., 2002; Tugade et al., 2004). Positive affect may reduce the magnitude of negative emotional responses as well as facilitate broadening of thought and action repertoire according to Fredrickson (2001). That the stressful impact of more intense pain is lessened by the presence of positive emotions may imply that interventions should not only focus on reducing negative emotional states but also highlight pleasures as well as sources of positive emotions in the patients' lives. This is one path to well-being for this patient group.

Those patients having a higher score on action/maintenance reported less pain in weeks when, also, positive affect was higher than usual. That positive affect makes a difference to the relationship between readiness to change, and pain may be because when patients report that they have "learned good ways to keep their pain problems from interfering with their life" or "use strategies to help them deal better with their pain," such attitudes are not enough to influence pain perception. It appears that without positive affect a readiness to change approach does not influence reports of weekly pain, and this may be due to the fact that positive emotions in itself promote action. The finding indicates that a combination of cognitive factors and positive affect is most effective in relation to pain reduction. To our knowledge, no other study has examined the relationship between readiness to change approach, positive affect, and pain. Thus, this model should be tested in further studies. In addition, this study lacks repeated measures on pain readiness to change, that could help in further examinations of relationships such as these over time.

The link between positive affect and less reported pain, as shown here, may be explained by physiological mechanisms such as release of endogenous opioids (Bendetti & Amanzio, 1997) and/or by psychological mechanisms such as lower symptom and pain reports at higher levels of positive emotions (Cohen & Williamson, 1991; Cohen et al., 2003).

There are many benefits of positive emotions that influence cognition (Ashby et al., 1999; Aspinwall, 1998), such as the appraisal of aversive experiences to view it in a more positive way. In turn, this may promote adjustment and more adaptive coping (Aspinwall, 1998; Fredrickson, 2001; Taylor et al., 2002; Zautra, 2003). The potential of positive emotions may encourage new approaches to improving quality of life for patients in chronic pain. Our findings invite further studies of, for example, how individual differences in emotional awareness and regulation as well as social resources and interpersonal relationships mean something to a person's capacity to experience as well as utilize benefits of positive emotions.

There are some limitations of the studies. Our sample consisted of RA patients already included in and recruited from a larger follow-up study. One-third took part in our study, and they compare favorably with the original sample on important variables such as pain and level of disability. Still, this may be a selected group of patients being more resilient than the random sample. The participants also were asked to report on last week's pain, affect and stress. Such retrospective reports may be sources of recall bias and influenced by the individual's pain or affective level at the moment of report of the prior week's pain as well as emotional experiences. In addition, we know that the variables examined may fluctuate frequently within a week and even within one day. Daily or within-day assessments should be encouraged in further studies. Results from the second study on relationships between pain, positive affect and action/maintenance may, even if consistent with results from other studies (Pressman & Cohen, 2005), be related to a small number of observations on patients with high action/maintenance. This study also lacks repeated data from the PSOCQ. Future studies should incorporate more frequent and more comprehensive measurements to examine these relationships.

The findings from our two studies on the impact of positive affect may inform clinical practice; we need to develop methods to experience more positive emotions more often and incorporate them into rehabilitation programs and other behavior change interventions for this group of chronic pain patients.

Remarks

The findings presented here are based on and described in more detail in two of the papers (Strand et al., 2006, 2007) in the author's doctoral thesis: "The impact of positive affect: A study of affect dynamics, pain, and interpersonal relationship in patients with musculoskeletal disorders" University of Oslo, 2006. The research was carried through at Department of Behavioral Sciences in Medicine, University of Oslo and funded by the Research Council of Norway, Grant #147831/320.

References

Affleck, G., Tennen, H., Urrows, S., & Higgins, P. (1992). Neuroticism and the pain-mood relation in rheumatoid arthritis: Insights from a prospective daily study. *Journal of Consulting and Clinical Psychology, 60*, 119–126.

Ashby, F. G., Isen, A. M., & Turken, U. A. (1999). Neuropsychological theory of positive affect and its influence on cognition. *Psychological Review, 106*, 529–550.

Astin, J. A., Beckner, W., Soeken, K., Hochberg, M. C., & Berman, B. (2002). Psychological interventions for Rheumatoid arthritis: A meta-analysis of randomized controlled trials. *Arthritis & Rheumatism, 47*, 291–302.

Aspinwall, L. G. (1998). Rethinking the role of positive affect in self-regulation. *Motivation and Emotion, 22*, 1–32.

Banks, S. M., & Kerns, R. D. (1996). Explaining high rates of depression and pain: Does the evidence support a relationship? *Psychological Bulletin, 97*, 18–34.

Beck, A. T., Steer, R. A., & Garbin, M. G. (1988). Psychometric Properties of the Beck Depression Inventory: Twenty-five years of evaluation. *Clinical Psychological Review, 8*, 77–100.

Bendetti, F., & Amanzio, M. (1997). The neurobiology of placebo analgesia: From endogenous opioids to cholecystokinin. *Progress in Neurobiology, 51*, 109–125.

Blumer, D., & Heilbronn, M. (1982). Chronic pain as a variant of depressive diseases: The pain-prone disorder. *Journal of Nervous and Mental Diseases, 170*, 381–406.

Bradley, L. A., & Alberts, K. R. (1999). Psychological and behavioral approaches to pain management for patients with rheumatic disease. *Rheumatic Disease Clinics of North America, 25*, 215–232.

Clark, N. M., Becker, M. H., Janz, N. K., Lorig, K., Rakowski, W., & Anderson, L. (1991). Self-management of chronic disease by older adults: A review and questions for research. *Journal of Aging and Health, 3*, 3–27.

Cohen, S., & Williamson, G. M. (1991). Stress and infection disease in humans. *Psychological Bulletin, 109*, 5–24.

Cohen, S., Doyle, W. J., Turner, R. B., Alper, C. M., & Skoner, D. P. (2003). Emotional style and susceptibility to the common cold. *Psychosomatic Medicine, 65*, 652–657.

Estrada, C. A., Isen, A. M., & Young, M. J. (1997). Positive affect facilitates integration of information and decreases anchoring in reasoning among physicians. *Organizational Behavior and Human Decision Processes, 72*, 117–135.

Fernandez, E., & Milburn, T. W. (1994). Sensory and affective predictors of overall pain and emotions associated with affective pain. *The Clinical Journal of Pain, 10*, 3–9.
Folkman, S., & Moskowitz, J. T. (2000). Positive affect and the other side of coping. *American Psychologist, 55*, 647–654.
Fredrickson, B. L., & Branigan, C. (2005). Positive emotions broaden the scope of attention and thought-action repertoires. *Cognition and Emotion, 19*, 313–332.
Fredrickson, B. L. (2001). The role of positive emotions in positive psychology. *The broaden-and-build theory of positive emotions. American Psychologist, 56*, 218–226.
Fredrickson, B. L., & Losada, M. F. (2005). Positive affect and the complex dynamics of human flourishing. *American Psychologist, 60*, 678–686.
Gaskin, M. E., Greene, A. F., Robinson, M. E., & Geisser, M. E. (1992). Negative affect and the experience of Chronic pain. *Journal of Psychosomatic Research, 36*, 707–713.
Heiberg, T., & Kvien, T. K. (2002). Preferences for improved health examined in 1024 patients with rheumatoid arthritis: Pain has highest priority. *Arthritis and Rheumatism, 15*, 391–397.
Isen, A. M., Daubman, K. A., & Nowicki, G. P. (1987). Positive affect facilitates creative problem solving. *Journal of Personality and Social Psychology, 52*, 1122–1131.
Isen, A. M. (1987). Positive affect, cognitive processes and social behavior. *Advances in Experimental Social Psychology, 20*, 203–253.
Isen, A. M., Rosenzweig, A. S., & Young, M. J. (1991). The influence of positive affect on clinical problem solving. *Medical Decision Making, 11*, 221–227.
Janssen, S. A. (2002). Negative affect and sensitization to pain. *Scandinavian Journal of Psychology, 43*, 131–137.
Katz, P. P. (1998). The stresses of rheumatoid arthritis: Appraisals of perceived impact and coping efficacy. *Arthritis Care and Research, 11*, 9–22.
Kerns, R. D., Bayer, L. A., & Findley, J. C. (1999). Motivation and adherence in the management of chronic pain. In A. R. Block, E. F. Kremer, & E. Fernandez (Eds.), *Handbook of pain syndromes: Biopsychosocial perspectives* (pp. 99–121). London: Lawrence Erlbaum.
Kerns, R. D., Rosenberg, R., Jamison, R. N., Caudill, M. A., & Haythornthwaite, J. (1997). Readiness to adopt a self-management approach to chronic pain: The Pain Stages of Change Questionnaire (PSOCQ). *Pain, 72*, 227–234.
Kerns, R. D., & Habib, S. A. (2004). Critical review of the pain readiness to change model. *Journal of Pain, 5*, 357–367.
Lazarus, R. S. (1999). *Stress and emotion: A new synthesis*. New York: Springer.
Lefebvre, J. C., Keefe, F. J., Affleck, G., Raezer, L. B., Starr, K., & Caldwell, D. S. (1999). The relationship of arthritis self-efficacy to daily pain, daily mood, and daily pain coping in rheumatoid arthritis patients. *Pain, 80*, 425–435.
Lorig, K. R., & Holman, H. (2003). Self-management education: History, definition, outcomes, and mechanisms. *Annals of Behavioral Medicine, 26*, 1–7.
Manne, S., & Zautra, A. (1989). Spouse criticism and support: Their association with coping and adjustment to rheumatoid arthritis. *Journal of Personality and Social Psychology, 56*, 608–617.
Newman, S., Steed, L., & Mulligan, K. (2004). Self management interventions for chronic illness. *Lancet, 364*, 1523–1537.
Pressman, S. D., & Cohen, S. (2005). Does positive affect influence health? *Psychological Bulletin, 131*, 925–971.
Prochaska, J. O., DiClemente, C. C., & Norcross, J. C. (1992). In search of how people change: Application to addictive behaviors. *American Psychologist, 47*, 1102–1114.
Prochaska, J., Norcross, J. C., & DiClemente, C. C. (1999). *Changing for good*. New York: Morrows.
Smestad, L. M., Vaglum, P., Moum, T., & Kvien, T. (1997). The relationship between psychological distress and traditional clinical variables: A 2 year prospective study of 216 patients with early rheumatoid arthritis. *British Journal of Rheumatology, 36*, 1–8.
Strand, E. B., Zautra, A. J., Thoresen, M., Ødegård, S., Uhlig, T., & Finset, A. (2006). Positive affect as a factor of resilience in the pain-negative affect relationship in patients with rheumatoid arthritis. *Journal of Psychosomatic Research, 60*, 477–484.

Strand, E. B., Kerns, R. D., Christie, A., Haavik-Nilsen, K., Klokkerud, M., & Finset, A. (2007). Higher levels of pain readiness to change and more positive affect reduce pain reports – A weekly assessment study on arthritis patients. *Pain, 137*, 204–213.
Taylor, S. E., Kemeny, M. E., Reed, G. M., Bower, J. E., & Gruenewald, T. L. (2002). Psychological resources, positive illusions, and health. *American Psychologist, 55*, 99–109.
Tugade, M. M., Fredrickson, B. L., & Barrett, L. F. (2004). Psychological resilience and positive emotional granularity: Examining the benefits of positive emotions on coping and health. *Journal of Personality, 72*, 1162–1190.
Turk, D. C., & Rudy, T. E. (1991). Neglected topics in the treatment of chronic pain patients: Relapse, noncompliance, and adherence enhancement. *Pain, 44*, 5–28.
Watson, D., Clark, L. A., & Tellegen, A. (1988). Development and validation of brief measures of positive affect: The PANAS scales. *Journal of Personality and Social Psychology, 54*, 1063–1070.
Watson, D. (2000). *Mood and temperament*. New York: The Guilford Press.
Zautra, A. J. (2003). *Emotion, stress and health* (p. 2003). New York: Oxford Press.
Zautra, A. J., Johnson, L., & Davis, M. C. (2005). Positive affect as a source of resilience for women in chronic pain. *Journal of Consulting and Clinical Psychology, 73*, 212–220.
Zautra, A. J., Smith, B., Affleck, G., & Tennen, H. (2001). Examinations of chronic pain and affect relationships: Applications of a dynamic model of affect. *Journal of Consulting and Clinical Psychology, 69*, 786–795.
Zautra, A. J., Guarnaccia, C. A., & Dohrenwend, B. P. (1986). Measuring small life events. *American Journal of Community Psychology, 4*, 625–655.

Chapter 8
Studying Predictors of Posttraumatic Growth in Cancer Patients

Marta Scrignaro, Sandro Barni, Maria Luisa Bonetti, and Maria Elena Magrin

The term "posttraumatic growth" (PTG) refers to positive psychological change in the perception of self, in the experience of relationships with others, and in one's general philosophy of life, experienced as a result of the person's struggle with highly challenging life circumstances (Tedeschi & Calhoun, 2004).

Now, a number of valuable psychological theories of posttraumatic growth have been proposed (Calhoun & Tedeschi, 2006; Christopher, 2004; Janoff-Bulman, 2006). However, theories of growth have tended to be descriptive rather than explanatory. The Organismic valuing theory of growth through adversity (Joseph & Linley, 2005) accounts for why people would be motivated to move toward growth. Moving from the assumption of Self-determination Theory, the model posits that human beings are active and growth-oriented, guided by an innate organismic valuing process that allows them to know their own best directions in life and to integrate their psychological experiences into a unified sense of self. However, this process is challenging and requires a supportive social environment that provides the nutriments for the satisfaction of the fundamental psychological needs of autonomy, competence, and relatedness (Deci & Ryan, 2000). The theory holds that it is natural for the subject to modify existing models of the world to positively accommodate new trauma-related information when the social environment provides the nutriments of basic psychological needs.

Traumas are shocks to personal inner assumptive worlds which provide a dramatic test of human coping abilities (Janoff-Bulman, 2006). The task for the survivors is to rebuild a viable assumptive world that is both valid and comfortable

M. Scrignaro (✉) • M.E. Magrin
Department of Psychology, University of Studies of Milan-Bicocca, Milan, Italy
e-mail: marta.scrignaro1@unimib.it

S. Barni • M.L. Bonetti
Hospital of Treviglio, Treviglio (BG), Italy

I. Brdar (ed.), *The Human Pursuit of Well-Being: A Cultural Approach*,
DOI 10.1007/978-94-007-1375-8_8, © Springer Science+Business Media B.V. 2011

through the re-examination of the pre-trauma goals and beliefs (Park & Folkman, 1997). Coherently, with the dual process model of goal pursuit and goal adjustment (Brandtstädter & Rothermund, 2002), the organismic valuing theory posits that moving toward growth requires accommodation of the new trauma-related information as opposed to assimilation. Assimilation and accommodation are two modes of coping with discrepancies between desired and factual circumstances of developmental outcomes (Brandtstädter & Renner, 1990). In the assimilative mode, the subject tries to reduce discrepancies through a purposeful modification of life circumstances. On the contrary, in the accommodative mode, goal discrepancies are removed by downgrading blocked goals and rescaling aspiration channeling of assimilative energies toward new, feasible goals. From the organismic theoretical perspective (Ryan, 1995), ruminative states appear as manifestation of a shift from assimilation toward accommodation (Brandtstädter & Rothermund, 2002).

Receiving a cancer diagnosis can be a frightening and unexpected event that nevertheless could act as a trigger to growth (Stanton, Bower & Low, 2006). Actually, 60% of patients report profound positive changes in themselves, their relationships, and other life domains after cancer experience (Bellizzi & Blank, 2006).

The main aim of the present research was to test the organismic valuing theory of growth in a group of cancer patients. Coherently, with the Organismic valuing theory of growth, the research firstly intended to verify the effectiveness of the pattern of accommodative versus assimilative strategies in predicting PTG; secondly, the research wants to verify the effectiveness of autonomy-supportive, posttrauma social environment in predicting accommodative versus assimilative strategies in a group of mixed cancer patients (Joseph & Linley, 2005).

Method

Procedure

A structured questionnaire was offered to 150 cancer patients recruited during their medical examination or chemotherapy in an Hospital in Northern Italy.

All patients gave their informed consent to participate in the study, which has been performed in accordance with the ethical standards laid down in the Declaration of Helsinki. The participation to the research was volunteer.

Participants

One hundred and thirty-one patients completed the questionnaire (87% of those offered). Of these, 78% were females, with a mean age of 52 years (SD = 7.70; range from 30 to 73), and with low educational level, 83% were married and 66%

were employed. The participants were prevalently diagnosed with Stage 1 (28%) or Stage 2 (28%) breast cancer (65%) or gastro-enteric cancer (27%). Average number of months since diagnosis was 35 (SD 37.21; range from 1 to 160). Ninety-one percentage of participants had undergone surgical procedures, and 79% received chemotherapy and/or radiotherapy.

Measures

The Italian version of the *Impact of Event Scale* (IES; Horowitz, Wilner, & Alvarez, 1979) is a self-report questionnaire that uses four-point scales (0 = not at all, through 5 = often) to measure symptoms of intrusion and avoidance related to PTSD. The IES consists of two conceptually distinct subscales: intrusion and avoidance. The measure in the present sample was bi-dimensional as shown by explanatory principal components factor analysis which yielded two factors accounting for 45% of the variance and the high internal consistency of the two subscale (intrusion α=.84; avoidance α=.73)

The impact scale (IMP) is a tailored version of the exploratory intensity measurement scale (Bellizzi & Blank, 2006). It is a four-item self-report questionnaire that uses ten-point scales (1 = no impact through 10 = highest impact) to measure the degree to which the traumatic event shattered the identity and, more specifically, the personal goals and purposes, the self-image and the relationship. The measure in the present sample was unidimensional as shown by an exploratory principal components factor analysis which yielded one factor accounting for 76% of the variance and the high internal consistency of the total scale (α=.85). Accordingly, responses to all IMS items were averaged to yield a single score.

The Italian version of the *Brief Cope Questionnaire* (Carver, 1997) is a self-report questionnaire that uses four-point scales (1 – I haven't been doing this at all, through 4 – I have been doing this a lot) to measure the extent to which the participants are currently coping with stress in their life associated with cancer. The Brief Cope consists of 14 conceptually distinct subscales. The measure in the present sample was bi-dimensional as shown by an exploratory principal components factor analysis which yielded two factors accounting for 56% of the variance and the moderate internal consistency of the two subscale (approach α=.76; avoidance α=.62). Accordingly, responses to active coping, planning, seeking instrumental social support, positive reinterpretation, turning to religion, humor subscales and to self-blame, self-distraction, acceptance, seeking emotional social support, focus on venting emotions, denial, behavioral disengagement, and alcohol and drug abuse subscales were averaged to yield double scores, respectively approach coping and avoidance coping.

The *Need Satisfaction in Relationship Scale* (NSRS; La Guardia, Ryan, Couchman, & Deci, 2000) is a self-report questionnaire that uses seven-point scales (1 – not at all true through 7 – very true) to assess the degree to which a person experiences basic need satisfaction while relating to his or her caregiver.

NSRS consists of three conceptually distinct subscales: autonomy, competence, and relatedness. The measure in the present sample was unidimensional as shown by an exploratory principal components factor analysis which yielded one factor accounting for 45% of the variance and the high internal consistency of the scale (α=82; avoidance). Accordingly, responses to all NSRS items were averaged to yield a single score.

The Posttraumatic Growth Inventory (PTGI) (Tedeschi & Calhoun, 1996) consists of 21 items answered on a six-point scale (1 – *I did not experience this change* through 6 – *I experienced this change to a very great degree*). A sample item is "I changed my priorities about what is important in life." Although the PTGI can be scored in terms of five subscales (relating to others, new possibilities, personal strength, spiritual change, and appreciation of life), the measure in the present sample was unidimensional as shown by an exploratory principal components factor analysis which yielded one factor accounting for 51% of the variance and the high internal consistency of the total scale (α=.95). Accordingly, responses to all PTGI items were averaged to yield a single score.

Coherently with the Organismic valuing theory (Joseph & Linley, 2005), intrusive symptoms, high impact on personal goals and purposes, self-image and relationship and the approach coping were categorized as accommodative strategies. On the contrary, avoidance symptoms, low impact on personal goals and purposes, self-image and relationship, and the avoidance coping were categorized as assimilative strategies.

Results

Participants' level of PTG was categorized into low, moderate, or high level on the basis of the average score obtained on the total item of the Posttraumatic Growth Inventory (PTGI). Moving from the response scale of the Post-traumatic Growth (PTGI) (1=I did not experience this change as a result of my crisis, 2=I experienced this change to a very small degree as a result of my crisis, 3=I experienced this change to a small degree as a result of my crisis, 4=I experienced this change to a moderate degree as a result of my crisis, 5=I experienced this change to a great degree as a result of my crisis, 6=I experienced this change to a very great degree as a result of my crisis), the PTG scores were computed into three different categories: low PTG level ranged from 1 to 3, moderate PTG level ranged from 3 to 4, and high PTG level ranged from 4 to 6. Coherently, with this categorization, 31.78% of participants identified a high level of growth as a result of the experience with cancer, 20.22% identified a moderate level, and 48.70% did not identify any growth.

We computed a one-way ANOVA examining PTG score as a function of some disease-related factors (time since diagnosis, severity of diagnosis, type of chemotherapy) and some personal and contextual factors (gender, age, marital status, educational level, profession). For all factors, there were no significant differences.

Table 8.1 Descriptive statistics and correlations of PTG with predictor variables

Variable	*M*	SD	*r*
Intrusion's symptoms	4.71	1.02	.27*
Avoidance's symptoms	4.25	1.00	.24*
Impact of diagnosis on identity	5.05	2.07	.47**
Approach coping	2.06	0.07	.54**
Avoidance coping	1.07	0.04	.26**
Autonomy-supportive caring	5.96	1.00	.04
Posttraumatic growth	3.26	1.27	–

*$p<.05$; **$p<.01$

Table 8.2 Correlations between autonomy-supportive caring and PTG, and its predictors

	1	2	3	4	5	6
1. Intrusion's symptoms	–					
2. Avoidance's symptoms	.59**	–				
3. Impact of diagnosis on identity	.56**	.42**	–			
4. Approach coping	.18*	.19*	.34**	–		
5. Avoidance coping	.44**	.46**	.46**	.29**	–	
6. Autonomy-supportive caring	–.15	–.19*	–.06	.07	–.18*	–
7. Posttraumatic growth	.27**	.24**	.47**	.54**	.26**	.04

*$p<.05$; **$p<.01$

Table 8.1 shows descriptive statistics and correlations between PTG and the hypothesized predictors. The subjective perception of the impact of event and the approach coping strategies strongly and positively correlates with PTG. On the contrary, symptoms of intrusion and avoidance coping strategies weakly correlate with PTG. Further Table 8.1 shows descriptive statistics for autonomy-supportive style of caring. All patients perceived their caregiver as supportive for the basic psychological needs of autonomy, relatedness, and competence.

Table 8.2 shows the correlation between autonomy-supportive style of caring, PTG, and its predictors. The level of the avoidance's symptoms and the avoidance coping style weakly correlated with autonomy-supportive caregiver. On the contrary, not one of the other predictors of growth significantly correlate with autonomy-supportive style of caring.

In order to test the effectiveness of the processes of accommodative versus assimilative strategies in predicting PTG, accommodative and assimilative strategies were simultaneously regressed onto PTG by stepwise method. Table 8.3 shows the results of the linear regression model. Only "approach coping" and "impact of diagnosis" played a direct effect on PTG scores. Both the approach coping stile and impact of diagnosis were respectively reliable predictors of PTG. Not one of the other dimensions played a significant direct effect on PTG.

In order to test the pattern of accommodative processes in promoting growth, a saturated path model was tested by path analysis, using multiple regression model. Figure 8.1 shows the results of path analysis. Symptoms of intrusion started up the

Table 8.3 Results of the linear regression model of predictors onto PTG

Predictors	R^2	*B*	*t*
Intrusion's symptoms	.00	.02	0.22
Avoidance's symptoms	.00	.03	0.37
Impact of diagnosis on identity	.09	.32	4.26**
Approach coping	.28	.42	5.49**
Avoidance coping	.00	–.02	0.25
Total	.37		

*p<.05; **p<.01

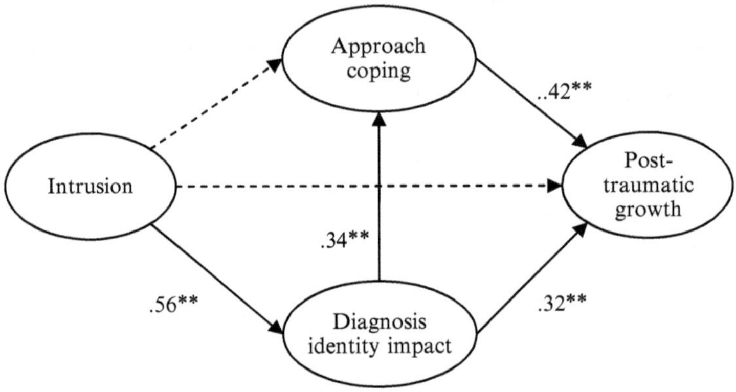

Fig. 8.1 Path model of accommodative processes in predicting growth (*Note:* **p<.01)

process toward growth by shattering the identity of patients that perceived a breakdown in their self-image, goals, and relationships (β=.56, p<.01); the breakdown in turn channeled the ruminative process toward an approach coping strategy (Sobel test, t=3.73, p<.01). The approach coping strategy was both a reliable predictor of PTG (β=.42, p<.01, r^2=.28) and a significant partial mediator (Sobel test, t=3.37, p<.01) of the effect of the impact on identity of diagnosis on PTG.

Discussion

This study captures not only direct influences of some predictors of PTG but also their indirect effects. Coherently, with the organismic valuing theory of growth, data suggest that growth does not occur as a direct result of trauma. An undesirable and intense turnover in the mind that dismantles the pre-trauma schema is necessary and functional to the shift toward the re-examination of the pre-trauma goals and beliefs about the self and the others (Park & Folkman, 1997). Thus, high level of initial intrusion is a predictor of successful growth via disorganization and reorganization of the self-structure and active problem-focused coping strategies. Congruent reintegration of the self with threat experience allows the subjects to go beyond their previous levels of functioning.

These results are coherent with the theoretical model of Tedeschi and Calhoun (2004, 2006) that highlighted the crucial role of "the turnover in the mind." Repeated thinking that includes reminiscing and a cognitive engagement are necessary to start up the process of growth. However, for the authors, it is needed that the early form of automatic and intrusive processing becomes more deliberate and reflective to produce growth. The content of this more deliberate ruminative process tends to be the rebuilding of the individual's general way of understanding oneself in the world. The mediating role of the diagnosis impact on personal identity could be explained in this direction. The perception of the necessity to redefine the personal aims and purposes, the self-image and the relationship with others (i.e., diagnosis impact on identity) could be interpreted as a shift from automatic intrusive processes to a more deliberate cognitive engagement that exerts a direct effect on post-traumatic growth, as assumed by Tedeschi and Calhoun's model.

The role of the diagnosis impact on identity is coherent with the assumptions of the Organismic valuing theory too. These results, indeed, could highlight the central distinction between meaning as comprehensibility (understanding the event and why it happened) and meaning as significance (understanding the existential implications of the event) for a deeper understanding of the process of growth. Initially, survivors may be concerned with questions of comprehension, but over time, they come to ask questions of significance and it is meaning as significance that is necessary for growth (Joseph & Linley, 2006). The mediating role of the diagnosis impact on personal aims and purposes could be explained as the necessary shift from meaning as comprehensibility to meaning as significance that enables the subject to move toward a positive accommodation of the event.

Further, these results are interesting with regard to coping process too. They confirmed the evidence of the scientific researches on the role of an active engagement with the stressors related to cancer (i.e., approach coping) to enhance a positive psychological change after trauma. In addition, this study consented to study the contribution of the coping strategies combined with the contribution of other psychological processes. The results underlined not only the direct effect of active coping strategies but also the role of deliberate cognitive engagement in promoting the selection of a more adaptive coping.

Coherently, with the evidence of the literature (Linley & Joseph, 2004), the role of the autonomy-supportive social context and, more specifically, of the caregiver is unclear. It seems that the satisfaction of the basic psychological needs of autonomy, competence, and relatedness primarily operates as factors of resilience, diminishing the avoidance symptoms and the use of avoidance strategies that both impede the cognitive engagement necessary for growth. However, a deeper understanding of the role of the social environment in promoting growth is still necessary. Some researchers highlight the relevance of the co-rumination and of the culture of the proximal and distal social context for a complete comprehension of the PTG process.

The present research relied on self-report, an obvious limitation. Like most studies of posttraumatic growth, the design of the present research was cross-sectional rather than longitudinal, leaving unclear the directionality of the associations. Further research should go beyond these limitations by examining samples of cancer patients in longitudinal designs.

Despite the above-mentioned limitations, in a clinical sense, the present study suggests that clinicians should not contain the distressful symptoms; on the contrary, they should support the accommodative processes of intrusion, re-evaluation of the personal identity, and the active coping strategy to promote the process of growth through adversity. Indeed, the process toward growth requires cognitive work (i.e., intrusion) and any intervention that impeded this work may, therefore, be damaging for growth. Moreover, personal growth after trauma seems to originate not from the event but from within the persons themselves, and this result stresses the central importance of the subject's inner resources for healing and for growth.

The study of growth seems a fruitful field of research for a positive psychology that would be a balance to mainstream psychology, which has been overly concerned with the negative aspects of human experience (Joseph & Linley, 2006).

References

Bellizzi, K. M., & Blank, O. B. (2006). Predicting posttraumatic growth in breast cancer survivors. *Health Psychology, 25*(1), 47–56.

Brandtstädter, J., & Renner, G. (1990). Tenacious goal pursuit and flexible goal adjustment: Explication and age-related analysis of assimilative and accommodative strategies of coping. *Psychology and Aging, 5*, 58–67.

Brandtstädter, J., & Rothermund, K. (2002). The life-course dynamics of goal pursuit and goal adjustment: A two-process framework. *Developmental Review, 22*, 117–150.

Calhoun, L. G., & Tedeschi, R. G. (2006). *Handbook of posttraumatic growth: Research and practice*. Mahwah, NJ: Erlbaum.

Carver, C. S. (1997). You want to measure coping but your protocol's too long: Consider the Brief COPE. *International Journal of Behavioural Medicine, 4*(1), 92–100.

Christopher, M. (2004). A broader view of trauma: A biopsychosocial-evolutionary view of the role of the traumatic stress response in the emergence of pathology and/or growth. *Clinical Psychology Review, 24*, 75–98.

Deci, E. L., & Ryan, R. M. (2000). The "What" and "Why" of goal pursuits: Human needs and the self-determination of behavior. *Psychological Inquiry, 11*(4), 227–268.

Horowitz, M., Wilner, N., & Alvarez, W. (1979). Impact of event scale: A measure of subjective stress. *Psychosomatic Medicine, 41*(3), 209–218.

Janoff-Bulman, R. (2006). Schema-change perspective on posttraumatic growth. In L. G. Calhoun & R. G. Tedeschi (Eds.), *Handbook of posttraumatic growth: Research and practice* (pp. 81–99). New York: Lawrence Erlbaum Associates.

Joseph, S., & Linley, P. A. (2005). Positive adjustment to threatening events: An organismic valuing theory of growth through adversity. *Review of General Psychology, 9*(3), 262–280.

Joseph, S., & Linley, P. A. (2006). Growth following adversity: Theoretical perspectives and implications for clinical practice. *Clinical Psychology Review, 26*, 1041–1053.

La Guardia, J. G., Ryan, R. M., Couchman, C. E., & Deci, E. L. (2000). Within-person variation in security of attachment: A Self-determination theory perspective on attachment, need fulfilment, and well-Being. *Journal of Personality and Social Psychology, 79*, 367–384.

Linley, P. A., & Joseph, S. (2004). Positive change following trauma and adversity: A review. *Journal of Traumatic Stress, 17*, 11–21.
Park, C. L., & Folkman, S. (1997). Meaning in the context of stress and coping. *Review of General Psychology, 1*(2), 115–144.
Ryan, R. M. (1995). Psychological needs and the facilitation of integrative processes. *Journal of Personality, 63*(3), 398–427.
Stanton, A. L., Bower, J. E., & Low, C. A. (2006). Posttraumatic growth after cancer. In L. G. Calhoun & R. G. Tedeschi (Eds.), *Handbook of posttraumatic growth: Research and practice* (pp. 138–175). New York: Lawrence Erlbaum Associates.
Tedeschi, R. G., & Calhoun, L. G. (1996). The posttraumatic growth inventory: Measuring the positive legacy of trauma. *Journal of Traumatic Stress, 9*, 455–471.
Tedeschi, R. G., & Calhoun, L. G. (2004). Posttraumatic growth: Conceptual foundations and empirical evidence. *Psychological Inquiry, 15*, 1–18.

Part II
Motivation and Goals

Chapter 9
It's All About Me: Maladaptive Self-focused Attention as a Mediator of the Relationship Between Extrinsic Goals and Well-Being

Mami Yamaguchi and Jamin Halberstadt

Subjective well-being or "happiness" is one of the most important goals for humans. Regardless of how people spend their time, whether working, pursuing hobbies, spending time with family, furthering their education, recreating, or volunteering, their choices are based on the belief that those choices will ultimately make them happier (Lyubomirsky, 2008). Indeed, the United States includes "the pursuit of happiness" as a fundamental human right in its Declaration of Independence (Lyubomirsky, Sheldon, & Schkade, 2005), while Bhutan has established the "gross national happiness indicator," placing individuals' happiness on par with economic development (Priesner, 1999). In psychology, the study of happiness, known as "positive psychology," is a relatively new and increasingly legitimized field. Positive psychologists study the pursuit of happiness – the characteristics associated with thriving individuals and communities and the qualities that make life worth living (Seligman & Csikszentmihalyi, 2000).

However, despite the ubiquitous use of the concept of subjective well-being, or maybe because of it, easy operationalization has been defied. Diener (1984), reviewing early definitions used by philosophers and social scientists, noted that those definitions can be divided into three groups. First, well-being has been regarded as the possession of particular socially and historically specific personal qualities (e.g., Aristotle's "eudaimonia," which can be obtained by living a virtuous life). Second, well-being has been regarded as a subjective evaluation of one's own life, reflecting satisfaction in various life domains relative only to one's personal standards. Third, well-being has been regarded as the balance of positive and negative affect experienced on a daily basis. Most modern researchers agree, though, that subjective well-being consists of both affective and cognitive components (Ryan & Deci, 2001), and that it

M. Yamaguchi (✉) • J. Halberstadt
University of Otago, Dunedin, New Zealand
e-mail: mamiy@psy.otago.ac.nz

I. Brdar (ed.), *The Human Pursuit of Well-Being: A Cultural Approach*,
DOI 10.1007/978-94-007-1375-8_9, © Springer Science+Business Media B.V. 2011

is evidenced not only by the absence of negative affect and the presence of positive affect, but also by the evaluation of one's life as satisfying as a whole (Diener, 1984).

However, the hybrid approach that relies on positive affect, negative affect, and life satisfaction indices as a composite measure of global subjective well-being has been criticized by Ryff (1989), who argued that it overlooks some important aspects of psychological health. She created a measure of "psychological well-being" based on theoretical constructs such as Maslow's (1968) "self-actualization" and Rogers' (1961) "fully functioning person." Ryff delineated psychological health and positive functioning in the following six categories: self-acceptance, positive relations with others, autonomy, environmental mastery, purpose in life, and personal growth. Ryff conducted a study in which three different age groups (i.e., young, middle-aged, and older adults) were assessed on a set of prior well-being indices (e.g., measuring affective balance and life satisfaction) and psychological well-being. Based on the weak relationships between some aspects of psychological well-being (particularly positive relations with others and personal growth) and traditional measures, Ryff argued that the traditional measures were not sufficient to capture the whole range of positive functioning.

Another way of understanding the differing perspectives on happiness is in terms of "hedonism" and "eudaimonism." Hedonism equates well-being with pleasure and happiness, and hedonic well-being is derived from experiences that maximize pleasure and that are devoid of pain and discomfort. Eudaimonism, on the other hand, defines well-being as self-actualization, and eudaimonic well-being is derived from fulfilling one's true self or potential (Ryan & Deci, 2001). Ryff's work is in line with the eudaimonic view, and her psychological well-being measure is often used to assess people's eudaimonic well-being.

Empirical support for a two-component view of well-being was provided by Keyes, Shmotkin, and Ryff (2002). They examined whether traditional well-being (i.e., hedonic well-being plus cognitive evaluation of life satisfaction – termed "subjective well-being" [SWB] in their study and eudaimoinc well-being – termed "psychological well-being" [PWB]) reflects empirically divergent constructs in a US sample of adults. The results showed that different combinations of well-being were associated with demographically different individuals. For example, the combination of low SWB and high PWB was observed more often in people who were younger, had higher education, and were higher on "openness to experience."

In addition to capturing different meanings of well-being, hedonic and eudaimonic well-being suggest distinct kinds of research questions, methodologies, and interpretations of data (Ryan & Deci, 2001). For example, past research has found that parents tend to score lower on happiness indicators, be it their life satisfaction, marital satisfaction, or mood (Umberson & Gove, 1989), than people without children, despite the positive comments often heard from parents regarding the value of parenthood. The discrepancy may be partly caused by the use of different measures of well-being: parents may find child rearing very eudaimonically satisfying, that it gives their life meaning, direction, and purpose, despite experiencing lengthy periods of hedonic displeasure. Furthermore, as Keyes, Shmotkin, and Ryff (2002) point out, hedonic and eudaimonic well-being can compensate or complement each other in situations where one can experience one type of well-being but not the other. Hence, it is imperative that both perspectives of well-being be considered in order to further the understanding of what promotes psychological health and optimal subjective well-being.

Life Goals and Well-being

A number of studies have examined various factors that affect well-being, with some surprising results. Some external circumstances, such as income and age, which intuitively should predict happiness, turned out to be only weakly related to it (Diener & Suh, 1998; Myers, 1993). These results have led to a greater focus on psychological factors such as personality and aspirations. For example, among the Big Five personality dimensions, extraversion and neuroticism have been found to be reliable predictors of well-being (Diener, 1998). Schmutte and Ryff (1997) examined the relationship between personality and well-being in middle-aged adult samples, measured by the NEO Five-Factor Inventory (Costa & McCrae, 1992) and the Psychological Well-Being scale (Ryff, 1989), respectively. They found that each personality characteristic was uniquely associated with the six facets of Psychological Well-Being. For example, neuroticism was negatively correlated with self-acceptance and environmental mastery. Conscientiousness was positively correlated with environmental mastery and purpose in life. Extraversion and agreeableness were positively correlated with all the six facets including personal growth and positive relations with others.

However, DeNeve and Cooper (1998), based on a meta-analysis study of the relationship between personality and subjective well-being, speculated that personal goals are more important than personality in determining subjective well-being. Chan and Joseph (2000) found that personality and life goals in combination predicted well-being better than either in isolation, and, in particular, that people high in extraversion, who did not value financial success, were happiest. Some evidence suggests that the relation between personality traits and well-being may in fact be mediated by their association with particular types of goals. For example, Elliot, Sheldon, and Church (1997) reported that people scoring high in neuroticism choose avoidance goals rather than approach goals, which in turn are associated with a worse subjective well-being.

Emmons (2002) eloquently explains the importance of goals, arguing that they "are the concretized expression of future orientation and life purpose, and provide a convenient and powerful metric for examining these vital elements of a positive life" (p. 106). That is, life goals provide a person's life with purpose and structure and contribute to well-being by guiding their thoughts and emotional states. Furthermore, personal goals are based on individual motivation, and they provide meaningful objectives toward which people strive in their daily lives (Salmela-Aro, Pennanen, & Nurmi, 2001).

Researchers have been particularly interested to how the content of people's goals predict their well-being. Kasser and Ryan (1993) distinguished two types of life goals: intrinsic and extrinsic. Intrinsic goals refer to goals that are inherently satisfying to pursue and are ends in themselves. They typically include goals such as meaningful relationships with others (i.e., emotional intimacy), personal growth and development and community service. Extrinsic goals, on the other hand, refer to goals that are dependent on others' approval or evaluation for their satisfaction. Furthermore, extrinsic goals are often means to other ends, with success measured only by their achievement, rather than by the process of attaining them. Extrinsic goals include such things as financial success, physical attractiveness, popularity and social status.

Similarly, Headey (2008) distinguishes "non-zero sum" and "zero-sum" goals, based on whether the goals involve competition with others. For example, non-zero sum goals such as building a good family, developing friendships, maintaining a long-term marital relationship, or contributing to a community typically have no negative implications on others' pursuit of these same ends; zero-sum goals such as building a successful career or amassing great wealth are necessarily achieved at others' expense. As a result, non-zero sum goals (which have much in common with intrinsic goals) allow for the enhancement and strengthening of relationships with others. Zero-sum (extrinsic) goals, in contrast, inherently revolve around the self and do not help in nurturing good relationships with others who become competitors that directly or indirectly lose as a consequence of one's success.

A number of studies have associated the pursuit of intrinsic (vs extrinsic) goals with greater well-being, although the cause of the relationship is debated. Schmuck (2001) has suggested that those who pursue intrinsic goals satisfy their needs for autonomy and relatedness, as intrinsic goal pursuit makes people engage in activities that directly satisfy those needs. People striving mainly for extrinsic goals have the same basic needs but try to fulfill them indirectly through rewards and positive evaluations from others. The reliance on others to obtain fulfillment is likely to make people more vulnerable to criticism and negative feedback from others, and the time and energy consumed to pursue extrinsic goals means that the fulfillment of their basic psychological needs is likely to be neglected.

Although such findings are robust and well replicated (Kasser & Ryan, 1993, 1996, 2001; Schmuck, 2001; Schmuck, Kasser, & Ryan, 2000; Sheldon, Ryan, Deci, & Kasser, 2004), there are some cultural differences in the extent to which extrinsic goal pursuit is associated with lower well-being. For example, Ryan et al. (1999) found that the negative relationship between extrinsic goals and well-being was weaker among Russian than among American women. Brdar, Rijavec, and Miljković (2008) reported a similar difference among Croatian college students. In our own data, Chinese participants who exerted more effort toward extrinsic goals showed greater well-being compared to those who exerted more effort toward intrinsic goals (Yamaguchi & Halberstadt, 2006). Brdar et al. (2008) suggested that extrinsic goals, such as financial success, might be regarded differently in transitional countries, where they may be necessary for survival and self-expression, than in affluent western societies. With the rapid spread of consumerism and capitalism, however, the relationships observed in western societies are likely to become increasingly common.

What Makes Extrinsic Goal Pursuit Detrimental to Well-being?

Why might the pursuit of extrinsic goals relative to intrinsic goals be detrimental to well-being? Kasser and Ryan (1996) propose three possible explanations. First, they argue that people who pursue extrinsic goals may have certain personalities such as neuroticism and emotional insecurity, which manifest in the need for securing one's self-worth by others' praise and approval. Second, extrinsic goal pursuit may cause people to spend more time in "controlled, ego-involving, and driven behaviors" (p. 286) and less in self-actualizing experiences. Since self-actualization supports personal growth, and personal growth is associated with happiness, those who have less of these experiences are likely to feel less happy. Third, extrinsic goals may be more difficult to attain, causing more stress and distress. This latter explanation is congruent with the results of a large correlational study in our own laboratory, which examined the relationship between well-being and various dimensions of life goals (i.e., importance, effort, attainment, perceived goal difficulty, and goal satisfaction). In that study, people who exerted more effort toward extrinsic goals reported that their goals were harder to attain, which was also reflected in greater negative affect. In contrast, people who exerted more effort toward intrinsic goals reported greater goal satisfaction and positive affect (Yamaguchi & Halberstadt, 2006).

Another explanation as to why extrinsic goals do not promote well-being is provided by self-determination theory (Deci & Ryan, 2000). It proposes that basic psychological needs (relatedness, competence, and autonomy) have to be met for a person to feel content. The attainment of extrinsic goals is likely to promote competition between people, which sabotages psychological closeness and intimacy, and exacerbates a sense of isolation and alienation. Furthermore, it may be getting more difficult to feel competent in extrinsic goal domains because of top achievers (e.g., billionaires, celebrities, and professional athletes) are increasingly salient in the media. Finally, autonomy may be undermined by extrinsic goals, as their achievement is dependent on others' evaluations and judgment, detracting from the sense of ownership and control over their pursuit.

Yet another characteristic of extrinsic goals that may interfere with their ability to enhance well-being is their suitability for social comparison. Such goals may be inherently more tangible and quantifiable than intrinsic goals, which in turn may facilitate comparison with others' performance. However, the relationship between social comparison and well-being is complex, as the direction (i.e., upward and downward), target domain, and underlying motivation of social comparison all influence its effects (Heidrich & Ryff, 1995). For example, Fry and Debats (2003) reported an interaction between social comparison (i.e., upward vs downward) and life domain on well-being. Specifically, they found that high levels of well-being in women were predicted by *upward* social comparison in the domains of social relationships and crisis coping, and in men by *downward* social comparison in the domains of physical, organizational, and intellectual functioning.

Based on the findings of the past studies, however, it appears that, in general, people who frequently engage in social comparisons tend to report negative affect (Fujita, 2008), particularly among people who are already unhappy. Lyubomirsky and Ross (1997), for example, found that chronically happy people are less affected by social comparisons than chronically unhappy people. In their study, participants were asked to solve anagrams in the presence of a confederate who either solved the questions at a slower or faster speed. Happy individuals maintained their positive mood regardless of a confederate's performance, but unhappy individuals were adversely affected by a confederate who solved the anagrams faster.

Kasser and Ryan (1996) also suggest that extrinsic goals may not be as beneficial for well-being even when they are attained. One reason may be that people quickly adapt to material improvements in their well-being, making the attainment of materialistic goals inherently unsatisfying. Easterlin (2005), for example, found that individuals in a national survey in the United States showed complete adaptation (no permanent change in well-being) in material domains, such as income and possessions. Nonmonetary domains, such as family and health, in contrast, resisted complete adaptation. For instance, persons with disabilities and people who stayed single reported less happiness over time compared with their counterparts. Easterlin posited social comparison as a possible explanation for the complete adaptation observed in material goal pursuit.

Self-focused Attention as a Cognitive Mediator?

As is evident in this brief and nonexhaustive review, there are various, nonmutually exclusive accounts of how well-being is influenced by extrinsic goals, including the personality characteristics associated with them, the competitive behavior they produce, their incompatibility with basic psychological needs, and the ease with which they promote social comparison. None of these explanations, however, includes evidence for the cognitive mechanisms involved in lowering affect. Such a mechanism would need to invoke a variable that is triggered by extrinsic goals but not intrinsic goals, and that is also detrimental to well-being.

One critical cognitive difference between extrinsic and intrinsic goal pursuit, we propose, is their attentional requirements. Although any type of goal pursuit involves self-awareness, as individuals have to monitor progress toward their goals, extrinsic goals, which revolve around personal gain and self-enhancement, require particular attention to oneself; indeed attention paid to others is largely for monitoring their progress in order to assess one's own. Intrinsic goal pursuit, in contrast, necessarily involves attention to others and awareness of their well-being. Because attention is a limited cognitive resource (Csikszentmihalyi, 1993), goal-driven attention to self comes at the expense of other opportunities or experiences that could add quality to life.

In addition to opportunity costs, heightened self-focused attention per se has been implicated in negative affect and psychological outcomes, including psychopathologies, such as dysphoria, anxiety, and depression (Ingram, 1990). Duval and Wicklund's (1972) objective self-awareness theory predicts that self-focus makes the discrepancy between one's actual and ideal selves more salient, which in turn elicits negative affect and discrepancy-reducing behaviors. Higgins' (1987) self-discrepancy theory similarly identifies types of discrepancies and their affective implications. In particular, the theory proposes that the gap between one's "actual self" and one's "ideal self" predicts feelings of dejection such as disappointment and dissatisfaction; the gap between one's "actual self" and one's "ought self" predicts feelings of agitation such as fear and restlessness. Scheier and Carver's (1983) self-control theory, on the other hand, argues that discrepancy does not automatically elicit negative affect, but that the expectation of success in reducing the discrepancy between the current self and standards is important. The degree of the expectancies, they argue, influences people's engagement or withdrawal from discrepancy-reducing behavior.

Thus, if extrinsic goal pursuit makes people focus more on themselves, and particularly the discrepancy between their actual and ideal self-representation, self-focused attention is likely to be deleterious to well-being. We conducted an exploratory experimental study to investigate whether the pursuit of extrinsic goals, relative to intrinsic goals, increases attention to the self, and whether this increase results in lower reported well-being. A goal manipulation was developed, which assumed the presence of both types of goals in any given individual, and it involved increasing the momentary accessibility of one over the other. Participants were asked to write for at least five minutes about their "most important extrinsic (intrinsic) goal" – what it was, why they wanted to achieve it, and how they were going to achieve it. Examples were provided for each type of goal (community contribution and personal growth as intrinsic goals; financial success and social status as extrinsic goals). Participants were instructed to take a moment and imagine "what their lives would be like if they achieved the goal" before writing about it.

Self-focused attention was measured implicitly in a novel target detection task, in which participants indicated as quickly as possible whether one of two letters – their own first initial or, as a control, the previous participant's first initial – was present in either a small or a large stimulus array. This task bears some superficial similarity to the "name-letter" phenomenon (Franck, De Raedt, & De Houwer, 2007) in which people express relatively more positive attitudes toward their own initials than toward other letters and which has been used as an implicit measure of self-esteem. Pretesting, however, showed that performance of the target detection task is not related to implicit self-esteem but rather represents a reflection of automatic attention to a symbol of the self.

Following the target detection task, participants were asked to respond to a set of well-being questionnaires: The PANAS, the Satisfaction with Life Scale, the Vitality Scale, and the Subjective Happiness Scale. The PANAS (Watson, Clark, & Tellegen, 1988) includes 20 mood states (10 negative and 10 positive) used to assess participants' present affective state. The Satisfaction with Life Scale (Diener, Emmons, Larson, & Griffin, 1985) is a five-item instrument designed to measure how satisfied one is with one's life based on global cognitive assessments. The Subjective Vitality Scale (Ryan & Frederick, 1997) assesses individual differences in the state of feeling alive, alert, and energetic. The Subjective Happiness Scale (SHS: Lyubomirsky & Lepper, 1999) is a four-item measure that assesses individuals' global subjective happiness.

The results indicated that extrinsic goal priming did indeed increase self-focused attention. All participants were faster to identify their own initial than a control initial, and faster to identify either initial in a small versus a large array of letters. However, for participants who wrote about their most important extrinsic goal, the advantage for self-initials was more pronounced in large arrays – a sign of an attentional mechanism. However, self-focused attention was not associated with a decline in reported well-being on any measure (Yamaguchi & Halberstadt, 2008).

Maladaptive Self-focused Attention

Why did self-focus not produce changes in affect or well-being? First, it is important to note that self-focused attention is not always maladaptive. Although it has been linked to higher levels of psychological distress, chronic negative affect, and depression (Ingram, 1990), some researchers argue that self-focused attention is also required for self-regulation, self-knowledge, and other adaptive cognitive functions (Carver & Scheier, 1981; Mullen & Suls, 1982; Nasby, 1989). These complex effects suggest that self-focus (and in turn goal pursuit) may only be maladaptive under some circumstances, or for some people.

For example, distinguishing pathological from healthful self-focus, Woodruff-Borden, Brothers, and Lister (2001) pointed out important differences in the nature and content of self-focus. They examined self-focus in three different clinical groups suffering from depression, panic disorder and anxiety disorder, using the Self-Focused Sentence Completion (SFSC; Exner, 1973). The SFSC consists of 30 sentence stems, many starting with a singular pronoun such as I, me, or my (e.g., I think; I wish), which participants are asked to complete. The responses are coded into different categories based on content (self, external, ambivalent, and other) and valence (positive, negative, and neutral). It was found that self-focus, regardless of valence, predicted all the three clinical pathologies. This relationship became even stronger when only negatively valenced self-focus was used in the analysis.

Ingram (1990) similarly argued that dysfunctional self-focus is determined by its degree, duration and flexibility, as well as by the valence of its cognitive content. Based on a review of studies on self-focused attention and psychopathology, he proposed the construct of "self-absorption," which is characterized by a combination of heightened self-focused attention and an inability to regulate that attention – an inability to readily "switch off" self-focus in order to allocate attention to something else. In an empirical study of self-absorption on well-being, Muraven (2005) asked normal participants to judge whether a list of personality words described themselves or (in a different within-subject condition) a close other. In each task, they were presented beeps to which they had to respond as quickly as possible. The slower response times for the beeps during the self-condition compared to the other condition were taken as an index of self-focus inflexibility. It was found that people high in private self-awareness showed difficulty in shifting their attention away from the self-reported anxiety and dysphoria compared to people who were low in self-awareness or people who were more adept at regulating their attention.

Penn and Witkin (1994) argue that six dimensions of self-focus (content, valence, intensity, duration, consistency and purpose) determine whether it elicits healthful or harmful effects. In a study of adolescents, whose rapid physical, psychological, and intellectual development produces corresponding changes in self-focus, Penn and Witkin found that adolescents who show self-focus inflexibility across a greater range of situations (i.e., high consistency) tend to have more problems with healthy functioning and well-being compared to peers who have inflexibility in specific situations.

Would chronic self-absorption or attentional inflexibility moderate the attention–well-being relationship reported in our goal priming study? Although we did not have a direct measure of self-focus inflexibility, we conducted a preliminary analysis using certain trials of the target detection task as a proxy. Specifically, we examined responses to control initials that followed self-initials, compared to responses to control initials that followed other control initials. The difference between these two was taken as a measure of the ease with which self-focus, once engaged, could be realigned to another stimulus. A multiple regression revealed that although neither self-focused attention nor self-focus flexibility predicted well-being independently, the combination of high self-focus and low self-focus flexibility did. Although this analysis used an ad hoc measure of flexibility, the interaction effect is consistent with Muravan's data, and with the proposal that extrinsic goals may lower well-being in those who lack the ability to regulate the self-focused attention those goals produce.

Conclusion

The findings of our study indicate that the combined effect of self-focused attention and self-focus inflexibility may be involved in the relationship between extrinsic goals and detrimental well-being. We propose that thinking about and planning for extrinsic goal pursuit produces a low-level attentional shift toward the self, which, among people who cannot easily disengage it, produces negative affect. Many questions, of course, remain unanswered. In addition to replicating the reported study with a new and independent measure of flexibility, it is important to study the implications of attentional shifts in the long term. What are the effects, for example, of repeated priming of extrinsic goals over a long period of time? Will small changes in laboratory-manipulated affect be manifest in differences in long-term chronic well-being? And if so, can the process be reversed by focusing individuals on intrinsic goal pursuits in order to take attention away from the self, and thereby *improve* well-being? Only when we fully understand the different ways goals are represented and implemented and the cognitive-affective consequences of these processes, might we gain some corresponding insight into the complex meaning of "well-being" and how to achieve it.

References

Brdar, I., Rijavec, M., & Miljković, D. (2008). Approaches to happiness, life goals, and well-being. In T. Freire (Ed.), *Understanding positive life. Research and practice on positive psychology*. Lisboa: Climepsi Editores.

Carver, C. S., & Scheier, M. F. (1981). *Attention and self-regulation: A control theory approach to human behavior*. New York: Springer.

Chan, R., & Joseph, S. (2000). Dimensions of personality, domains of aspiration, and subjective well-being`. *Personality and Individual Differences, 28*, 347–354.

Costa, P. T., & McCrae, R. R. (1992). *Revised NEO Personality Inventory (NEO-PI-R) and NEO Five-Factor Inventory (NEO-FFI) professional manual*. Odessa, FL: Psychological Assessment Resources.

Csikszentmihalyi, M. (1993). *The evolving self*. New York: HarperCollins.

Deci, E. L., & Ryan, R. M. (2000). The "What" and "Why" of goal pursuits: Human needs and the self-determination of behavior. *Psychological Inquiry, 11*, 227–268.

DeNeve, K. M., & Cooper, H. (1998). The happy personality: A meta-analysis of 137 personality traits and subjective well-being. *Psychological Bulletin, 124*, 197–229.

Diener, E. (1984). Subjective well-being. *Psychological Bulletin, 95*, 542–575.

Diener, E. (1998). Subjective well-being and personality. In D. F. Barone, M. Hersen, & V. B. Van Hasselt (Eds.), *Advanced personality* (pp. 311–334). New York, NY: Plenum Press.

Diener, E., Emmons, R. A., Larson, R. J., & Griffin, S. (1985). The satisfaction with life scale. *Journal of Personality Assessment, 49*, 71–75.

Diener, E., & Suh, M. E. (1998). Subjective well-being and age: An international analysis. In K. W. Schaie & M. P. Lawton (Eds.), *Annual review of gerontology and geriatrics* (Focus on emotion and adult development, Vol. 17, pp. 304–324). New York, NY: Springer.

Duval, S., & Wicklund, R. A. (1972). *A theory of objective self-awareness*. New York: Academic.

Easterlin, R. A. (2005). Building a better theory of well-being. In L. Bruni & P. L. Porta (Eds.), *Economics & happiness: Framing the analysis*. New York: Oxford University Press.

Elliot, A. J., Sheldon, K. M., & Church, M. A. (1997). Avoidance personal goals and subjective well-being. *Personality and Social Psychology Bulletin, 23*, 915–927.

Emmons, R. A. (2002). Personal goals, life meaning, and virtue: Wellsprings of a positive life. In C. L. M. Keyes & J. Haidt (Eds.), *Flourishing: Positive psychology and the life well-lived* (pp. 105–128). Washington, DC: American Psychological Association.

Exner, J. E. (1973). The self focus sentence completion: A study of egocentricity. *Journal of Personality Assessment, 37*, 437–455.

Franck, E., De Raedt, R., & De Houwer, J. (2007). Implicit but not explicit self-esteem predicts future depressive symptomatology. *Behaviour Research and Therapy, 45*, 2448–2455.

Fry, P. S., & Debats, D. L. (2003). Domain-specific social comparison orientations as predictors of health-related quality of life, life satisfaction, and general optimism in late life functioning. *Journal of Mental Health and Aging, 9*, 243–269.

Fujita, F. (2008). The frequency of social comparison and its relation to subjective well-being. In M. Eid & R. J. Larsen (Eds.), *The science of subjective well-being* (pp. 239–257). New York: Guilford Press.

Headey, B. (2008). Life goals matter to happiness: A revision of set-point theory. *Social Indicators Research, 86*, 213–231.

Heidrich, S. M., & Ryff, C. D. (1995). Health, social comparisons, and psychological well-being: Their cross-time relationships. *Journal of Adult Development, 2*, 173–186.

Higgins, E. T. (1987). Self-discrepancy: A theory relating self and affect. *Psychological Review, 94*, 319–340.

Ingram, R. E. (1990). Self-focused attention in clinical disorders: Review and a conceptual model. *Psychological Bulletin, 107*, 156–176.

Kasser, T., & Ryan, R. M. (1993). A dark side of the American-dream: Correlates of financial success as a central life aspiration. *Journal of Personality and Social Psychology, 65*, 410–422.

Kasser, T., & Ryan, R. M. (1996). Further examining the American dream: Differential correlates of intrinsic and extrinsic goals. *Personality and Social Psychology Bulletin, 22*, 280–287.
Kasser, T., & Ryan, M. R. (2001). Be careful what you wish for: Optimal functioning and the relative attainment of intrinsic and extrinsic goals. In P. Schmuck & M. K. Sheldon (Eds.), *Life goals and well-being: Towards a positive psychology of human striving* (pp. 116–131). Seattle: Hogrefe & Huber Publishers.
Keyes, C. L. M., Shmotkin, D., & Ryff, C. D. (2002). Optimizing well-being: The empirical encounter of two traditions. *Journal of Personality and Social Psychology, 82*, 1007–1022.
Lyubomirsky, S. (2008). *The how of happiness: A scientific approach to getting the life you want.* New York: Penguin Press.
Lyubomirsky, S., & Lepper, S. H. (1999). A measure of subjective happiness preliminary reliability and construct validation. *Social Indicators Research, 46*, 137–155.
Lyubomirsky, S., & Ross, L. (1997). Hedonic consequences of social comparison: A contrast of happy and unhappy people. *Journal of Personality and Social Psychology, 73*, 1141–1157.
Lyubomirsky, S., Sheldon, K. M., & Schkade, D. (2005). Pursuing happiness: The architecture of sustainable change. *Review of General Psychology, 9*, 111–131.
Maslow, A. H. (1968). *Toward a psychology of being* (2nd ed.). New York: Van Nostrand.
Mullen, B., & Suls, J. (1982). The effectiveness of attention and rejection as coping styles: A meta-analysis of temporal differences. *Journal of Psychosomatic Research, 26*, 43–49.
Muraven, M. (2005). Self-focused attention and the self-regulation of attention: Implications for personality and pathology. *Journal of Social and Clinical Psychology, 24*, 382–400.
Myers, D. G. (1993). *The pursuit of happiness*. New York: Avon.
Nasby, W. (1989). Private self-consciousness, self-awareness, and the reliability of self-reports. *Journal of Personality and Social Psychology, 56*, 950–957.
Penn, M. L., & Witkin, D. J. (1994). Pathognomic versus developmentally appropriate self-focus during adolescence: Theoretical concerns and clinical implications. *Psychotherapy: Theory, Research, Practice, Training, 31*, 368–374.
Priesner, S. (1999). Gross national happiness: Bhutan's vision of development and its challenges. In S. Kinga (Ed.), *Gross national happiness* (pp. 24–52). Thimphu: The centre for Bhutan studies.
Rogers, C. R. (1961). *On becoming a person*. Boston: Houghton Mifflin.
Ryan, R. M., Chirkov, V. I., Little, T. D., Sheldon, K. M., Timoshina, E., & Deci, E. L. (1999). The American dream in Russia: Extrinsic aspirations and well-being in two cultures. *Personality and Social Psychology Bulletin, 25*, 1509–1524.
Ryan, R. M., & Deci, E. L. (2001). On happiness and human potentials: A review of research on hedonic and eudaimonic well-being. *Annual Review of Psychology, 52*, 141–166.
Ryan, R. M., & Frederick, C. (1997). On energy, personality, and health: Subjective vitality as a dynamic reflection of well-being. *Journal of Personality, 65*, 529–565.
Ryff, C. D. (1989). Happiness is everything, or is it: Explorations on the meaning of psychological well-being. *Journal of Personality and Social Psychology, 57*, 1069–1081.
Salmela-Aro, K., Pennanen, R., & Nurmi, J.-E. (2001). Self-focused goals: What they are, how they function, and how they relate to well-being. In P. Schmuck & M. K. Sheldon (Eds.), *Life goals and well-being: Towards a positive psychology of human striving* (pp. 148–166). Seattle: Hogrefe & Huber Publishers.
Scheier, M. F., & Carver, C. S. (1983). Self-directed attention and the comparison of self with standards. *Journal of Experimental Social Psychology, 19*, 205–222.
Schmuck, P. (2001). Intrinsic and extrinsic life goals preference as measured via inventories and via priming methodologies: Mean differences and relations with well-being. In P. Schmuck & M. K. Sheldon (Eds.), *Life goals and well-being: Towards a positive psychology of human striving* (pp. 132–147). Seattle: Hogrefe & Huber Publishers.
Schmuck, P., Kasser, T., & Ryan, R. M. (2000). Intrinsic and extrinsic goals: Their structure and relationship to well-being in German and us college students. *Social Indicators Research, 50*, 225–241.
Schmutte, P. S., & Ryff, C. D. (1997). Personality and well-being: Reexamining methods and meanings. *Journal of Personality and Social Psychology, 73*, 549–559.

Seligman, M. E. P., & Csikszentmihalyi, M. (2000). Positive psychology: An introduction. *American Psychologist, 55*, 5–14.

Sheldon, K. M., Ryan, R. M., Deci, E. L., & Kasser, T. (2004). The independent effects of goal contents and motives on well-being: It's both what you pursue and why you pursue it. *Personality and Social Psychology Bulletin, 30*, 475–486.

Umberson, D., & Gove, W. R. (1989). Parenthood and psychological well-being. *Journal of Family Issues, 10*, 440–462.

Watson, D., Clark, L. A., & Tellegen, A. (1988). Development and validation of brief measure of positive and negative affect: The panas scales. *Journal of Personality and Social Psychology, 54*, 1063–1070.

Woodruff-Borden, J., Brothers, A. J., & Lister, S. C. (2001). Self-focused attention: Commonalities across psychopathologies and predictors. *Behavioural and Cognitive Psychotherapy, 29*, 169–178.

Yamaguchi, M., & Halberstadt, J. (2006). *The relationship between life goals and well-being in Western and non-Western samples*. Unpublished data, University of Otago, Otago.

Yamaguchi, M., & Halberstadt, J. (2008). *Self-focused attention: A possible mediator of the relationship between life goals and well-being*. Paper presented at the the Fourth European Positive Psychology Conference.

Chapter 10
The Relation of Intrinsic and Extrinsic Aspirations to Adolescent Life Satisfaction

Marina Merkaš, Zora Raboteg-Šarić, and Dubravka Miljković

Researchers exploring the components of subjective well-being conceptualize it as comprising an emotional (positive and negative affect) and a cognitive (life satisfaction) component (Diener, Suh, Lucas, & Smith, 1999). Life satisfaction has been defined as a cognitive, subjective evaluation of one's overall life and/or major facets (domains) of one's life (Diener, Emmons, Larsen, & Griffin, 1985; Diener et al., 1999). Benefits of experiencing high levels of life satisfaction include a variety of positive outcomes in interpersonal, intrapersonal, health, vocational, and educational areas (see Ryan & Deci, 2001, for a review). Research with children and adolescents has been focused on correlates of life satisfaction (Huebner, 1991; Huebner, Suldo, & Valois, 2006), and a variety of correlates has been revealed, including psychopathological symptoms, risk behavior, and physical health indices (see Huebner, 2004, for a review). Demographic variables appear to be weakly related to satisfaction with life among children and adolescence (Huebner, 2004). Boys reported higher life satisfaction in comparison to girls in samples of Portuguese (Neto, 1993) and Turkish (Verkuyten, 1986) students. Reports of satisfaction with life as a whole among American (Gilman & Huebner, 2003; Huebner, 2004) and Australian (Gullone & Cummins, 1999) children appear to be invariant across age and gender. These inconsistent findings point to the need for further studies to understand clearly gender differences in life satisfaction among children and adolescents living in different cultures.

According to Huebner (2004), the theoretical models of life satisfaction, including unidimensional and multidimensional ones, can be organized into three major conceptual frameworks. The two unidimensional models (general and global) are

M. Merkaš (✉) • Z. Raboteg-Šarić
Ivo Pilar Institute of Social Sciences, Zagreb, Croatia
e-mail: Marina.Merkas@pilar.hr

D. Miljković
Faculty of Teacher Education, University of Zagreb, Zagreb, Croatia

I. Brdar (ed.), *The Human Pursuit of Well-Being: A Cultural Approach*,
DOI 10.1007/978-94-007-1375-8_10, © Springer Science+Business Media B.V. 2011

similar in the assumption that a single result can represent different levels of satisfaction with life and are dissimilar in the aggregation method of the total result. The total result within the general model should consist of the sum of satisfaction judgments across different life domains, while within the global model, life satisfaction reports are best assessed through items that are context-free. The multidimensional models focus more on profiles of one's satisfaction with specific life domains. Huebner (1994) proposed a hierarchical life satisfaction model in which a general life satisfaction higher-order factor is composed of five specific second-order life domains (family, friends, school, self, living environment). Some authors have proposed multidimensional models in which domain-specific reports are moderated by the importance rating given to each life domain (Seligson, Huebner, & Valois, 2003). Compared to unidimensional models and measures of life satisfaction, the multidimensional models and measures that target specific life satisfaction domains yield more differentiated information and enable more focused diagnostic, prevention, and intervention strategies (Huebner, 1994, 2001; Huebner, Laughlin, Ash, & Gilman, 1998).

Adolescents report personal goals in a variety of life domains (Massey, Gebhardt, & Garnefski, 2008). Goal content, goal pursuit, and goal attainment are related to adolescent behaviors, health, and well-being. Therefore, to understand adolescents' well-being, it seems important to understand adolescent goals. The most common adolescent goals relate to occupation and education; other important goals include those relating to relationships, while goals like fame, money, and power appear less important (Massey et al., 2008). Many studies have found gender differences in adolescent goal content (see Massey et al., 2008; Nurmi, 1991). While girls are more oriented toward interpersonal goals (Anderman & Anderman, 1999; Kasser & Ryan, 1993; Kasser, Ryan, Zax, & Sameroff, 1995), boys rate social status (Anderman & Anderman, 1999) and financial aspirations as more important (Kasser & Ryan, 1993).

The self-determination theory (SDT) posits that within any life domain, opportunities to experience basic psychological needs (autonomy, competence, and relatedness) are necessary in promoting well-being (Deci & Ryan, 2000; Ryan & Deci, 2002). The content of goals and the reasons why people pursue them can affect well-being. Life goals can be classified into intrinsic and extrinsic ones on the basis of their content (Kasser & Ryan, 1996). Grouzet et al. (2005) provided evidence for the generalizability of the intrinsic-extrinsic goal distinction by showing that it holds up in 15 different cultures. Different types of life goals have different behavioral and emotional consequences (Deci & Ryan, 2000). Research findings suggest that college students who are especially focused on intrinsic goals have higher well-being (e.g., vitality, self-actualization), whereas the reverse is true for a focus on the extrinsic goals (Kasser & Ryan, 1993, 1996; Ryan & Deci, 2001; Schumuck, Kasser, & Ryan, 2000). Studies have shown that individuals who pursue intrinsic life goals are generally more satisfied with their life (Rijavec, Brdar, & Miljković, 2006; Ryan & Deci, 2002). Adolescents who especially value extrinsic goals are more involved in the health-risk behaviors (Williams, Cox, Hedberg, & Deci, 2000). Females rate the importance of intrinsic aspirations higher than males

(Chan & Joseph, 2000; Kasser & Ryan, 1996), and the reverse is true for the importance of extrinsic aspirations (Kasser & Ryan, 1996).

Previous studies in Croatia on the relationship between well-being and aspirations reported findings that college students' well-being is related to both intrinsic and extrinsic goals (see Rijavec, 2007, for a review). Rijavec et al. (2006) found that extrinsic aspirations have an indirect effect on life satisfaction through fulfillment of the need for competence. They also showed that placing importance on intrinsic aspirations will lead to greater well-being both directly and indirectly, through satisfaction of two psychological needs (relatedness and competence). Brdar (2006) found that intrinsic goals have an indirect effect on college students' well-being, mediated by satisfaction of the basic psychological needs, while extrinsic goals have a direct effect on students' well-being.

The aim of the present research was to examine the relationships between aspirations and life satisfaction in high school students. Specifically, we have tried to determine to what extent different life goals predict adolescent overall life satisfaction as well as satisfaction with different life domains (family, friends, and school). Based on previous studies with adolescents, we hypothesized that students will generally value intrinsic goals at a higher level than extrinsic goals. Also, we hypothesized that students who especially value intrinsic goals have higher life satisfaction, whereas the reverse is true for a focus on extrinsic goals. The final purpose of this study was to examine potential differences between adolescent girls and boys in terms of their life goals and satisfaction with life.

Method

Participants

The sample comprised 468 students. There were 259 girls and 209 boys attending secondary school classes (grades 9–12). The students ranged in age from 14 to 20 years with a mean of 16.4 years (SD = 1.17).

Measures

Global life satisfaction

The Satisfaction with Life Scale (SWLS; Diener et al., 1985) is a short, five-item instrument designed to measure global cognitive judgments of one's life. Participants reported how much they agreed with particular statements on five-point scales (1 – "strongly disagree"; 5 – "strongly agree"). A higher score indicates higher level of global life satisfaction. In this study, the internal consistency of the SWLS was acceptable (see Table 10.1).

Table 10.1 Descriptive statistics for the importance of aspirations, global life satisfaction, and domain-specific life satisfaction scales

	Scale	*M*	SD	Range	α
Aspirations	Affiliation	6.09	0.94	1–7	.62
	Community feeling	5.38	1.21	1–7	.83
	Physical fitness	6.44	0.72	1–7	.74
	Financial success	4.62	1.31	1–7	.84
	Social recognition	3.49	1.60	1–7	.88
	Appearance	4.47	1.37	1–7	.78
	Intrinsic aspirations	6.00	0.73	1–7	.83
	Extrinsic aspirations	4.17	1.21	1–7	.91
Satisfaction	Satisfaction with family	4.29	1.05	1–6	.88
	Satisfaction with school	3.51	1.11	1–6	.81
	Satisfaction with friends	5.21	0.79	1–6	.86
	Satisfaction with life	3.27	0.78	1–5	.71

Satisfaction with life domains

Three subscales of the Multidimensional Students' Life Satisfaction Scale (MSLSS; Huebner, 1994, 2001) were used to assess adolescents' satisfaction with specific life domains (family, school, friends). The MSLSS has been used with youth from different countries (Gilman, Huebner, & Laughlin, 2000; Gilman et al., 2008; Huebner & Gilman, 2002), including Croatia (Gilman, Ashby, Šverko, Florell, & Varjas, 2005; Roth & Gilman, 2006). In this study, a six-point agreement format was used (1 – "strongly disagree"; 6 – "strongly agree"). Scoring of each domain is obtained by summing the relevant items and then dividing them by the number of items comprising each domain. Negatively worded items are reversed-keyed, so a higher score indicates higher levels of satisfaction. The three subscales of the MSLSS showed good internal consistency among the sample of Croatian students (see Table 10.1).

Importance of aspirations

Adapted version of the Aspiration Index (Kasser & Ryan, 1996) was used to assess adolescents' aspirations (life goals). Participants rated the importance, to themselves, of each aspiration on a seven-point scale (1 – "not at all"; 7 – "very"). Principal component analysis yielded six factors that were identical to six types of life goals assessed by the Aspiration Index: social recognition (fame), appealing appearance (image), financial success (wealth), affiliation (relatedness), community feeling (helpfulness), and physical fitness (health). Items measuring self-acceptance (growth) loaded on several factors in the current sample and were excluded from further analysis. The internal consistency of the subscales was generally satisfactory, except for somewhat low internal consistency of the affiliation subscale (see Table 10.1). Similar findings have been reported in Kasser et al. (1995) study.

Background information about respondents' characteristics included students' gender and age (years).

Procedure

Approval to collect data was first secured from the school principal and counselor. Likewise, a prior consent from the students was obtained before administering the questionnaire. The questionnaire was administered by the researcher in regular classroom setting during a single session. Data were collected and coded anonymously.

Results

Descriptive Statistics

The means and standard deviations on independent variables that measure six different types of the students' goals and dependent variables that measure global and domain-specific life satisfaction are presented in Table 10.1.

Physical fitness (e.g., being healthy), affiliation (e.g., close relationships) and community feeling (e.g., helping the world be a better place) are found to be the most important aspirations for adolescents. Students placed less importance on the attaining extrinsic goals of financial success (e.g., having many material possessions and much wealth), attractive appearance (e.g., being good-looking) and social recognition (e.g., being popular and admired). The mean response rating for the SWLS indicates a moderate level of overall life satisfaction among the student sample. The means on the subscales of the MSLSS indicate a high level of satisfaction with friends and a moderately high level of satisfaction with family. Finally, the mean of the satisfaction with school indicates that respondents were slightly more likely to be satisfied than dissatisfied with their school experiences.

Gender Differences

We performed t-tests to examine gender differences in the importance ratings of different aspirations and life satisfaction scores (Table 10.2). Girls rated the importance of community feeling, affiliation and health significantly higher than boys. Boys were more oriented toward financial success, while girls placed higher importance on attractive image. Generally, girls valued more intrinsic goals than boys, while gender differences in the overall importance of extrinsic goals were not significant. Gender differences in global life satisfaction and satisfaction with family were not significant. Girls reported higher satisfaction with their friends and school than boys.

Table 10.2 Gender differences in the importance of aspirations, global life satisfaction, and satisfaction with specific life domain

	Scale		Boys	Girls	*t*
Aspirations	Affiliation	*M*	5.88	6.27	4.44**
		SD	1.03	0.82	
	Community feeling	*M*	5.10	5.61	4.56**
		SD	1.35	1.03	
	Physical fitness	*M*	6.38	6.50	2.04*
		SD	0.81	0.64	
	Financial success	*M*	4.77	4.51	2.07*
		SD	1.34	1.28	
	Social recognition	*M*	3.60	3.41	1.21
		SD	1.64	1.57	
	Appearance	*M*	4.19	4.68	3.77**
		SD	1.39	1.31	
	Intrinsic aspirations	*M*	5.79	6.15	5.13**
		SD	0.83	0.59	
	Extrinsic aspirations	*M*	4.16	4.18	0.19
		SD	1.20	1.22	
Satisfaction	Satisfaction with family	*M*	4.27	4.31	0.37
		SD	1.12	0.99	
	Satisfaction with school	*M*	3.37	3.62	2.43*
		SD	1.18	1.03	
	Satisfaction with friends	*M*	5.13	5.28	2.01*
		SD	0.86	0.71	
	Satisfaction with life	*M*	3.28	3.27	0.13
		SD	0.79	0.76	

*$p<.05$; **$p<.01$

Correlational and Regression Analyses

Older students were less satisfied with family, friends, school and their life in general than younger students (Table 10.3). Correlations among the importance of health (physical fitness) and life satisfaction measures were all significant and positive. Placing more importance on community contribution correlated positively with satisfaction with family and school as well as with global life satisfaction. Adolescents who placed higher value on affiliation were more satisfied with their life, friends and school. In general, students' overall life satisfaction and satisfaction with specific life domains were more strongly related to intrinsic than to extrinsic life goals (Table 10.3). The importance of extrinsic aspiration for financial success was negatively related to satisfaction with school while the importance of attractive appearance was positively associated with life satisfaction and satisfaction with family. Aspiration for social recognition was not related to any of the life satisfaction domains.

Table 10.3 Correlations between demographic variables, the importance of aspirations, overall life satisfaction, and domain-specific life satisfaction scores

	1	2	3	4	5	6	7	8	9	10	11	12	13
1. Age	–												
2. Gender[a]	–.10*	–											
3. Affiliation	.01	–.21**	–										
4. Community feeling	–.04	–.21**	.40**	–									
5. Physical fitness	.00	–.10*	.39**	.43**	–								
6. Financial success	.00	.10*	.09	–.03	.20**	–							
7. Social recognition	–.08	.06	.16**	.16**	.10*	.54**	–						
8. Appearance	.02	–.18**	.33**	.23**	.28**	.53**	.60**	–					
9. Intrinsic aspirations	.00	–.25**	.74**	.85**	.71**	.06	.15**	.33**	–				
10. Extrinsic aspirations	–.05	.00	.25**	.14**	.24**	.81**	.86**	.85**	.22**	–			
11. Satisfaction with family	–.13**	–.02	.09	.25**	.15**	.03	.08	.11*	.23**	.09	–		
12. Satisfaction with school	–.12*	–.11*	.10*	.28**	.14**	–.19**	–.03	–.01	.24**	–.10	.33**	–	
13. Satisfaction with friends	–.14**	–.10*	.18**	.05	.13**	–.01	–.03	.09	.18**	.02	.25**	.21**	–
14. Satisfaction with life	–.10*	.01	.14**	.17**	.25**	.04	.06	.16**	.24**	.09	.49**	.33**	.31**

*p<.05; **p<.01
[a]*Girls* 1, *boys* 2

Table 10.4 Hierarchical regression analyses for global and domain-specific life satisfaction scores

	Satisfaction							
	Life		Family		Friends		School	
Variables	β	ΔR^2	β	ΔR^2	β	ΔR^2	β	ΔR^2
Step 1		.01[b]		.02*		.03*		.03*
Age	–.10*		–.13**		–.15*		–.13*	
Gender[a]	.00		–.03		–.11[b]		–.13*	
Step 2		.08**		.06**		.05*		.10**
Affiliation	.01		–.04		.15**		–.02	
Community feeling	.06		.23**		–.08		.23**	
Physical fitness	.20**		.05		.09		.08	
Financial success	–.08		.00		–.04		–.21*	
Social recognition	–.03		.00		–.10		.03	
Appearance	.16*		.07		.11		.01	
Full model		.09**		.08**		.08**		.13**

*$p<.05$; **$p<.01$
[a] *Girls* 1, *boys* 2
[b] Significant at the $p<.10$ level

To examine the relationship between aspiration content and students' well-being, four sets of hierarchical regression analyses were conducted on the life satisfaction measures (Table 10.4). The scores on the six subscales of the Aspiration Index were entered as a block in the second step of each regression analysis, after controlling for students' gender and age. Adding the second block of predictor variables to the regression equation demonstrated that students' aspirations added significantly to the predictability of life satisfaction and satisfaction with family, school and friends.

Inspection of the individual variables within this block indicated that students' global life satisfaction was significantly predicted by a higher importance of intrinsic aspiration of health and extrinsic aspiration of attractive appearance. Satisfaction with friends was related to students' orientation toward affiliation. Placing more importance on community feeling and less on aspirations for financial success was associated with higher satisfaction with school. Students whose life goals were more focused on community contribution were also more satisfied with their family experiences.

Discussion

Placing more importance on intrinsic aspirations than on extrinsic aspirations has been well documented in the past research with adults and college students (Kasser & Ryan, 1996; Rijavec et al., 2006; Schmuck et al., 2000). This study also demonstrates that students have stronger intrinsic aspirations than extrinsic ones. Goal content is typically age-graded and adolescents aspire to goals which are, according to their social context and resources, open to them (Massey et al., 2008). Placing more importance on intrinsic goals is also in accordance with adolescents' reports about personal goals and the type of goals that their typically strive (Massey et al., 2008).

In the present study, girls rated the overall importance of intrinsic goals significantly higher than boys. This finding is consistent with previous findings on gender differences in the overall importance of intrinsic aspirations (Kasser & Ryan, 1996; Rijavec et al., 2006; Schmuck et al., 2000). In this study, we did not find gender differences in the overall importance of extrinsic aspirations, while previous research showed that males rated the overall importance of extrinsic aspirations more highly than females (Kasser & Ryan, 1996). Rijavec et al. (2006) also did not find significant gender differences in the overall importance of extrinsic aspirations among college students. The results of our study show that girls placed more importance on affiliation and community feeling than boys, which is in accordance with previous findings among college students (Kasser & Ryan, 1993) and teenagers (Kasser et al., 1995). In addition, like in some other studies (Kasser & Ryan, 1993), boys rated the importance of aspiration for financial success higher than girls. Extrinsic aspiration for appearance in the current study was more important to girls than boys. It is possible that, in accordance with their traditional gender role, girls are more concerned with their physical appearance as an important part of their self-concept in adolescence (Kiang & Harter, 2006). Girls also report greater importance of interpersonal goals (Massey et al., 2008; Nurmi, 1991), while boys are more oriented toward material aspects of life (Nurmi, 1991), their success, and competence. The discrepancies between the aspirations of boys and girls in adolescence could partly be attributed to contextual factors such as school setting, socialization, and culture (Massey et al., 2008).

In accordance with the adolescent life satisfaction literature (Huebner, Drane, & Valois, 2000), adolescents in this study view their overall life positively. Students' global life satisfaction reports did not differ as a function of gender, as in previous research (Huebner et al., 2000). Girls reported higher satisfaction with school and with friends, and this is consistent with the results of previous studies (Huebner et al., 2000; Roth & Gilman, 2006). Although the effect size of gender differences in these domains is modest, future studies should focus more on understanding why these gender differences appear (Huebner et al., 2000) since little is known about gender differences in adolescent life satisfaction (Goldbeck, Schmitz, Besier, Herschbach, & Henrich, 2007). In the present study, older students were less satisfied with their life as well as with the specific life domains. According to Goldbeck et al. (2007), decreasing life satisfaction between 11 and 16 years has to be considered as a normal developmental phenomenon consistent with developmental theories. Decreasing life satisfaction could be, partly, explained by the different challenges (e.g., somatic and psychosocial changes) that adolescents face during their transitional process from childhood to adulthood, which may lead to dissatisfaction and vulnerability (Steinberg, 2005). According to Gilman and Huebner (2003), global life satisfaction remains invariant across age, which is inconsistent with developmental theories that emphasize the "storms and stresses" of adolescence. Longitudinal data are needed to effectively determine the stability of overall and domain-specific life satisfaction reports across age (Goldbeck et al., 2007; Huebner et al., 2000).

In the current sample of adolescents, global life satisfaction was more strongly related to satisfaction with family than to satisfaction with friends and school. Research has revealed that different family characteristics are very important correlates of adolescents' life satisfaction (Antaramian, Huebner, & Valois, 2008; Suldo & Huebner, 2004). In previous studies, positive family experiences correlated strongly with adolescent overall life satisfaction, even more strongly than positive peer experiences (Dew & Huebner, 1994; Huebner, 1991). Dew and Huebner (1994) also found that measures of family-related self-concept were greater predictors of life satisfaction than were peer and academic self-concept measures across adolescence. Franc, Šakić, and Ivičić (2002) showed that family values were among the highest rated values for Croatian youth, so this finding could partly explain why satisfaction with family, in comparison to other specific life satisfaction domains, had the highest correlation to overall satisfaction with life in this study.

This research showed that adolescents who reported high importance of intrinsic goals also reported about more global and domain-specific life satisfaction. Similarly, the relative centrality of intrinsic goals was associated with greater well-being and less distress in other studies (Kasser & Ryan, 1993, 1996), and it was shown that present achievement of intrinsic goals has direct and indirect (through satisfaction of basic needs) effects on life satisfaction (Rijavec et al., 2006). Several tentative explanations of these findings are possible. First, according to SDT, success at intrinsic goals is associated with fulfillment of basic needs and enhancement of well-being. Second, a person's well-being might depend on his or her profile of value priorities. The goals of the value types such as self-direction, universalism, and benevolence largely correspond with the innate needs or intrinsic goals postulated by the SDT, and the priority given to those values is likely to correlate positively with well-being (Sagiv & Schwartz, 2000). Third, the reverse direction of casual inference, from well-being to intrinsic goals, is also possible. For example, individuals who are satisfied with their lives may be more likely to have emotional resources to improve the world through activism or generativity and to focus on the welfare of close others (Sagiv & Schwartz, 2000).

In the current study, adolescents who value wealth and material success were especially dissatisfied with their school experiences. The negative association between financial success goal and well-being is consistent with previous research (Kasser & Ryan, 1993) and predictions of SDT. The positive association between overall life satisfaction and importance of extrinsic aspiration for appearance is inconsistent with our prediction based on the SDT. The match perspective and the aspiration theory could be used to explain positive relation between extrinsic goals and well-being (see Vansteenkiste, Soenens, & Duriez, 2008, for a review). According to the match perspective, the impact of extrinsic aspirations for well-being depends on the extent to which adolescents' own aspirations match with the aspirations prompted within the immediate social context and their environment.

In line with the aspiration theory, the negative affect of extrinsic aspirations (e.g., appealing image) is limited to the pursuit of such aspirations but could be inverse once adolescents are able to attain these aspirations (e.g., attain attractive image). Huebner, Gilman, and Laughlin (1999) found that adolescents' perception of their physical appearance was related to their global life satisfaction, and it seems that appearance is a highly salient aspect of adolescent identity (Shapka & Keating, 2005).

There are several limitations of this study. All data are cross-sectional, so no conclusion regarding causality can be made between aspirations and life satisfaction. In addition, we used only six aspirations (life goals) and therefore, restricted the range of important goals that adolescents may hold. Likewise, we used only three life domains and there are other possible important domains of a human life (e.g., self, living environment) that could also be related to different aspirations in adolescence. Additional studies are needed to clarify the nature of association between aspirations and specific domains of life satisfaction in adolescence. Future progress in the study of adolescent life satisfaction and aspirations would particularly benefit from longitudinal research on goal attainment.

Despite the limitations, the results of this research confirm the notion that placing more importance on intrinsic goals is associated with higher life satisfaction. Our findings highlight the importance of examining differential effects of the content of adolescent life goals on satisfaction with specific life domains.

References

Anderman, L. H., & Anderman, E. M. (1999). Social predictors of changes in students' achievement goal orientations. *Contemporary Educational Psychology, 24*(1), 21–37.

Antaramian, S. P., Huebner, E. S., & Valois, R. F. (2008). Adolescent life satisfaction. *Applied Psychology: An International Review, 57*, 112–126.

Brdar, I. (2006). Životni ciljevi i dobrobit: Je li za sreću važno što želimo? [Life goals and well-being: Are aspirations important for happiness?]. *Društvena istraživanja, 15*(4–5), 671–691.

Chan, R., & Joseph, S. (2000). Dimensions of personality, domains of aspiration, and subjective well-being. *Personality and Individual Differences, 28*(2), 347–354.

Deci, E. L., & Ryan, R. M. (2000). The "what" and "why" of goal pursuits: Human needs and the self-determination of behavior. *Psychological Inquiry, 11*, 227–268.

Dew, T., & Huebner, E. S. (1994). Adolescents' perceived quality of life: An exploratory investigation. *Journal of School Psychology, 32*, 185–199.

Diener, E., Emmons, R. A., Larsen, R. J., & Griffin, S. (1985). The satisfaction with life scale. *Journal of Personality Assessment, 49*, 71–75.

Diener, E., Suh, E. M., Lucas, R. E., & Smith, H. L. (1999). Subjective well–being: Three decades of progress. *Psychological Bulletin, 125*, 276–302.

Franc, R., Šakić, V., & Ivičić, I. (2002). Vrednote i vrijednosne orijentacije adolescenata: hijerarhija i povezanost sa stavovima i ponašanjima [Values and value orientations of adolescents: Hierarchy and correlation with attitudes and behaviour]. *Društvena istraživanja, 11*(2–3), 215–238.

Gilman, R., Ashby, J., Šverko, D., Florell, D., & Varjas, K. (2005). A study of perfectionism among Croatian and American youth. *Personality and Individual Differences, 39*, 155–166.

Gilman, R., & Huebner, E. S. (2003). A review of life satisfaction research with children and adolescents. *School Psychology Quarterly, 18*(2), 198–205.
Gilman, R., Huebner, E. S., & Laughlin, J. (2000). A first study of the multidimensional students' life scale with adolescents. *Social Indicators Research, 52*, 135–160.
Gilman, R., Huebner, E. S., Tian, L., Park, N., O'Byrne, J., Schiff, M., et al. (2008). Cross-national adolescent multidimensional life satisfaction reports: Analyses of mean scores and response style differences. *Journal of Youth and Adolescence, 37*, 142–154.
Goldbeck, L., Schmitz, T., Besier, T., Herschbach, P., & Henrich, G. (2007). Life satisfaction decreases during adolescence. *Quality of Life Research, 16*(6), 969–979.
Grouzet, F. M. E., Kasser, T., Ahuvia, A., Fernandez-Dols, J. M., Kim, Y., Lau, S., et al. (2005). The structure of goal contents across 15 cultures. *Journal of Personality and Social Psychology, 89*, 800–816.
Gullone, E., & Cummins, R. (1999). The comprehensive quality of life scale: A psychometric evaluation with an adolescent sample. *Behaviour Change, 16*(2), 127–139.
Huebner, E. S. (1991). Correlates of life satisfaction in children. *School Psychology Quarterly, 6*(2), 103–111.
Huebner, E. S. (1994). Preliminary development and validation of a multidimensional life satisfaction scale for children. *Psychological Assessment, 6*, 149–158.
Huebner, E. S. (2001). *Manual for multidimensional students' life satisfaction scale.* 2001 *Version.* Retrieved November 4, 2008, from University of South Carolina, Web site (http://www.cla.sc.edu/psyc./pdfdocs/huebslssmanual.doc)
Huebner, E. S. (2004). Research on assessment of life satisfaction of children and adolescents. *Social Indicators Research, 66*, 3–33.
Huebner, E. S., Drane, J. W., & Valois, R. F. (2000). Levels and demographic correlates of adolescent life satisfaction reports. *School Psychology International, 21*, 281–292.
Huebner, E. S., & Gilman, R. (2002). An introduction to the multidimensional students' life satisfaction scale. *Social Indicators Research, 60*(1–3), 115–122.
Huebner, E. S., Gilman, R., & Laughlin, J. (1999). The multidimensionality of children's well-being reports: Discriminant validity of life satisfaction and self-esteem. *Social Indicators Research, 46*, 1–22.
Huebner, E. S., Laughlin, J. E., Ash, C., & Gilman, R. (1998). Further validation of the multidimensional students' life satisfaction scale. *Journal of Psychological Assessment, 16*, 118–134.
Huebner, E. S., Suldo, S. M., & Valois, R. F. (2006). Children's life satisfaction. In K. A. Anderson & L. H. Lippman (Eds.), *What do children need to flourish? Conceptualizing and measuring indicators of positive development* (pp. 41–59). New York: Springer.
Kasser, T., & Ryan, R. M. (1993). A dark side of the American dream: Correlates of financial success as a central life aspiration. *Journal of Personality and Social Psychology, 65*, 410–422.
Kasser, T., & Ryan, R. M. (1996). Further examining the American dream: Differential correlates of intrinsic and extrinsic goals. *Personality and Social Psychology Bulletin, 22*(3), 280–287.
Kasser, T., Ryan, R. M., Zax, M., & Sameroff, A. J. (1995). The relations of maternal and social environments to late adolescents' materialistic and prosocial values. *Developmental Psychology, 31*, 907–914.
Kiang, L., & Harter, S. (2006). Sociocultural values of appearance and attachment processes: An integrated model of eating disorder symptomatology. *Eating Behaviors, 7*, 134–151.
Massey, E. M., Gebhardt, W. A., & Garnefski, N. (2008). Adolescent goal content and pursuit: A review of the literature from the past 16 years. *Developmental Review, 28*, 421–460.
Neto, F. (1993). The satisfaction with life scale: Psychometric properties in an adolescent sample. *Journal of Youth and Adolescence, 22*, 125–134.
Nurmi, J. E. (1991). How do adolescents see their future? A review of the development of future orientation and planning. *Developmental Review, 11*, 1–59.
Rijavec, M. (2007). Životni ciljevi mladih i psihološka dobrobit [Life goals of young people and psychological welfare]. *Dijete i društvo, 9*(2), 355–366.
Rijavec, M., Brdar, I., & Miljković, D. (2006). Extrinsic vs. intrinsic life goals, psychological needs and life satisfaction. In A. Delle Fave (Ed.), *Dimensions of well-being: Research and intervention* (pp. 91–103). Milano: Franco Angeli.

Roth, N., & Gilman, R. (2006). Analysis of response style differences on the multidimensional students' life satisfaction scale between Croatian and American youth. *Review of Psychology, 13*(1), 19–25.

Ryan, R. M., & Deci, E. L. (2001). On happiness and human potentials: A review of research on hedonic and eudaimonic well-being. *Annual Review of Psychology, 52*, 141–166.

Ryan, R. M., & Deci, E. L. (2002). Overview of self-determination theory: An organismic dialectical perspective. In E. L. Deci & R. M. Ryan (Eds.), *Handbook of self-determination research* (pp. 3–33). Rochester: University of Rochester Press.

Sagiv, L., & Schwartz, S. H. (2000). Values priorities and subjective well-being: Direct relations and congruity effects. *European Journal of Social Psychology, 30*, 177–198.

Schmuck, P., Kasser, T., & Ryan, R. M. (2000). The relationship of well-being to intrinsic and extrinsic goals in Germany and the U.S. *Social Indicators Research, 50*, 225–241.

Seligson, J. L., Huebner, E. S., & Valois, R. F. (2003). Preliminary validation of the brief multidimensional students' life satisfaction scale. *Social Indicators Research, 61*, 121–145.

Shapka, J. D., & Keating, D. P. (2005). Structure and change in self-concept during adolescence. *Canadian Journal of Behavioural Sciences, 37*, 83–96.

Steinberg, L. (2005). Cognitive and affective development in adolescence. *Trends in Cognitive Sciences, 9*, 69–74.

Suldo, S. M., & Huebner, E. S. (2004). The role of life satisfaction in the relationship between authoritative parenting dimensions and adolescent problem behavior. *Social Indicators Research, 66*, 165–195.

Vansteenkiste, M., Soenens, B., & Duriez, B. (2008). Presenting a positive alternative to materialistic strivings and the thin-ideal: Understanding the effects of extrinsic relative to intrinsic goal pursuits. In S. J. Lopez (Ed.), *Positive psychology: Exploring the best in people* (Vol. 4, pp. 57–86). Westport, CT: Greenwood Publishing Company.

Verkuyten, M. (1986). The impact of ethnic and sex differences on happiness among adolescents in the Netherlands. *Journal of Social Psychology, 126*, 259–260.

Williams, G. C., Cox, E. M., Hedberg, V. A., & Deci, E. L. (2000). Extrinsic life goals and health-risk behaviors in adolescents. *Journal of Applied Social Psychology, 30*(8), 1756–1771.

Chapter 11
Where Does the Motivation for the Antiretroviral Therapy Come From? Assessing Existential Meaning, Personal Growth, and Motivation Toward Antiretroviral Therapy in People Affected by HIV/AIDS

Krzysztof Szadejko and Gabriele Covotta

Where does the motivation for the antiretroviral (ARV) therapy come from and what are the factors that promote such motivation? The positive psychology of growing through the illness is a very fascinating topic for study, because such knowledge can help to understand individual perception of meaning in life and motivation toward treatment. The purpose of this chapter is to examine the relevance of considering personal growth and meaningfulness in assessing outcomes from clinical treatment of HIV/AIDS disease.

Motivation toward treatment. Motivation is considered an important factor of a person's readiness to participate in interventions intended to change behavior (Deci & Ryan, 1985). The Self-Determination Theory (SDT) differentiates types of behavioral regulation in terms of the degree to which they represent autonomous or self-determined (vs controlled) functioning. Intrinsic motivation is the prototype of autonomous activity. When people are intrinsically motivated, they are, by definition, self-determined (Deci & Ryan, 2002). SDT also differentiates types of extrinsic motivation based on the degree to which the behavioral regulation has been internalized, suggesting that the more it is fully internalized and integrated with one's self, the more it will represent autonomous functioning. SDT posits four types of extrinsic regulatory styles (from the least to the most autonomous): *external regulation*, *introjected regulation*, *identified regulation*, and *integrated regulation* (Deci & Ryan, 2000). External regulation represents the common view of extrinsic motivation, i.e., doing an activity to seek a reward or to avoid punishment. Introjected regulation refers to taking in a regulation but not accepting it as one's own. Identified regulation refers to accepting the value of the activity as personally important. Integrated regulation refers to integrating that identification with other aspects of one's self. External and introjected regulations are considered relatively controlled forms of extrinsic motivation, whereas identified and integrated regulations are

K. Szadejko (✉) • G. Covotta
Institute for Advanced Study "Donald J. Ottenberg", Modena, Italy
e-mail: sciadeico@libero.it

I. Brdar (ed.), *The Human Pursuit of Well-Being: A Cultural Approach*,
DOI 10.1007/978-94-007-1375-8_11, © Springer Science+Business Media B.V. 2011

considered relatively autonomous. Finally, SDT posits that Amotivation represents the relative absence of intentional behavioral regulation, i.e., the person is neither intrinsically nor extrinsically motivated to engage in a particular behavior (Ryan, Plant, & O'Malley, 1995).

Meaningfulness. Because AIDS can be a life-threatening infection, it appears that existential issues could be important factors to consider with respect to assessing the impact of antiretroviral (ARV) therapy. For instance, having a strong sense of existential meaning is associated with salutary health-related outcomes in physical, mental and physiological domains (Zika & Chamberlain, 1992). Studies have associated a positive sense of meaning in life to different positive health outcomes (Berg & Sarvimäki, 2003; Fry, 2000; Lyon & Younger, 2005). Viktor Emmanuel Frankl was the first who talked about "searching for meaning" – a hypothesized human will to find meaning in existence (Frankl, 1959, 1969). Based on his theories, Crumbaugh and Maholick (1964) developed the *Purpose in Life* (PIL) questionnaire to measure experience of meaning in life. Even though the PIL has been used in different studies (Crumbaugh & Henrion, 1988), it has several limitations. One of the most important problems is the fundamental difference between the experience of *purpose* in life and the experience of *meaning* in life. Consequently, Battista and Almond (1973) developed a new questionnaire, the *Life Regard Index* (LRI), based on their conceptualization of meaningful life. Several other existing instruments incorporated existential meaning as part of a more complex construct like *Seeking of Noetic Goal* (Reker & Cousins, 1979; Dyck, 1987), *Spiritual Well-Being* (Ellison, 1983), *Life Attitude Profile* (Reker, Peacock, & Wong, 1987) and *Sense of Coherence* (Antonovsky, 1993). However, it appears that the *Existential Meaning Scale* (Lyon & Younger, 2005) is the only published instrument that measures existential meaning as a single conceptual entity.

Posttraumatic growth. Even in the best of times, achieving personal growth is not an easy task. It is even more difficult to "grow" and to experience meaning in life when facing traumatic events. However, traumatic events do not always lead to negative outcomes. People may experience positive inner changes following stressful events (Somerfield & McCrae, 2000), such as a positive reinterpretation of the trauma (Scheier, Weintraub, & Carver, 1986) and posttraumatic growth (Tedeschi, Park, & Calhoun, 1998). The idea that positive psychological consequences could result from coping with stressful events has been recognized in the psychotherapy literature since Frankl (1969) first discussed the search for meaning as a means to alleviate suffering. In their definition of posttraumatic growth, Tedeschi et al. (1998) underlined how personal growth represents a shift in perception that may happen when people begin to take stock of the effects of a traumatic event. This kind of cognitive evaluation enables individuals to make positive changes in their life, values, attitudes, and beliefs (Tedeschi et al., 1998).

Subjective well-being. Subjective well-being (SWB) refers to how and why people experience their lives in positive ways, and includes both cognitive and affective reactions (Diener, 1984; Diener, Emmons, Larson, & Griffin, 1985). Although subjective well-being has been construed as a subjective experience within the individual (Campbell, Converse, & Rodgers, 1976), positive cognitive evaluations of one's life and a global assessment of all aspects of a person's life, it is more commonly viewed as an integrated judgment of the person's life (Diener, 1984; Diener & Biswas-Diener, 2008).

In recent years, there has been a widening interest in research from a eudaimonic perspective of subjective well-being associated with positive health (Ryff, 1989; Ryff & Keyes, 1995; Ryff & Singer, 2006; Ryff, Singer, & Love, 2004). Research initiatives on the eudaimonic perspective of subjective well-being, often referred to as psychological well-being (PWB), has been complemented by a heightened interest in how well people perceive aspects of their functioning (i.e., the extent to which they feel they are in control of their lives, feel that what they do is meaningful and worthwhile), and how they value having good relationships with others (Ryan & Deci, 2001). We included this new focus in our study in order to assess not only the level of individual satisfaction of patients in their very peculiar situation of health, but also to verify if the subjective well-being could be a predictor of self-determined motivation toward ARV therapy. The theoretical construct as well as questionnaire items we employed to measure psychological well-being derives from Diener approach (Diener, 1984).

Present study. One of the main objectives in this research was to define the role of making meaning of the illness and to shed light on the processes that can explain the relationships among personal growth, perception of meaning in life and motivation toward antiretroviral therapy. More specifically, we hypothesized that persons with the HIV/AIDS disease, who attain a greater degree of positive growth, would be more likely to perceive stronger sense of existential meaning and higher motivation toward the ARV therapy.

The following hypotheses were proposed: (1) Perception of existential meaning will be positively associated with both personal growth and life satisfaction; (2) Personal growth will relate positively to self-determined motivation for ARV therapy; and (3) Perception of meaningful life and personal growth will both predict self-determined motivation toward ARV treatment.

Method

Participants and Procedure

HIV/AIDS affected participants ($n = 117$) were recruited from 23 residential care houses in 13 regions of Italy. A total of 176 questionnaires were distributed, accompanied by a letter emphasizing the confidentiality and anonymity of responses. Completion of the questionnaire was voluntary and anonymous. A total of 117 completed questionnaires were returned (overall response rate = 65.1%). Among those who did not participate, 48 patients (28.4%) were not able to answer because of the advanced phase of illness, six patients (3.6%) were absent, and five patients (3%)

refused to participate in the research. The age of participants ranged from 26 to 59 years, with an average of 44 years. The vast majority (82%) were male.

Measures

Treatment Motivation Questionnaire (*TMQ*). Self-determined motivation toward the ARV therapy (26 items) was assessed with the Treatment Motivation Questionnaire (TMQ), developed by Ryan et al. (1995). Sample items include "If I remain in treatment, it will probably be because: I'll get in trouble if I don't" (external reasons), "I started the therapy because: I really want to make some changes in my life" (internalized reasons), "I want to openly relate with others in the therapy" (help seeking), "I am confident this therapy will work for me" (confidence). Evaluating internal consistency of constructs with Cronbach's alpha, we observed that External Reasons scale was not reliable ($\alpha = .41$); for this reason, we did not consider this scale in the future data analysis. We suspect that items of this subscale were not appropriate for this specific sample or that it is caused by various unknown reasons. The other three scales of TMQ indicated good reliability ($\alpha = .81$; $M = 45.26$, SD = 7.29, range from 11 to 55) for the Internalized Reasons (self-determined motivation), $\alpha = .82$ ($M = 21.78$, SD = 5.78, range from 6 to 30) for the Help Seeking and $\alpha = .72$ ($M = 18.28$, SD = 4.63, range from 5 to 25) for the Confidence scale.

Existential Meaning Scale (*EMS*). Perception of meaningful life (10 items) was assessed with the Existential Meaning Scale (EMS), developed by Lyon and Younger (2005). Sample items are "My day-to-day life has meaning" and "My life is empty." Two items of the EMS were modified majoring this study in an attempt to improve the reliability of the scale. The observed Cronbach's alpha indicated good reliability $\alpha = .82$ ($M = 36.03$, SD = 8.11, range from 10 to 50).

Posttraumatic Growth Inventory (*PTGI*). Personal positive changes (21 items) were assessed with the Posttraumatic Growth Inventory (PTGI), developed by Tedeschi and Calhoun (1996). Sample items were "Following the illness … I developed new interests" (new possibilities), "… I perceive greater sense of closeness with others" (relating to others), "… I have greater feeling of self- reliance" (personal strength), "… I have better understanding of spiritual matters" (spiritual change), "… I better appreciate each day" (appreciation of life). The observed Cronbach's alpha, for the personal positive changes scale (total score of *PTGI*), indicated very good reliability $\alpha = .92$ ($M = 69.44$, SD = 18.70, range from 21 to 105).

Satisfaction with Life Scale (*SWLS*). Subjective well-being (global cognitive judgments of one's own life – five items) was assessed with the Satisfaction with Life Scale (SWLS), developed by Diener (1984). A sample item was "I'm satisfied with my life." The observed Cronbach's alpha indicated good reliability $\alpha = .80$ ($M = 12.91$, SD = 5.31, range from 5 to 25).

The impact of illness on a patient's lifestyle was measured with a simple question: "Generally the HIV/AIDS illness has a positive or a negative impact on your lifestyle?"

All items were on a five-point Likert response scale ranging from 1 (strongly disagree) to 5 (strongly agree).

Control variables. Variables that could affect the hypothesized relationships were included as controls. In order to protect anonymity, and thereby reduce the risk of social desirability bias (Podsakoff, MacKenzie, Lee, & Podsakoff, 2003), most of the control variables were measured by way of categories. How the person became infected with the HIV virus was measured by four categories: sexual intercourse, exchange of syringe, blood transfusion, and "I don't know." The sexual orientation was measured by four categories: heterosexual, homosexual, bisexual, and transsexual. The time spent in antiretroviral therapy was measured in terms of weeks, months, and years.

Results

Table 11.1 presents positive correlations between the measured constructs. As hypothesized, the existential meaning was significantly correlated to personal growth, subjective well-being, and internalized motivation toward ARV therapy. Similarly, significant correlations were observed also between personal growth and both internalized motivation toward ARV therapy and life satisfaction. The results did not support significant correlations between subjective well-being and internalized motivation, as well as between confidence in treatment and both personal growth and subjective well-being.

Table 11.1 Spearman rank correlations among Meaningfulness, Personal growth, Subjective well-being, and Internalized motivation toward ARV therapy

	Meaningfulness	Personal growth
Personal growth	.52**	
Subjective well-being	.55**	.42**
Internalized motivation	.23*	.44**

*$p<.05$; **$p<.01$

We constructed a structural equation model to test the key hypothesis focusing to explain internalized motivation toward ARV therapy. Paths in the model were set according to previous multiple regression. The AMOS Version 16.0 software was used. The models were tested using maximum likelihood.

Figure 11.1 presents the results for the final model. The Root Mean Square Error of Approximation (RMSEA) was .00, Chi-square was .24 ($df=1, p<.05$), the Normed Fit Index (NFI) was .998, and Goodness Fit Index (GFI) was .999. Overall, these indices suggest that the final model is a good fit for the data. The Chi-square was moderate, but this is common with small samples. All paths were significant, except one between existential meaning and self-determined motivation (.07, $p = .47$).

The key findings were the strong associations between personal growth and motivation for the therapy (beta = .47), between existential meaning and personal

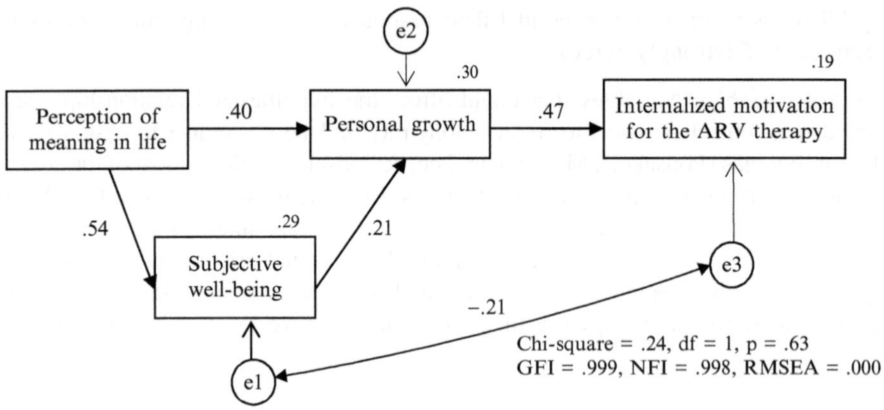

Notes: Each path is shown with the standardized path coefficients. Circles represent latent traits and rectangles represent measured variables

Fig. 11.1 Path analysis: Predictors of the internalized motivation for ARV therapy

growth (beta=.40), and between existential meaning and subjective well-being (beta=.54). According to the best-fitting model, internalized motivation for the therapy is predominantly predicted by the personal growth ($R^2 = .19$, $p < .05$), while the exogenous variables (i.e., existential meaning and subjective well-being) have both indirect effects (through personal growth) on motivation.

Table 11.2 The effect of HIV/AIDS illness on patient's lifestyle

	Impact of HIV/AIDS illness on patient's lifestyle		
	Positive	Negative	$F_{1,116}$
Meaningfulness	38.73	34.07	10.15**
Personal growth	76.31	64.49	12.50**
Subjective well-being	14.39	11.84	6.91**
Internalized motivation	46.63	44.24	3.16

**$p \leq .01$

One unexpected finding of this study was that 42% of patients declared a positive impact of the HIV/AIDS illness on their lifestyle and 58% reported a negative impact. The impact of the illness on a patient's lifestyle was measured with a simple question: "Generally the HIV/AIDS illness has a positive or a negative impact on your lifestyle?" A one-way ANOVA was conducted to determine differences between the two types of impact in four dependent variables: Meaningfulness, Personal growth, Subjective well-being, and Self-determined motivation. The tests revealed that perceptions of meaningfulness ($F_{1,116} = 10.15$, $p < .01$), personal growth ($F_{1,116} = 12.50$, $p < .01$), and subjective well-being ($F_{1,116} = 6.91$, $p = .01$) were significantly higher for participants with positive impact of illness on their life compared with the negative one. However, there was nonsignificant difference between the two types of impact in internalized motivation toward ARV therapy (see Table 11.2).

Discussion

A primary purpose of the study was to examine where does the motivation for the ARV therapy in people affected by HIV/AIDS come from. To examine this issue, we attempted to measure constructs like perception of existential meaning, personal growth, and subjective well-being. Since the present study supports the main hypothesis, it confirmed the usefulness of the theory of self-determination to understand some processes which foster the motivation during the course of antiretroviral therapy.

Specifically, from the results, we wish to draw attention on three points. First, the results suggest that personal growth positively influences the internalized motivation for ARV therapy. It appears that patients affected by HIV/AIDS who come through (fulfill) the positive changes in their life also find higher inner motivation to live and to undertake the therapy. Contrarily, individuals with lower personal growth reported lower self-motivation toward treatment. This result can be compared with the results of Tedeschi et al. (1998), who found that cognitive evaluation of events facilitates individuals to make positive changes in their attitudes and beliefs.

Second, the results suggest that making meaning of the illness is the first step toward personal growth, which relates to the person's inner motivation. For the patients in this tough situation in their life, it is not easy at all to make meaning of the HIV/AIDS disease, especially because the social context thwarts the natural tendencies toward active engagement and psychological growth. In many cases, HIV-affected persons are just rejected by their families. However, positive impact of the HIV/AIDS on a patient's lifestyle was observed among those who made positive sense of meaning in life from having the illness (42%). There are several studies on impact of illness on a patient's lifestyle (Schwartz, Devine, Schechter, & Bender, 1991; Devins et al., 2001; Knodel & VanLandingham, 2002; Lyon & Younger, 2005). It would be useful to examine, in longitudinal studies, perception of meaning in life, personal growth, and coping strategies in relation to the motivation toward the treatment. A need for a qualitative research to define the real nature and meaning of the meaningfulness in HIV/AIDS disease context has emerged too. It would be a further contribution for the studies already done by researchers on meaningfulness and personal growth.

Third, and perhaps most important, is that making meaning together with the perception of subjective well-being helps a person to grow internally. Results from the path analysis suggest that personal growth is a mediator between both existential meaning and subjective well-being, and internalized motivation for the therapy. The environment of Care Houses (Case Alloggio), where data were collected, is characterized by a "family climate" that differs from the typical atmosphere of a hospital. It helps the patients to increase their general well-being, especially when patients live for a longer period of time.

One of the central tenets of the self-determination theory is that the quality of social contexts influences the motivation, performance, and well-being of individuals who operate within them (Deci & Ryan, 1985, 2002; Osbaldiston & Sheldon, 2003). The theory uses the concept of autonomy support versus control to characterize the quality of social environments. In future researches with HIV-affected patients, it would be interesting to study how this welcoming and pleasant climate (supportive environment) influences self-determined motivation toward treatment, course of therapy, and adherence to long-term medical regimens.

When interpreting the present findings, some limitations must be considered. First, the small number of participants ruled out the possibility of extending results on wider groups of patients affected by HIV/AIDS. Second, the sample seems to be biased: The patients were mostly males (82%). Thus, it is possible that the results would have emerged differently if more females were included in the analysis. Finally, the sample is very homogenous: Everyone was recruited from the same program at the same network of treatment centers (Case Aloggio).

In sum, what we tried to find in this study was the answer for the question: "Where does the motivation for the antiretroviral therapy come from?" We are aware of the many limitations of this study. What was found is only a small part of the answer. Hopefully, this will encourage other investigations to further explore the motivational dynamics as well as other domains. This modest study helped us to realize that while taking care of the patient, we must remember that, in addition to prescribing medication, it is also important to facilitate the person's discovery of an existential meaning from having the illness. Helping patients to find meaning in their suffering heals their soul and helps them to grow. It increases their motivation to exist and, in consequence, to be self-determined toward the therapy.

References

Antonovsky, A. (1993). The structure and properties of the sense of coherence scale. *Social Science Medicine, 36*, 725–733.

Battista, J., & Almond, R. (1973). The development of meaning in life. *Psychiatry, 36*, 409–427.

Berg, G. V., & Sarvimäki, A. (2003). A holistic-existential approach to health promotion. *Scandinavian Journal of Caring Sciences, 17*(4), 384–391.

Campbell, A., Converse, S. E., & Rodgers, W. L. (1976). *The quality of American life*. New York: Russell Sage Foundation.

Crumbaugh, J. C., & Henrion, R. (1988). The PIL test: Administration, interpretation, uses, theory, and critique. *International Forum for Logotherapy, 11*, 76–88.

Crumbaugh, J. C., & Maholick, L. T. (1964). An experimental study in existentialism: The psychometric approach to Frankl's concept of noogenic neurosis. *Journal of Clinical Psychology, 20*, 200–207.

Deci, E. L., & Ryan, R. M. (1985). *Intrinsic motivation and self-determination in human behavior*. New York: Plenum.

Deci, E. L., & Ryan, R. M. (2000). The "what" and "why" of goal pursuits: Human needs and the self-determination of behavior. *Psychological Inquiry, 11*, 227–268.

Deci, E. L., & Ryan, R. M. (Eds.). (2002). *Handbook of self-determination research*. Rochester, NY: University of Rochester Press.

Devins, G. M., Dion, R., Pelletier, L. G., Shapiro, C. M., Abbey, S., Raiz, L. R., et al. (2001). Structure of lifestyle disruptions in chronic disease: A confirmatory factor analysis of the Illness Intrusiveness Ratings Scale. *Medical Care, 39*(10), 1097–1104.

Diener, E. (1984). Subjective well-being. *Psychological Bulletin, 95*(3), 542–575.

Diener, E., & Biswas-Diener, R. (2008). *Happiness: Unlocking the mysteries of psychological wealth*. Oxford: Blackwell.

Diener, E., Emmons, R. A., Larson, R. J., & Griffin, S. (1985). The satisfaction with life scale. *Journal of Personality Assessment, 49*, 71–75.

Dyck, M. J. (1987). Assessing logotherapeutic constructs: conceptual and psychometric status of the purpose in life and seeking of noetic goals tests. *Clinical Psychology Review, 7*, 439–447.

Ellison, C. W. (1983). Spiritual well-being: Conceptualization and measurement. *Journal of Psychology and Theology, 11*, 330–340.

Frankl, V. (1959). *Man's search for meaning*. New York: Simon & Schuster.

Frankl, V. (1969). *The will to meaning*. New York: New American Library.

Fry, P. S. (2000). Religious involvement, spirituality, and personal meaning for life: Existential predictors of psychological well-being in community residing and institutional care elders. *Aging and Mental Health, 4*, 375–387.

Knodel, J., & VanLandingham, M. (2002). The impact of the AIDS epidemic on older persons. *AIDS, 16*, 77–83.

Lyon, D. E., & Younger, J. (2005). Development and preliminary evaluation of the existential meaning scale. *Journal of Holistic Nursing, 23*(1), 54–65.

Osbaldiston, R., & Sheldon, K. M. (2003). Promoting internalized motivation for environmentally responsible behavior: A prospective study of environmental goals. *Journal of Environmental Psychology, 23*, 349–357.

Podsakoff, P. M., MacKenzie, S. B., Lee, J. Y., & Podsakoff, N. P. (2003). Common method biases in behavioral research: A critical review of the literature and recommended remedies. *Journal of Applied Psychology, 88*(5), 879–903.

Reker, G. T., & Cousins, J. B. (1979). Factor structure, construct validity and reliability of the seeking of noetic goals (SONG) and purpose in life (PIL) tests. *Journal of Clinical Psychology, 35*, 85–91.

Reker, G. T., Peacock, E. J., & Wong, P. T. (1987). Meaning and purpose in life and well-being: A life-span perspective. *Journal of Gerontology, 42*, 44–49.

Ryan, R. M., & Deci, E. L. (2001). On happiness and human potentials: A review of research on hedonic and eudaimonic well-being. *Annual Review of Psychology, 52*, 141–166.

Ryan, R. M., Plant, R. W., & O'Malley, S. (1995). Initial motivations for alcohol treatment: Relations with patient characteristics, treatment involvement and dropout. *Addictive Behaviors, 20*, 279–297.

Ryff, C. D. (1989). Happiness is everything, or is it? Explorations on the meaning of psychological well-being. *Journal of Personality and Social Psychology, 57*(6), 1069–1081.

Ryff, C. D., & Keyes, C. L. (1995). The structure of psychological well-being revisited. *Journal of Personality and Social Psychology, 69*, 719–727.

Ryff, C. D., & Singer, B. H. (2006). Best news yet on the six-factor model of well-being. *Social Science Research, 35*, 1102–1118.

Ryff, C. D., Singer, B. H., & Love, G. D. (2004). Positive health: Connecting well-being with biology. *Philosophical Transactions of the Royal Society of London, B, 359*, 1383–1394.

Scheier, M. F., Weintraub, J. K., & Carver, C. S. (1986). Coping with stress: Divergent strategies of optimists and pessimists. *Journal of Personality and Social Psychology, 51*, 1257–1264.

Schwartz, L. B., Devine, P. A., Schechter, C. B., & Bender, A. N. (1991). Impact of illness on lifestyle. *Loss, Grief & Care, 4*, 3–21.

Somerfield, M. R., & McCrae, R. R. (2000). Stress and coping research: Methodological challenges, theoretical advances and clinical applications. *American Psychologists, 55*, 620–625.

Tedeschi, R. G., & Calhoun, L. G. (1996). The posttraumatic growth inventory: Measuring the positive legacy of trauma. *Journal of Traumatic Stress, 9*, 455–471.

Tedeschi, R. G., Park, C. L., & Calhoun, L. G. (1998). Posttraumatic growth: Conceptual issues. In R. G. Tedeschi & L. G. Calhoun (Eds.), *Posttraumatic growth: Positive changes in the aftermath of crisis* (pp. 1–22). Mahwah: Erlbaum.

Zika, S., & Chamberlain, K. (1992). On the relation between meaning in life and psychological well-being. *British Journal of Psychology, 83*, 133–145.

Part III
Personality

Chapter 12
The Relationships Between Temperament, Character Strengths, and Resilience

Ann-Marie K. Hutchinson, Anita D. Stuart, and Hester G. Pretorius

While in the past psychology has typically focused on identifying and treating mental illness, psychological deficits, and disabilities, a number of psychologists and researchers have initiated a paradigm shift to one of positive psychology which emphasizes enhancing personal strengths, developing and maintaining well-being, and encouraging positive emotions. Positive psychology is concerned with identifying, measuring, and enhancing human strengths and happiness and should be viewed as a complementary framework for the deficit-based medical model.

Seligman (2002, 2003) indicates that although psychology originated as an approach to identifying genius and nurturing talents prior to World War II, in the aftermath of the war, psychology became a science devoted to identifying and treating mental illness utilizing the disease model. This view may, however, represent an American perspective. Strümpfer (2006) notes that this view of psychology as focusing on pathology only, may be an extreme one because, as he points out, many other advancements that were not necessarily purely focused on pathology were developing in the field of psychology at the same time. He acknowledges, however, that the general emphasis in psychology at the time was on psychopathology. Many theorists and psychologists operating out of this problem-orientated framework have begun to question the usefulness of such a paradigm.

The strengths perspective encapsulates "assumptions and attributions about health, motivation, capacities, potential and social functioning" (Strümpfer, 2006, p. 12). Martin Seligman (2002) is considered to be the founding father of the field of positive psychology and is often credited with coining the term "positive psychology" (Strümpfer, 2006). However, Abraham Maslow already used the phrase "positive psychology" in 1954 (Maslow, 1954, p. 353) while Seligman only began using the

A.-M.K. Hutchinson (✉) • A.D. Stuart • H.G. Pretorius
University of Johannesburg, Johannesburg, South Africa
e-mail: annmarie.hutchinson@gmail.com

I. Brdar (ed.), *The Human Pursuit of Well-Being: A Cultural Approach*,
DOI 10.1007/978-94-007-1375-8_12, © Springer Science+Business Media B.V. 2011

term in 1997 (Strümpfer, 2006). It should thus be noted that positive psychology, rather than being a new paradigm, is instead a return to some of the ideas of previous psychologists who have encouraged focusing on human strengths. For example, many theorists proposing positive psychology concepts (e.g., Bohart & Greening, 2001; McLafferty & Kirylo, 2001; Murphy & Moriarty, 1976; Ryff & Keyes, 1995; Strümpfer, 1990, 1995; Werner & Smith, 1982; Wissing & Van Eeden, 2002) occurred before Seligman's (2002) emphasis on creating a "paradigm shift" to positive psychology. In addition, a number of papers dealing with resilience in childhood is collated in Anthony and Cohler (1987). Similarly, much research in the realm of well-being and other aspects of positive psychology are explored in the various studies compiled by Snyder and Lopez (2002). The current movement in positive psychology, therefore, can be viewed as a return to this focus on human strengths and potentialities as originally proposed by Maslow and the humanistic psychology movement.

Cowen and Kilmer (2002) point out that although some positive psychology theories outside of Seligman's have been acknowledged by various positive psychology researchers, the current trends in the positive psychology field seem isolated from the original thinkers and contributors to the field (Strümpfer, 2006). Nevertheless, a valuable contribution to the field of positive psychology is the attempt by Peterson and Seligman (2004) to operationalize human strengths and virtues by creating a classification system on the same principles as the DSM-IV for mental illness, referred to as the "un-DSM" for measuring psychological wellness. This classification system is referred to as the Values in Action Inventory of Strengths (VIA-IS) (Peterson & Seligman, 2004).

Seligman (2002) states that although the strengths identified in the VIA-IS are considered to be fairly consistent traits, they can be nurtured and developed. This statement refers to the nature vs. nurture debate which has played a great role in psychology literature in the past. Although most modern psychologists and researchers tend to agree that both nature and nurture play a role in the development of individuals, most research has focused on the role of nature and nurture in mental illness. The focus in research thus far has not been to investigate the interface of nature vs. nurture in psychological wellness. The study of epigenetics in particular has brought new developments regarding the biological genetic basis of some mental illnesses. Although this vastly contributes to knowledge regarding identifying and treating mental illness, it does not give an indication as to whether biology plays a role in the development of psychological wellness. One psychological construct that focuses on the biological aspect of individuals is temperament. Temperament refers to the biological aspect of personality that is defined as a stable, enduring aspect impacting the thoughts, feelings, and behaviors of an individual which appears in the formative years of life (Buss & Plomin, 1984).

While much research has been conducted on the biological basis of mental illness (e.g., a collection of studies by various researchers compiled by Strelau, Farley & Gale (1986); a compilation of studies by Bates & Wachs (1994)), very little research has been conducted in the realm of biology and psychological well-being, with the exception of Steger, Hicks, Kashdan, Krueger, & Bouchard, 2007. The current study aims to address this question.

There are a number of theories that focus on psychological well-being. One particular theory which focuses on well-being by highlighting an individual's resilience is salutogenesis, and Aaron Antonovsky (1987) is well-known for his work in this area, especially his focus on what is known as *sense of coherence*. While the pathogenic paradigm focuses on why and how illness occurs, the salutogenic paradigm focuses on the origins and development of health and wellness, and this paradigm looks at the functioning of the individual in various life circumstances. Sense of coherence is a global orientation which consists of three aspects namely comprehensibility, manageability, and meaningfulness (Antonovsky, 1987). This theory contends that some people are more resilient and have higher levels of well-being than others. For example, although a number of people may experience a similar event (such as an earthquake), the theory maintains that everyone's psychological responses will differ; some people will develop healthy outcomes while others will develop pathology.

Although research has considered the personality variables associated with salutogenesis, very little research has explored the strengths of individuals in terms of their relationship to resilience. In addition to exploring the possible biological basis of well-being, the current study aims to investigate this relationship between character strengths and resilience.

The specific aim of this study is to investigate whether the biological construct of temperament predicts character strengths and resilience in the late adolescence–young adulthood life span phase.

A more general aim is to assess the extent to which there are relationships between temperament, character strengths, and resilience, by critically evaluating literature in previous fields. This information will be analyzed and integrated systematically on a component basis in order to expound the nature of these relationships.

Furthermore, this research aims to make a contribution to the integration and systematization of information regarding the nature of the relationships among temperament, character strengths, and resilience.

The possible value of conducting the present study is that an understanding of these relationships may be advanced, thereby, fostering an appreciation of the factors surrounding strengths and positive characteristics in individuals. In this way, interventions that not only take into account strengths and resilience but that, in fact, focus on these positive characteristics, may be used as preventative models in the lives of individuals. Thus, preventative intervention strategies including wellness-enhancing programs may be developed for individuals in various contexts. Importantly, investigating temperament, character strengths, and resilience in young adults may result in specific intervention strategies aimed at assisting young people in managing the turbulence and transitional nature of this life stage (Santrock, 2003).

Method

Participants

Using quantitative research methodology, a convenience sample of male and female young adults ($N = 620$) was selected from a tertiary institution. The participants' ages ranged between 17 and 30 years, with 42% of the sample being male. The language distribution of valid and relevant responses was as follows: African 36.7%, European 63.3%, other 6.5% of the sample. The participants all met the requirements for admission to a tertiary institution, which conducts all certificate, diploma, or degree courses in English and thus participants were assumed to be linguistically competent enough to complete the questionnaires in English.

All participants were in the process of completing or had already completed a tertiary education and were under the age of 30 and thus considered to be young adults exploring life roles, becoming independent and experiencing a transitional life phase. Therefore, all participants were deemed to meet the criterion of having experienced stressors and consequently the opportunity to demonstrate resilience and different character strengths.

Procedure

The researcher presented a short five-minute information session on the aims of the study and other issues, such as informed consent, but potential participants were not given any directives that may jeopardize the results of the research. Participants were assured of anonymity and confidentiality and were instructed to not put their names, surnames, or student numbers on the questionnaires. The researcher gave verbal instructions at every session and instructions for the various questionnaires were also printed above the questionnaire. The researcher was present at each of the testing sessions. Participants were encouraged to answer as quickly as possible, as per instructions in the individual questionnaires, as they were informed that the first answer that comes to their mind is usually the most accurate one.

Instruments

The four questionnaires used were all self-report measures. In order to assess individual temperament, the *Zuckerman–Kuhlman Personality Questionnaire* (Zuckerman, Kuhlman, Teta, Joireman, & Kraft, 1993) was used, which is founded on and aimed at measuring temperament as a biologically based construct. It consists of 99 questions based on a true or false scale. Reliability coefficients for the overall questionnaire range between .72 and .83; thus, indicating acceptable Cronbach

Alphas (Aluja, Garcia, & Garcia, 2002). The scale comprises five subscales, namely neuroticism–anxiety (19 items), activity (17 items), sociability (17 items), impulsive sensation seeking (19 items) and aggression–hostility (17 items). The remaining 10 items represent an infrequency scale, used as a validity measure. The current study confirmed good reliability for the subscales of this questionnaire, with alpha coefficients ranging from .71 to .81 for the various subscales.

To ascertain an individual's particular character strengths, the VIA-IS (Peterson & Seligman, 2004) has been referred to as the positive psychology complement to the DSM-IV (APA, 1994). It consists of 240 questions based on a five-point Likert scale, with responses ranging from 1 to 5. This measure has been shown to be reliable and valid, with alpha coefficients greater than .70 by the authors (Peterson & Seligman, 2004). Establishing reliability of this measure in a South African context was part of this study. The scale posits 24 character strengths, which are further categorized into six categories labeled as *virtues*. Factor analysis conducted on this questionnaire did not confirm the six categories or virtues as they have been defined, and this, as such, may indicate that these are not appropriate for the South African context. The current study, however, utilizes the six theoretical virtue categories for the purposes of analyses, for their theoretical interpretation. Further studies should be conducted on the applicability of these theoretical factors for South Africa.

The *Sense of Coherence Scale* (Antonovsky, 1987) and the Resilience Scale (Wagnild & Young, 1993) were used to measure resilience and Cronbach alpha coefficients for these questionnaires range from .82 to .95 for the Sense of Coherence Scale (Antonovsky, 1987; Erikkson & Lindstrom, 2005) and .91 for the Resilience Scale (Wagnild & Young, 1993). The current study confirmed high alpha coefficients for both of these questionnaires. The Sense of Coherence Scale consists of 29 questions based on a seven-point Likert scale with responses ranging from 1 to 7, while the Resilience Scale consists of 26 questions based on a seven-point Likert scale with responses ranging from 1 to 7. All of the above-mentioned measuring instruments have been used in previous research and were deemed culturally fair. The Sense of Coherence Scale (Antonovsky, 1987) is published in English but is also available in Afrikaans and Tswana (Antonovsky, 1993). However, this questionnaire was presented in English due to the fact that all the participants were fluent in English, and since the Zuckerman-Kuhlman Personality Questionnaire (Zuckerman et al., 1993), VIA-IS (Peterson & Seligman, 2004) and Resilience Scale (Wagnild & Young, 1993) are only available in English.

Results

As part of the investigation into the distribution of the variables in the present study, the first four moments are inspected to assess on a high level the extent to which the variables violate the assumption of normality. Table 12.1 shows these moments for the variables in question.

Table 12.1 Descriptive statistics of the dimensions of temperament, character strengths, and resilience

		Mean	Median	SD	Skewness	Kurtosis
Temperament (ZKPQ)	Impulsive Sensation-Seeking	0.52	0.53	0.20	−0.12	−0.44
	Neuroticism–Anxiety	0.48	0.47	0.23	0.16	−0.73
	Aggression–Hostility	0.40	0.35	0.21	0.28	−0.64
	Activity	0.48	0.47	0.20	0.02	−0.54
	Sociability	0.47	0.47	0.22	−0.08	−0.75
Virtues of character strengths (VIA-IS)	Wisdom and knowledge	2.26	2.26	0.47	−0.00	−0.22
	Courage	2.14	2.18	0.44	0.15	0.08
	Humanity	2.06	2.03	0.45	0.41	0.30
	Justice	2.09	2.10	0.48	0.25	−0.02
	Temperance	2.35	2.33	0.44	0.14	0.20
	Transcendence	2.09	2.08	0.47	0.31	−0.05
Resilience (SOC & RS)	Sense of Coherence Scale	4.41	4.35	0.64	0.32	0.20
	Resilience Scale	5.19	5.35	1.02	−1.07	1.56

As can be inferred from Table 12.1, inspection of the skewness and kurtosis of the distributions of the variables did not seem to indicate non-normality. Formalized tests of normality (i.e., the Kolmogorov–Smirnov test and the Shapiro–Wilk's test) did, however, indicate that the hypothesis that these scales are normally distributed would be rejected at the 5% level. It is acknowledged though that these tests may be too conservative or sensitive for data with samples as large as that being considered in the current study.

Any potential differences attributable to age or gender were accounted for in the logistic regression analyses. Pearson product moment correlations indicating relationships between variables are depicted in Table 12.2.

From Table 12.2, it can be seen that resilience, represented by both the Sense of Coherence and Resilience Scales, exhibits statistically significant correlations with the neuroticism–anxiety, aggression–hostility and activity subscales of temperament on the Zuckerman–Kuhlman Personality Questionnaire. Furthermore, the Sense of Coherence construct is statistically correlated with the sociability subscale of temperament.

Many of the virtue categories of character strengths displayed statistically significant correlations with the various subscales of temperament. Temperance was significantly correlated with all subscales of temperament. Furthermore, the impulsive sensation seeking subscale of temperament was not associated with any virtues of character strengths other than temperance. Neuroticism–anxiety was correlated with all virtues other than that of justice, while aggression–hostility was correlated with all virtues except courage. The activity subscale of temperament exhibited statistically significant correlations across all virtues of character strengths. The sociability subscale showed correlations with humanity, temperance, and transcendence.

Table 12.2 Pearson's correlation coefficients between temperament, character strengths, and resilience

		Resilience		Character strengths					
		1.	2.	3.	4.	5.	6.	7.	8.
Resilience	Sense of coherence	–	.46**	.33**	.42**	.36**	.30**	.23**	.32**
	Resilience		–	.32**	.41**	.38**	.36**	.27**	.38**
Character strengths	Wisdom and knowledge			–	.75**	.68**	.63**	.57**	.72**
	Courage				–	.73**	.65**	.61**	.71**
	Humanity					–	.76**	.55**	.75**
	Justice						–	.70**	.67**
	Temperance							–	.62**
Temperament	Impulsive sensation-seeking	–.05	–.05	.03	.02	.06	–.05	–.23**	–.04
	Neuroticism–Anxiety	–.46**	–.12**	–.17**	–.24**	–.09*	–.08	–.12**	–.06
	Aggression–Hostility	–.22**	–.09*	–.16**	–0.06	–.12**	–.27**	–.35**	–.21**
	Activity	.18**	.09*	.35**	.40**	.21**	.20**	.21**	.20**
	Sociability	.08*	–.07	.06	.02	.15**	.03	–.19**	–.08*

** $p<.01$; * $p<.05$

Canonical correlations involve forming linear combinations of variables and investigating the relationship between these groups of variables. A canonical correlation of .53 was established between the virtues of character strengths and the subscales of temperament. The canonical correlation between resilience and the virtues of character strengths was .51 and that between temperament and resilience was .49. In addition, logistic regression analyses were utilized to further investigate relationships between variables.

Logistic regression is a technique which does not rely on the assumption of normality in terms of variable distributions and is useful where responses are binary in nature. The variables pertaining to sense of coherence, resilience and character strengths were all dichotomized for the purposes of this explanatory model. This was achieved by excluding the interquartile range. In other words, the upper 25% of responses indicate a high level of that variable, while the lower 25% indicate a low level. The resulting binary responses are well suited to logistic regression analysis. Different models were fitted for temperament and sense of coherence, temperament, and resilience and temperament and character strengths. In each model, the explanatory variables were selected in a step-wise forward manner. Variables eligible for inclusion in the models were the five temperament variables, age and gender. The results table, showing percentage correctly predicted for each of the models fitted, is depicted in Table 12.3.

As can be seen from Table 12.3, the logistic regression models using temperament as the independent variable were able to correctly predict high and low scores

Table 12.3 Accuracy of logistic regression models applied to each observed dependent variable

		Predicted values		
Observed	Groups	Low	High	% Correct
Sense of coherence	Low	116	37	75.8
	High	36	116	76.3
	Overall			76.1
Resilience	Low	91	52	63.6
	High	46	112	70.9
	Overall			67.4
Knowledge	Low	110	42	72.4
	High	42	110	72.4
	Overall			72.4
Courage	Low	121	38	76.1
	High	35	114	76.5
	Overall			76.3
Humanity	Low	121	44	73.3
	High	53	101	65.6
	Overall			69.6
Justice	Low	109	46	70.3
	High	56	89	61.4
	Overall			66.0
Temperance	Low	125	34	78.6
	High	41	101	71.1
	Overall			75.1
Transcendence	Low	108	43	71.5
	High	59	78	56.9
	Overall			64.6

on sense of coherence with 76.1% accuracy and high and low scores on resilience with 67.4% accuracy. Regarding the virtues associated with character strengths, the logistic regression models predicted high and low scores of knowledge with 72.4% accuracy, courage with 76.3% accuracy, humanity with 69.6% accuracy, justice with 66% accuracy, temperance with 75.1% accuracy and transcendence with 64.6% accuracy. Interestingly, gender was a significant independent variable for five of the eight models.

Discussion

Results indicate that there are relationships between temperament, character strengths, and resilience. This points to the possibility that positive emotionality such as character strengths and resilience do indeed have a biological component.

During young adulthood, individuals may be faced with difficult decisions and a general sense of change and turbulence, but enhancing personal character strengths and resilience may assist young people in sustaining psychological health and well-being.

There is a real need to find practical ways to implement intervention programs aimed at identifying character strengths and aspects of resilience and, in turn, developing and enhancing psychological well-being. Results indicate that intervention strategies aimed at encouraging individuals to identify and develop personal strengths and resilience are likely to be effective in facilitating psychological well-being. Sense of coherence, an aspect of resilience as it is defined in the present study, is a global orientation which indicates the extent to which an individual perceives the world as understandable, manageable, and meaningful. Therefore, how one perceives the environment could impact a person's sense of psychological well-being. If individuals in the late adolescence-young adulthood life phase can develop character strengths and resilience at this early age, they may already begin to develop a strong sense of coherence which will persist into their adult lives. Indeed, Antonovsky (1987) states that sense of coherence is stable and is unlikely to change at all after the age of 30. Early intervention, therefore, could identify and enhance personal strengths in order to assist individuals in successfully managing their own psychological health throughout the lifespan.

Temperament has been shown in the present study to predict high and low levels of resilience and character strengths with reasonable accuracy. Since temperament is stable and biologically based (Zuckerman, 2002), the research findings suggest psychological well-being may well have some origin in biology. Knowledge of an individual's temperament may provide an indication of that person's level of resilience as well as their key character strengths. Interventions aimed at improving psychological well-being may, therefore, be aimed at leveraging these unique strengths.

One of the more significant correlations identified in the present study is that between the activity subscale of temperament and the virtues of character strengths. Activity displayed positive, statistically significant correlation with all virtues. This suggests that a proactive lifestyle may be associated with the development of all character strengths.

Furthermore, it was found that there are relationships between the neuroticism–anxiety and aggression–hostility subscales of temperament and resilience and character strengths. Higher levels of neuroticism–anxiety and aggression–hostility are associated in general with lower levels of resilience and character strengths. While these correlations are statistically significant, most of the correlation coefficients are not very large in magnitude. Furthermore, correlations between the impulsive sensation seeking and sociability subscales do not exhibit statistically significant correlations with resilience and most character strengths. This implies that individuals who score high on the subscales of temperament are not precluded from developing their character strengths, and although the regressions indicate that resilience and character strengths may be predicted with reasonable accuracy, the correlations indicate that there is scope for the development of character strengths despite any potential biological predispositions.

Limitations of the Study

These results should, however, be interpreted with caution as the sample was fairly homogeneous. A second limitation of the study is that a large number of responses were omitted from the logistic regression as a result of the reclassification of the VIA-IS (Peterson & Seligman, 2004), the Sense of Coherence Scale (Antonovsky, 1987) and the Resilience Scale (Wagnild & Young, 1993) into dichotomous variables for the logistic regression models. One way to address this may be to include the omitted responses in a group classified as "neutral". It should also be noted that the choice of how much data to eliminate will have an effect on the results of the logistic regression, with the more data eliminated and the more extreme the groups, the greater the effects on the model. In addition, although the current study investigated temperament as a biologically based construct, other biological variables such as genetics and neurochemistry were beyond the scope of this research project. It should be noted that although based on the current study's results, it is implied that character strengths and resilience are predicted by temperament, this link cannot be assumed to be causal, and it cannot be ruled out that an additional third factor could have influenced the results.

It was indicated under the discussion of the VIA-IS that the current study did not find support for the theoretical factors used in the current study, and it was noted that this may indicate that these factors may not be appropriate in the South African context. A growing number of studies, however, have failed to validate the theoretical factor structure, providing evidence for factors ranging from one factor to four factors (Macdonald, Bore, & Munro, 2008; Brdar & Kashdan, 2009; Shryack, Steger, Krueger, & Kallie, 2010). Further studies casting doubt onto the theoretical factors should potentially indicate the need to review the theoretical factors indicated in the original formulation of the questionnaire.

Future Research

Future research could investigate whether the relationships between temperament, character strengths, and resilience are specific to young adults in the South African context or whether findings would be similar for young people all over the world. That is, research aimed at identifying the specific nature of psychological well-being in various contexts could be valuable. Researchers should employ similar statistical techniques using the same variables with diverse samples in order to ascertain differences among individuals. It would also be beneficial for future researchers to focus on the implementation of intervention strategies that enhance psychological well-being, including character strengths and resilience. Despite a biological propensity to behave in a particular way, Peterson & Seligman (2004) as well as Wissing & Van Eeden (2002) state that behavior can be shaped and character strengths and resilience can thus be developed and enhanced. Finally, researchers should investigate other biological concomitants of psychological well-being, such as genetics and neurochemical markers.

Conclusion

Overall, it can be concluded that there are relationships between temperament, character strengths, and resilience. In line with the positive psychology paradigm, it may be beneficial to teach young people strategies to develop and enhance character strengths and resilience as preventative measures for addressing psychological difficulties and mental illness. Intervention strategies that enhance psychological well-being (including character strengths and resilience) could be valuable in schools and tertiary education institutions, e.g., career guidance, psychological counseling, workshops, training courses, case studies, self-exploration activities, individual and group therapy, role modeling and mentoring, and community involvement projects.

It is possible that programs aimed at enhancing wellness will begin to attract as much attention from parties interested in the healthcare professions as mental illness has done in the past. It is the task of psychologists to address psychological well-being as well as psychological illness in an integrated manner, in order to facilitate a preventative model aimed at enhancing health and wellness in individuals.

References

Aluja, A., Garcia, O., & Garcia, L. F. (2002). A comparative study of Zuckerman's three structural models for personality through the NEO-PI-R, ZKPQ-III-R, EPQ-RS and Goldberg's 50-bipolar adjectives. *Personality and Individual Differences, 33*, 713–725.

Anthony, E. J., & Cohler, B. J. (Eds.). (1987). *The invulnerable child.* New York: Guildford.

Antonovsky, A. (1987). *Unravelling the mystery of health: How people manage stress and stay well.* San Francisco: Jossey-Bass.

Antonovsky, A. (1993). Complexity, conflict, chaos, coherence, coercion, and civility. *Social Science and Medicine Journal, 37*(8), 969–981.

Bates, J. E., & Wachs, T. D. (1994). *Individual differences at the interface of biology and behavior.* Washington: American Psychological Association.

Bohart, A. C., & Greening, T. (2001). Humanistic psychology and positive psychology. *American Psychologist, 56*, 81–82.

Brdar, B., & Kashdan, T. (2009). Character strengths and well-being in Croatia: An empirical investigation of structure and correlates. *Journal of Research in Personality, 44*(1), 151–154.

Buss, A. H., & Plomin, R. (1984). *Temperament: Early developing personality traits.* Hillsdale, NJ: Lawrence Erlbaum.

Cowen, E. L., & Kilmer, R. P. (2002). "Positive psychology": Some plusses and some open issues. *Journal of Community Psychology, 30*, 449–460.

Erikkson, M., & Lindstrom, B. (2005). Validity of Antonovsky's sense of coherence scale: A systematic review. *Journal of Epidemiology and Community Health, 59*(6), 460–466.

MacDonald, C., Bore, M., & Munro, D. (2008). Values in action scale and the Big 5: An empirical indication of structure. *Journal of Research in Personality, 42*, 787–799.

Maslow, A. H. (1954). *Motivation and personality*. New York: Harper & Row.

McLafferty, C. L., & Kirylo, J. D. (2001). Prior positive psychologists proposed personality and spiritual growth. *American Psychologist, 56*, 84–85.

Murphy, L. B., & Moriarty, A. (1976). *Vulnerability, coping and growth: From infancy to adolescence*. New Haven, CT: Yale University Press.

Peterson, C., & Seligman, M. E. P. (2004). *Character strengths and virtues: A handbook and classification*. New York: Oxford University Press.

Ryff, C. D., & Keyes, C. L. (1995). The structure of psychological well-being revisited. *Journal of Personality and Social Psychology, 69*(4), 719–727.

Santrock, J. W. (2003). *Adolescence* (9th ed.). New York: McGraw-Hill.

Seligman, M. E. P. (2002). *Authentic happiness*. New York: Free Press.

Seligman, M. E. P. (2003). Positive psychology: Fundamental assumptions. *The Psychologist, 16*, 126–127.

Shryack, J., Steger, M. F., Krueger, R. F., & Kallie, C. S. (2010). The structure of virtue: An empirical investigation of the dimensionality of the virtues in action inventory of strengths. *Personality and Individual Differences, 48*(6), 714–719.

Snyder, C. R., & Lopez, S. J. (Eds.). (2002). *Handbook of positive psychology*. Oxford: Oxford University Press.

Steger, M. F., Hicks, B. M., Kashdan, T. B., Krueger, R. F., & Bouchard, T. J., Jr. (2007). Genetic and environmental influences on the positive traits of the values in action classification: Findings from a twin study. *Journal of Research in Personality, 41*, 524–539.

Strelau, J., Farley, F. H., & Gale, A. (Eds.). (1986). *The biological bases of personality and behaviour* (Vol. I). Washington: Hemisphere.

Strümpfer, D. J. W. (1990). Salutogenesis: A new paradigm. *South African Journal of Psychology, 20*(4), 265–276.

Strümpfer, D. J. W. (1995). The origins of health and strength: From 'salutogenesis' to 'fortigenesis'. *South African Journal of Psychology, 25*(2), 81–87.

Strümpfer, D. J. W. (2006). The strengths perspective: Fortigenesis in adult life. *Social Indicators Research, 77*, 11–36.

Wagnild, G. M., & Young, H. M. (1993). Development and psychometric evaluation of the Resilience Scale. *Journal of Nursing Measurement, 1*, 165–178.

Werner, E. E., & Smith, R. S. (1982). *Vulnerable but invisible: A study of resilient children*. New York: McGraw-Hill.

Wissing, M. P., & Van Eeden, C. (2002). Empirical clarification of the nature of psychological well-being. *South African Journal of Psychology, 32*, 32–44.

Zuckerman, M. (2002). Zuckerman–Kuhlman Personality Questionnaire (ZKPQ): An alternative five-factor model. In B. De Raad & M. Perugini (Eds.), *Big five assessment* (pp. 377–396). Toronto: Hogrefe/Huber.

Zuckerman, M., Kuhlman, D. M., Teta, P., Joireman, J., & Kraft, M. (1993). A comparison of three structural models of personality: The big three, the big five and the alternative five. *Journal of Personality and Social Psychology, 65*, 757–768.

Chapter 13
Character Strengths and Well-Being: Are There Gender Differences?

Ingrid Brdar, Petra Anić, and Majda Rijavec

For most people, the pursuit of happiness is the pursuit of a life worth living. In the last decade, there have been a number of studies which investigated positive human functioning (Seligman & Chikszentmihalyi, 2000). Characteristics of positive individuals like interests, values, and the strengths of character increase opportunities for positive experiences and the probability of desired personal, social, and physical outcomes (Peterson & Seligman, 2004). Character strengths might be grounded in biology through an evolutionary process that selected for predispositions toward moral excellence as means of solving the important tasks necessary for survival of the species (Bok, 2002; Schwartz, 1994). The values in action model (VIA; Peterson & Seligman, 2004) is the most systematic approach to studying virtue and character strengths from a psychological perspective. This model includes 24 strengths, embedded in six virtues that are valued across cultures. However, recent studies cast doubt on the number of virtues, finding support for one-, three-, or four-dimensional models (Brdar & Kashdan, 2009; Macdonald, Bore, & Munro, 2008; Shryack et al., 2010).

Character strengths are important in their own right but also because they promote the individual's well-being and happiness. As expected, the VIA character strengths are, on the whole, associated with life satisfaction, given their definition as psychologically fulfilling (Park, Peterson & Seligman, 2004; Peterson, Ruch, Beermann, Park, & Seligman, 2007; Peterson & Seligman, 2004; Shimai, Otake, Park, Peterson, & Seligman, 2006). The higher a given character strength, the more life satisfaction reported.

I. Brdar (✉) • P. Anić
Department of Psychology, Faculty of Humanities and Social Sciences,
University of Rijeka, Rijeka, Croatia
e-mail: ibrdar@ffri.hr

M. Rijavec
Faculty of Teacher Education, University of Zagreb, Zagreb, Croatia

I. Brdar (ed.), *The Human Pursuit of Well-Being: A Cultural Approach*,
DOI 10.1007/978-94-007-1375-8_13,

Some strengths nevertheless appear to be more satisfying than others. Strengths of the heart (zest, gratitude, hope, and love) are more robustly associated with life satisfaction than more intellectual strengths such as appreciation of beauty, creativity, judgment, love of learning, or creativity (Park et al., 2004; Peterson et al., 2007). Among all character strengths, modesty had the weakest association with life satisfaction (Park et al., 2004; Shimai et al., 2006). In a study by Miljković and Rijavec (2008), similar results were reported. Hope, vitality, gratitude, humor, love/intimacy, and curiosity had the most robust link with life satisfaction, while the lowest correlations were found for prudence, modesty, judgment/critical thinking, fairness, and love for learning.

Several questions guided our research. First, we sought to explore the relationship between character strengths and life satisfaction in a large sample of people in Croatia, a transitional European country. Second, we wanted to examine gender differences in character strengths and their relation to life satisfaction.

So far, four studies examined gender differences in character strengths (Biswas-Diener, 2006; Linley et al., 2007; Miljković & Rijavec, 2008; Shimai et al., 2006). These studies confirmed the existence of gender differences in character strengths. However, it is not possible to find a consistent pattern in these gender differences. The only difference that was found in all four studies concerns higher ratings on kindness for women. In addition, women reported higher ratings for love in three studies (Linley et al., 2007; Miljković & Rijavec, 2008; Shimai et al., 2006). The authors explained the gender differences as differences in specific gender roles prevalent in specific culture.

In spite of a large number of studies, origins of gender differences in human behavior are still not fully explained. In psychology, most theorists who have studied this question have taken an essentialist or a social constructionist perspective. Essentialist perspectives emphasize that basic, stable gender differences arise from causes that are inherent to human species, such as biologically based, evolved psychological dispositions. Social constructionist perspectives, in contrast, emphasize the variation in gender differences across social contexts emerging from the meaning of male and female within particular contexts (Wood & Eagly, 2002). According to evolutionary psychology, the essential attributes responsible for gender-differentiated social behavior are psychological dispositions specific for each gender, that presumably were built into the human species through adaptation to primeval conditions (Buss, 1990). Based on the evolutionary explanation, it is expected that women endorse strengths such as kindness and love more highly then men, because these strengths are associated with their evolutionary role in nurturing the young. On the other hand, it is expected that men endorse strengths such as valor (bravery), which might be associated with their evolutionary role as hunter-gatherers (Eagly & Wood, 1999).

In addition to evolutionary explanations, gender differences could be associated with different expectations society has for men and women. Social structuralists view these differences as accommodations to the differing restrictions and opportunities that a society maintains for men and women (Eagly & Wood, 1999).

Obviously, men and women socialize differently (Block, 1983), starting within family from the moment the child is born and continuing in schools and peer groups (Fagot, Rodgers, & Leinbach, 2000). Characteristics which are most adaptive for nurturing are often encouraged in females – girls get direct practical training in nurturant and prosocial behavior – they are expected to look after younger children. On the other hand, boys are trained to suppress tears or feeling pain – they are taught to be tough and invulnerable; traits like autonomy and self-reliance are supported and valued (Šikić-Mićanović, 1997). In today's industrial and postindustrial economies, women are more likely to endorse domestic roles of homemakers and primary children caretakers, whereas men are more likely to assume roles in the paid economy and to be primary family providers (Padavic & Reskin, 2002; Shelton & John, 1996). The roles typically occupied by women and men in the Western society also differ in terms of emotional experience. Caretaker roles, which are typically women's roles in the home (e.g., wife, mother) and in employment settings (e.g., nurse, teacher, educator), are likely to involve sensitivity to the needs of others and emotional expression. Whereas men's roles are less likely to emphasize emotional experience (Wood, Rhodes, & Whelan, 1989).

A third perspective is the biosocial perspective: gender differences may arise as a result of biosocial interactions. The biosocial approach treats the psychological attributes of men and women as emergent, given the evolved characteristics of the sexes, developmental experiences, and situated activity in society (Wood & Eagly, 2002).

Beyond the question of relationship between character strengths and life satisfaction, another important research question is whether this relationship is similar for men and women. Women typically score higher on so-called strengths of heart while men excel at more intellectual strengths. Therefore, it may be hypothesized that these character strengths will be differently associated with life satisfaction in male and female sample. For females, higher correlations are expected between life satisfaction and strengths of heart, while for males intellectual strengths will also be highly related to life satisfaction. In the current study, we examined gender differences in the relationship between character strengths and life satisfaction.

Method

Participants

The sample consisted of 818 students (488 females and 330 males), aged from 18 to 28 years ($M = 20.95$; SD = 1.81). The participants attended seven faculties at two Croatian universities. The faculties represented all sciences (natural sciences, social sciences and technology). Data were gathered during regular classes by trained research assistants. All students agreed to complete the questionnaires.

Measures

VIA-IS (Peterson & Seligman, 2004) is a 240-item questionnaire that requires participants to assess their strengths using a five-point scale ("not like me at all" to "very much like me"). Each of the 24 strengths of character is measured by ten items. For instance, originality is assessed by items like "I like to think of new ways to do things", valor is measured by items like "I always stand up for my beliefs" and zest is assessed by items such as "I cannot wait to get started on a project."

The items were translated independently by three researchers with advanced knowledge of the English language. In the second stage, these translations were compared and the differences were resolved through joined discussion. The final translation was reviewed and refined by the language expert in both English and Croatian languages.

Only two scales had relatively low reliability (Cronbach's alpha coefficient was .69 for prudence and .67 for self-regulation). All other scales had satisfactory reliabilities – alpha coefficients ranged from .73 (modesty) to .84 (humor and perseverance).

SWLS (Diener, Emmons, Larsen, & Griffin, 1985) measures the cognitive component of subjective well-being. Participants rate their life satisfaction on five items, using a seven-point rating scale (ranging from "strongly disagree" to "strongly agree"). Sample items are "In most ways, my life is close to my ideal" and "I am satisfied with my life." The reliability of the scale was satisfactory ($\alpha = .74$).

Results

Descriptive statistics for each of the 24 strengths for the whole sample, and separately for females and males, are presented in Table 13.1. The means range from 3.43 (love of learning for men) to 4.14 (honesty for women), indicating some degree of negative skew, as has been reported in other studies (Linley et al., 2007; Peterson et al., 2007). Standard deviations ranged from 0.46 (intelligence and honesty for men) to 0.73 (spirituality for men and the whole sample). As for gender differences, women scored higher on eight strengths, while men scored higher only on self-regulation.

All strengths were rank ordered to see if men and women report higher scores on same strengths (Table 13.2). There is considerable consistency between the signature strengths of both genders. The top nine strengths were the same for both genders, although there were minor differences in ranks. Similarities can also be found in the strengths with lowest rank, with love of learning at the very bottom of the table.

Correlations between Strengths and Life Satisfaction

Correlations between character strengths and life satisfaction are presented in Table 13.3. Zest, hope, gratitude, and curiosity are substantially related to life satisfaction, regardless of participants' gender.

Table 13.1 VIA strengths in whole sample and across gender

	Whole sample		Women		Men		
	Mean	SD	Mean	SD	Mean	SD	*t*
Curiosity	3.91	0.52	3.91	0.53	3.92	0.50	0.29
Learning	3.46	0.64	3.48	0.66	3.43	0.62	1.27
Judgment	3.82	0.50	3.83	0.50	3.82	0.50	0.15
Originality	3.66	0.52	3.64	0.52	3.70	0.51	1.78
Intelligence	3.75	0.47	3.75	0.47	3.74	0.46	0.11
Perspective	3.79	0.52	3.80	0.52	3.78	0.51	0.76
Valor	3.79	0.53	3.77	0.54	3.81	0.52	0.90
Perseverance	3.77	0.57	3.77	0.56	3.78	0.59	0.34
Honesty	4.10	0.47	4.14	0.47	4.06	0.46	2.42*
Kindness	4.03	0.49	4.11	0.47	3.91	0.49	5.94*
Love	4.03	0.51	4.11	0.49	3.91	0.52	5.70*
Teamwork	3.82	0.49	3.82	0.49	3.83	0.50	0.33
Fairness	4.01	0.51	4.06	0.50	3.93	0.53	3.72*
Leadership	3.80	0.51	3.83	0.52	3.76	0.51	2.09*
Self-regulation	3.55	0.53	3.49	0.51	3.67	0.54	5.02*
Prudence	3.54	0.51	3.55	0.52	3.51	0.51	1.16
Beauty	3.64	0.58	3.74	0.54	3.48	0.60	6.54*
Gratitude	4.02	0.50	4.07	0.49	3.95	0.49	3.58*
Hope	3.95	0.54	3.96	0.54	3.95	0.54	0.48
Spirituality	3.55	0.73	3.58	0.72	3.53	0.73	0.96
Modesty	3.61	0.55	3.62	0.54	3.59	0.54	0.61
Humor	3.96	0.57	3.95	0.58	3.97	0.52	0.31
Zest	3.85	0.53	3.84	0.53	3.88	0.54	0.89
Forgiveness	3.75	0.57	3.79	0.56	3.70	0.57	2.29*

*$p < .05$; Instead of correction for multiple comparisons, only the .05 significance level is presented

Discussion

Mean scores on character strengths in our study were somewhat higher than those reported in previous research (e.g., Linley et al., 2007; Shimai et al., 2006). The highest rated strengths were honesty, kindness, love, gratitude, and fairness, and the lowest (in order from the bottom) were love of learning, prudence, self-regulation, spirituality, and modesty. Park, Peterson, and Seligman (2006) have found similar rankings in their extensive cross-cultural research. Our results are in correspondence with universal values necessary for viable society, as identified by Bok (2002). These are positive duties of mutual support, loyalty, and reciprocity, negative injunctions against violence, deceit and betrayal, and norms for fairness and procedural justice in cases of conflict regarding positive duties and negative injunctions. Character strengths of kindness, love, and gratitude constitute positive duties; honesty enables negative injunctions, while fairness underlies norms of equality and procedural justice.

Table 13.2 Character strengths rank-ordered by gender

Rank	Women	Mean	Rank	Men	Mean
1	Honesty	4.14	1	Honesty	4.06
2	Kindness	4.11	2	Humor	3.97
3	Love	4.11	3	Gratitude	3.95
4	Gratitude	4.07	4	Hope	3.95
5	Fairness	4.06	5	Fairness	3.93
6	Hope	3.96	6	Curiosity	3.92
7	Humor	3.95	7	Kindness	3.91
8	Curiosity	3.91	8	Love	3.91
9	Zest	3.84	9	Zest	3.88
10	Judgment	3.83	10	Teamwork	3.83
11	Leadership	3.83	11	Judgment	3.82
12	Teamwork	3.82	12	Valor	3.81
13	Perspective	3.80	13	Perspective	3.78
14	Forgiveness	3.79	14	Perseverance	3.78
15	Valor	3.77	15	Leadership	3.76
16	Perseverance	3.77	16	Intelligence	3.74
17	Intelligence	3.75	17	Originality	3.70
18	Beauty	3.74	18	Forgiveness	3.70
19	Originality	3.64	19	Self-regulation	3.67
20	Modesty	3.62	20	Modesty	3.59
21	Spirituality	3.58	21	Spirituality	3.53
22	Prudence	3.55	22	Prudence	3.51
23	Self-regulation	3.49	23	Beauty	3.48
24	Learning	3.48	24	Learning	3.43

Strengths with lowest rankings, as previously mentioned, were love of learning, prudence, self-regulation, spirituality, and modesty. Low ranking for love of learning can be attributed to the characteristics of our sample: all participants were students. Perhaps, they are overwhelmed with demands imposed to them by rather extensive curricula, so they perceive learning as something that has to be done and not something worth doing for itself. Findings of Steen, Kachorek, and Peterson (2003) support this premise: they found that it is not uncommon for students to state that they used to love learning, but that boredom and monotony of classroom activities had caused this trait to decrease. Similarly, low rankings of prudence and self-regulation, results also obtained in the study of Peterson et al. (2007), can be explained by age of our respondents and the life period they are in. This is the period of transition to adulthood, perhaps the last few years for trying out different things, taking risks, etc. High school students perceive prudence as a particularly unappealing strength, associated with timidity and lack of adventurousness, often responsible for missing out interesting and valuable experiences (Steen et al., 2003). We can assume that the same is true for college students. Low rank order of modesty is rather common in studies of character strengths (e.g., Biswas-Diener, 2006; Linley et al., 2007; Peterson et al., 2007), a finding confirmed in our study. Steen et al. (2003) attribute this result partially to the fact that modesty, amongst several other

Table 13.3 Correlations between strengths and life satisfaction

	Whole sample	Women	Men
Curiosity	.40*	.40*	.37*
Learning	.24*	.24*	.24*
Judgment	.23*	.23*	.22*
Originality	.30*	.31*	.28*
Intelligence	.35*	.31*	.40*
Perspective	.33*	.30*	.38*
Valor	.33*	.29*	.37*
Perseverance	.34*	.33*	.34*
Honesty	.29*	.28*	.30*
Kindness	.28*	.27*	.34*
Love	.36*	.37*	.36*
Teamwork	.26*	.22*	.30*
Fairness	.18*	.19*	.18*
Leadership	.24*	.23*	.27*
Self-regulation	.29*	.26*	.29*
Prudence	.19*	.20*	.17*
Beauty	.23*	.21*	.30*
Gratitude	.42*	.43*	.44*
Hope	.45*	.48*	.41*
Spirituality	.31*	.30*	.32*
Modesty	.15*	.12*	.19*
Humor	.35*	.32*	.40*
Zest	.47*	.47*	.45*
Forgiveness	.25*	.27*	.24*

*$p < .05$. Instead of correction for of multiple comparisons, only the .05 significance level is presented

character strengths, is not a strength often attributed to oneself. Besides this explanation, it is possible that modesty once was an important value, but that in present time, behaviors related to modesty function mostly as social harmonizers, a task not so important in individualistic societies (Biswas-Diener, 2006). Spirituality in our sample was also among strengths with lowest rankings. Similar results for spirituality were found in UK and Swiss samples but not in American sample (Linley et al., 2007; Peterson et al., 2007).

Gender Differences in Character Strengths

Rank order of character strengths for men and women showed some similarities for both genders: honesty, gratitude, and fairness were in top five signature strengths for both genders. Similarities are also evident on the other end of rank order: love of learning, prudence, spirituality, and modesty received lowest ratings by both genders.

In a research done by Linley and his collaborators (Linley et al., 2007), women scored higher on all character strengths except creativity. In our study, a similar pattern emerged: women scored higher than men on majority of character strengths, with significant differences for strengths of honesty, kindness, love, fairness, leadership, appreciation of beauty, gratitude, and forgiveness. Men scored significantly higher only on self-regulation. Similar results have been obtained in a Japanese sample (Shimai et al., 2006), where women scored higher on strengths of kindness, love, gratitude, teamwork, and appreciation of beauty, whereas men had higher scores on judgment, perspective, creativity, valor and self-regulation. Higher scores of women on strengths of love, kindness, gratitude, and forgiveness once again support the nurturing hypothesis (Eagly & Wood, 1999), but only partially, since we did not find that men scored higher on valor. Although gender differences are examined in only few studies until now, it seems reasonable to conclude that there is consistency in finding that women score higher on so-called nurturing strengths, whereas results for men differ from study to study. Those differences in men samples are hard to explain since all studies are done in modern Western societies, where similar roles for men are expected, regardless of the country they live in. The results did not confirm our hypothesis about gender differences in valor. Valor is a phasic strength which comes and goes, because it is relevant only in some settings. The measure used in this research asks for typical responses rather than those related to specific settings (Peterson & Seligman, 2004). It is possible that participants in our study gave only typical appraisals, not referring to specific situation in which valor could be expressed.

Evidently, there are more similarities than differences between our results and findings reported by Linley et al. (2007) and Shimai et al. (2006), which can be indicative of a universal human nature (Park et al., 2006).

Character Strengths and Life Satisfaction

Second aim of our research was to explore relationship between character strengths and life satisfaction. Life satisfaction in the whole sample was positively related to all character strengths, except modesty. In a study by Shimai et al. (2006), modesty showed strong negative correlations with happiness among both Americans and Japanese participants. Young adults who rated their own modesty as high were less likely to be happy. Harvey (2001) raised the interesting possibility that for modesty to be related to life satisfaction, an individual may need to have experienced some setbacks or losses in life. Since our participants were rather young, it is possible that they did not yet have experiences that could contribute to this relationship.

The highest correlations were found for zest, hope, gratitude, and curiosity. Other studies revealed similar results. For example, Park et al. (2004) found highest correlations between life satisfaction and strengths of hope and zest, as well as gratitude, love, and curiosity. The strengths most strongly correlated with life satisfaction in Swiss sample were zest, hope, love, curiosity, and perseverance, and in the US sample zest, hope, love, gratitude, and curiosity (Peterson et al., 2007). It can be assumed that high correlation between gratitude and life satisfaction comes from satisfaction with the past, with good things that have happened in someone's life. Similarly, but with different time perspective, positive relation of hope and life satisfaction can be explained with expectations of good outcomes in the future. The association between curiosity and life satisfaction might be explained through satisfaction of basic psychological needs. The innate needs to be competent and autonomous are manifested through curiosity and interest (Deci & Ryan, 1992), and the satisfaction of these needs is related to enhanced well-being (e.g., Reis, Sheldon, Gable, Roscoe, & Ryan, 2000; Sheldon, Ryan, & Rice, 1996). It is not surprising that zest was strongly linked to life satisfaction – zestful people are enthusiastic, vital, and full of energy, so it is hard to imagine that they are unhappy. Strength of love manifests itself in close relationships with others. Having good, satisfying interpersonal relationships is one of the main variables that differentiate happy and unhappy people (Diener & Seligman, 2002), so it is not surprising that strong association between life satisfaction and strength of love was found.

Humor, prudence, and fairness were least related with life satisfaction. This is not in line with previous studies that showed stronger positive relationship between humor and life satisfaction (Park et al., 2004; Peterson et al., 2007). Even though some studies have shown positive links between prudence and well-being (Digman, 1989; Marshall, Wortman, Vickers, Kusulas, & Hervig, 1994), in our sample, this link was rather weak. Prudence and life satisfaction might increase with age, and our participants were rather young. At their age, being prudent may lead to missing interesting and valuable experiences in life. The benefits of prudence may be obvious only later in life. When considering fairness, it is without doubt a fulfilling strength, but it is not always fun to be fair. Sometimes, the costs of being fair are too high, and people will not exhibit this strength (Peterson & Seligman, 2004). In some periods, fairness might be differently valued in specific cultures. The recent transition to market economy in Croatia has shown that fair and prudent people are not the most successful. It is interesting to note that fairness was amongst five strengths with highest ranking, but on the other hand, it is rather weakly related to life satisfaction. Our students obviously see themselves as fair, but this does not contribute to their life satisfaction.

Gender Differences in the Relationship between Character Strengths and Life Satisfaction

When a person's gender role characteristics come into conflict with his or her actual life situation, the person will experience reduction in psychological well-being (Grimmell & Stern, 1992). Different patterns of correlations between strengths and life satisfaction was expected for males and females. It was hyphothesized that life satisfaction will be more robustly linked with: (a) the strengths of heart for females and (b) intellectual strengths for males.

In both samples, gratitude, hope, and zest had the highest correlations with life satisfaction, while correlations of humor and modesty with life satisfaction were the lowest. Zest and gratitude are, obviously, universal predictors of life satisfaction, a finding which is in accordance with results of other studies (e.g., Park et al., 2004; Peterson et al., 2007).

Life satisfaction was linked stronger with intelligence, perspective, valor, kindness, teamwork and appreciation of beauty in male sample. For females, life satisfaction had higher link only with hope.

More robust links of life satisfaction and intellectual strengths (intelligence, perspective and valor) were expected for men. We also expected that strengths of heart (kindness, teamwork, and appreciation of beauty) will be more linked with life satisfaction for women. Findings confirmed only the first hypothesis – intellectual strengths were more strongly related to life satisfaction in male sample than in female, but this was also true for some strengths of heart. Although women score higher on kindness and appreciation of beauty, this makes them less satisfied than their male counterparts. One of the possible explanations of these findings is that women are expected to show more kindness and appreciation of beauty. They might sometimes express these behaviors without real feelings, while males possibly do it out of authentic need. At the same time, other people can see men as more honest when they express kindness and appreciation of beauty, therefore these behaviors might contribute to better relationships. Of course, it is also possible that typical gender roles are changing. Certain character strengths may have different meaning for students than for older adults.

Conclusions

The character strengths in our study proved to be psychologically fulfilling, as defined by Peterson and Seligman (2004). The higher a given character strength, the more life satisfaction was reported in both male and female samples. However, some strengths were found to bc more satisfying than others. In both samples, gratitude, hope, and zest were the most robust correlates of life satisfaction, while humor and modesty were strengths with the lowest correlations with life satisfaction. It was hypothesized that the link between strengths of heart and life satisfaction will be more robust for females, but this was found only for the strength of hope. As expected, intellectual strengths were more correlated with life satisfaction for males. Contrary to our hypothesis, higher correlations of some strengths of heart and life satisfaction were found for males. These results indicate that gender differences in the relationship between character strengths and life satisfaction need further research.

There are several limitations to the present study. Because participants were college students, the generalization to general population is not possible. It is important to note that the results are correlational and do no impute causality. For example, it may be that kindness leads to more life satisfaction, but it is also possible that satisfied people are more kind to others. Next, the data were based on self-reports and, therefore, suffer from the interpretative issues linked with such approaches.

Future work can focus on the relationship between character strengths and well-being in other contexts, beyond the college life, and in other cultures. Culture might have greater impact on gender differences for some strengths than for others. In addition, it would be interesting to explore gender differences in broader, higher-level strengths and their relationship with life satisfaction.

References

Biswas-Diener, R. (2006). From the equator to the North Pole: A study of character strengths. *Journal of Happiness Studies, 7*, 293–310.

Block, J. H. (1983). Differential premises arising from differential socialization of the sexes: Some conjectures. *Child Development, 54*, 1335–1354.

Bok, S. (2002). *Common values*. Columbia, MO: University of Missouri Press.

Brdar, B., & Kashdan, T. (2009). Character strengths and well-being in Croatia: An empirical investigation of structure and correlates. *Journal of Research in Personality, 44*(1), 151–154.

Buss, D. M. (1990). Evolutionary social psychology: Prospects and pitfalls. *Motivation and Emotion, 14*(4), 265–286.

Deci, E. L., & Ryan, R. M. (1992). The initiation and regulation of intrinsically motivated learning and achievement. In A. K. Boggiano & T. S. Pittman (Eds.), *Achievement and motivation: A social-developmental perspective* (pp. 9–36). New York: Cambridge University Press.

Diener, E., & Seligman, M. E. P. (2002). Very happy people. *Psychological Science, 13*, 80–83.

Diener, E., Emmons, R. A., Larsen, R. J., & Griffin, S. (1985). The satisfaction with life scale. *Journal of Personality Assessment, 49*(1), 71–75.

Digman, J. M. (1989). Five robust personality dimensions: Development, stability, and utility. *Journal of Personality, 57*, 195–214.

Eagly, A. H., & Wood, W. (1999). The origins of sex differences in human behavior: Evolved dispositions versus social roles. *The American Psychologist, 54*, 408–423.

Fagot, B. I., Rodgers, C. S., & Leinbach, M. D. (2000). Theories of gender socialization. In T. Eckes & H. M. Trautner (Eds.), *The developmental social psychology of gender* (pp. 65–89). Mahwah, NJ: Lawrence Erlbaum.

Grimmell, D. W., & Stern, G. S. (1992). The relationship between gender role ideals and psychological well-being. *Sex Roles, 27*, 487–497.

Harvey, J. H. (2001). The psychology of loss as a lens to a positive psychology. *The American Behavioral Scientist, 44*, 835–853.

Linley, P. A., Maltby, J., Wood, A. M., Joseph, S., Harrington, S., Peterson, C., et al. (2007). Character strengths in the United Kingdom: The VIA Inventory of Strengths. *Personality and Individual Differences, 43*, 341–351.

Macdonald, C., Bore, M., & Munro, D. (2008). Values in action scale and the Big 5: An empirical indication of structure. *Journal of Research in Personality, 42*, 787–799.

Marshal, G. N., Wortman, C. B., Wickers, R. R., Kusulas, J. W., & Hervig, L. K. (1994). The five-factor model of personality as a framework for personality-health research. *Journal of Personality and Social Psychology, 67*, 278–286.

Miljković, D., & Rijavec, M. (2008). What makes us happy: Strengths of mind, strengths of heart or self-control? In M. Cindrić, V. Domović, & M. Matijević (Eds.), *Pedagogy and the knowledge society* (pp. 241–250). Zagreb: Učiteljski fakultet.

Padavic, I., & Reskin, B. F. (2002). *Women and men at work*. Thousand Oaks, CA: Pine Forge Press.

Park, N., Peterson, C., & Seligman, M. E. P. (2004). Strengths of character and well-being. *Journal of Social and Clinical Psychology, 23*(5), 603–619.

Park, N., Peterson, C., & Seligman, M. E. P. (2006). Character strengths in fifty-four nations and the fifty US states. *Journal of Positive Psychology, 1*(3), 118–129.

Peterson, C., & Seligman, M. E. P. (2004). *Character strengths and virtues: A handbook and classification*. New York: Oxford University Press.

Peterson, C., Ruch, W., Beermann, U., Park, N., & Seligman, M. E. P. (2007). Strengths of character, orientations to happiness, and life satisfaction. *Journal of Positive Psychology, 2*(2), 1–8.

Reis, H. T., Sheldon, K. M., Gable, S. L., Roscoe, J., & Ryan, R. M. (2000). Daily well-being: The role of autonomy, competence, and relatedness. *Personality and Social Psychology Bulletin, 26*, 419–435.

Schwartz, S. H. (1994). Are there universal aspects in the structure and contents of human values? *Journal of Social Issues, 50*(4), 19–45.

Seligman, M. E. P., & Chikszentmihalyi, M. (2000). Positive psychology: An introduction. *The American Psychologist, 55*, 5–14.

Sheldon, K. M., Ryan, R. M., & Reis, H. T. (1996). What makes for a good day? Competence and autonomy in the day and in the person. *Personality and Social Psychology Bulletin, 22*, 1270–1279.

Shelton, B. A., & John, D. (1996). The division of household labor. *Annual Review of Sociology, 22*, 299–322.

Shimai, S., Otake, K., Park, N., Peterson, C., & Seligman, M. E. P. (2006). Convergence of character strengths in American and Japanese young adults. *Journal of Happiness Studies, 7*, 311–322.

Shryack, J., Steger, M. F., Krueger, R. F., & Kallie, C. S. (2010). The structure of virtue: An empirical investigation of the dimensionality of the virtues in action inventory of strengths. *Personality and Individual Differences, 48*(6), 714–719.

Šikić-Mićanović, L. (1997). Socialization and gender: The significance of sociocultural contexts. *Društvena istraživanja, 6*(4–5), 577–595.

Steen, T. A., Kachorek, L. V., & Peterson, C. (2003). Character strengths among youth. *Journal of Youth and Adolescence, 32*(1), 5–16.

Wood, W., & Eagly, A. M. (2002). A cross-cultural analysis of the behavior of women and men: Implications for the origins of sex differences. *Psychological Bulletin, 129*, 699–727.

Wood, W., Rhodes, N., & Whelan, M. (1989). Sex differences in positive well-being: A consideration of emotional style and marital status. *Psychological Bulletin, 106*(2), 249–264.

Part IV
Academic Performance and Coping

Chapter 14
Optimistic Attributional Style as a Predictor of Well-Being and Performance in Different Academic Settings*

Tamara O. Gordeeva and Evgeny N. Osin

Attributional style (or explanatory style) is a specific way people explain the causes of different events in their lives. Seligman and his colleagues introduced the concept of attributional style with three parameters (internality, stability and globality) and proposed a distinction between optimistic and pessimistic attributional styles (Seligman, Abramson, Semmel, & Von Baeyer, 1979). Attributional style became the central notion within the reviewed learned helplessness theory (Abramson, Seligman, & Teasdale, 1978) and its more recent revision, the theory of hopelessness (Abramson, Metalsky, & Alloy, 1989).

Attributional style was originally proposed as a cognitive factor of depression (Seligman et al., 1979). Meta-analytic studies of the relationship between explanatory style and depression (Mezulis, Abramson, Hyde, & Hankin, 2004; Sweeney, Anderson, & Bailey, 1986) have confirmed a strong association between uni-polar depression and pessimistic explanation of negative events (using internal, permanent, and pervasive causes), as well as positive events (using external, unstable, and local causes), although the association was weaker in the latter case.

Recently, the focus in attributional style research has shifted from helplessness, depression, and pessimism toward the relationship between optimistic attributional style and psychological well-being (Cheng & Furnham, 2001, 2003; Sanjuan & Magallares, 2009). A number of studies have revealed better health and increased longevity in people with optimistic attributional style (Peterson, 2000; Peterson & Seligman, 1987; Peterson, Seligman, & Vaillant, 1988).

---

*The preparation of this paper was partially supported by a Visiting Research Fellowship from the Leverhulme Trust to the second author.

T.O. Gordeeva
Moscow State University, Moscow, Russia

E.N. Osin (✉)
State University, Higher School of Economics, Moscow, Russia
e-mail: keen-psy@mail.ru

I. Brdar (ed.), *The Human Pursuit of Well-Being: A Cultural Approach*,
DOI 10.1007/978-94-007-1375-8_14, © Springer Science+Business Media B.V. 2011

Attributional Style Questionnaire (ASQ) is the most widely used psychometric instrument for measuring attributional style (Peterson et al., 1982; Seligman et al., 1979). Initial studies were done with three parameters of attributional style: internality, stability, and globality. However, the internal consistency of the scales measuring internality ranged from moderate (Peterson et al., 1982) to low (Cutrona, Russell, & Jones, 1985; Furnham, Sadka, & Brewin, 1992; Tennen & Herzberger, 1985; Xenikou, Furnham, & McCarrey, 1997), and for this reason, the internality parameter was abandoned in more recent studies (Martin-Krumm, Sarrazin, Peterson, & Famose, 2003; Peterson & Vaidya, 2001; Peterson et al., 2001) and theoretical works (Abramson et al., 1989; Peterson, 2000; Seligman, 2002).

Instead, serious arguments were proposed in favor of a controllability parameter, since it was shown that experienced inability to control the events leads to helplessness and depression (Seligman, 1975). The studies which used the controllability parameter provided sound evidence for its importance: it was found to be a reliable predictor of depression, loneliness, and anxiety, as well as of positive emotional reactions and positive future expectations and performance (Deuser & Anderson, 1995). A number of new questionnaires measuring attributional style include controllability scales (ASAT, Anderson & Arnoult, 1985; WASQ, Ashforth & Fugate, 2006; ASAT-III, ASAT-IY, Anderson & Riger, 1991; CDS, Russel, 1982; SFASQ, Gordeeva, Osin, & Shevyakhova, 2009).

The Attributional Style for Positive and Negative Events and Achievement in Different Domains

The studies exploring the relation of attributional style to achievement in different domains have produced contradictory results. The association of explanatory style for *negative events* with professional success was first shown by Seligman and Shulman (1986) in an insurance agent sample. The research exploring the association of attributional style for negative events with academic and sports achievement was most extensive and also the most contradictory in terms of outcomes. In several studies, optimistic attributional style was found to be associated with *higher* grades (Martinez & Sewell, 2000; Peterson & Barrett, 1987; Rowe & Lockhart, 2005; Yates & Yates, 1995) and better sport performance (Seligman, Nolen-Hoeksema, Thornton, & Thornton, 1990); other studies, in contrast, have revealed its association with *lower* levels of academic achievement (LaForge & Cantrell, 2003; Yee, Pierce, Ptacek, & Modzelesky, 2003) and sport performance (Davis & Zaichkowski, 1998), and some studies failed to reveal any significant association (Bridges, 2001; Hale, 1993; Musgrave-Marquart, Bromley, & Dalley, 1997; Satterfield, Monahan, & Seligman, 1997; Ward, 2003; Yee et al., 2003).

Optimistic attribution style for negative events may have both advantages and disadvantages. Optimistic thinking (viewing negative events as external, unstable, specific) may promote hope and lead to increased persistence, but it may also lead to relaxation and withdrawal of effort. In turn, pessimistic thinking (viewing negative events as internal, stable, and global) may entail helplessness and passivity, but it may also result in investing more effort and energy into activity. For instance, students who gave pessimistic explanations to their poor examination performance tended to make more plans to study for the next examination (Follette & Jacobson, 1987).

In their early work testing the reformulated helplessness theory, Seligman et al. (1979) reported that scores for internality and stability of *positive events* on the ASQ were inversely associated with depression, but the relationship was weaker than that found for negative situations. A meta-analysis of 104 studies (Sweeney et al., 1986) confirmed this finding, and it became a common practice to measure attributional style using only negative events or to calculate a composite difference score by subtracting positive event scores from negative event ones.

However, the results of empirical studies indicate that attributional styles for positive and negative events are distinct variables. For instance, it was shown that workers who rated positive events highly on a single dimension of attributional style did not necessarily rate negative events low on the same dimension (Xenikou et al., 1997). Low correlations between attributional scales for positive and negative events have been reported by other researchers as well (Peterson & Seligman, 1984; Zautra, Guenther, & Chartier, 1985). These results suggest that discounting positive events or calculating a single composite score is a questionable practice which leads to the confounding of these distinct constructs, resulting in a blurred overall picture.

Needles and Abramson (1990) proposed a model of recovery from depression, hypothesizing that depressed persons who tend to attribute positive life events to global and stable causes ("enhancing" attributional style) are likely to become hopeful (and thus less depressed) when positive events occur; the model was supported in a longitudinal study using depressed college students (Needles & Abramson, 1990). Several other studies have produced consistent findings, indicating the important role of positive event attributions in the recovery from depression. For instance, optimistic attributional style for positive events was associated with lower level of depression symptoms in people with clinical depression (Johnson, Crofton, & Feinstein, 1996; Johnson, Han, Douglas, Johannet, & Russell, 1998; Voelz, Haeffel, Joiner, & Wagner, 2003), as well as in male prisoners with no depression history prior to imprisonment (Peterson & Seligman, 1984). More recently, explanations of positive events were shown to be important predictors of psychological well-being, self-esteem, and effective coping strategies (Cheng & Furnham, 2003; Rigby & Huebner, 2005; Sanjuan & Magallares, 2009; Sanjuan, Perez Garcia, Rueda, & Ruiz, 2008).

The association between attributional style for positive events and achievement has received relatively little research attention so far, although the findings are promising. For instance, in the domain of professional achievement, it was found that attributional style for positive events (in contrast to the negative ones) predicted work performance in British insurance company salespeople (Corr & Gray, 1996) and work adjustment in pharmaceutical company managers (Ashforth & Fugate, 2006). In the academic domain, it was found that higher mathematics achievement in elementary schoolchildren is associated with optimistic explanatory style for positive events (Yates & Yates, 1995), but in a sample of law school students, its association with performance was negative (Satterfield et al., 1997). Clearly, more research is needed to replicate this finding in different age groups and educational and professional contexts.

A few reasons can be addressed in order to explain the seeming contradictions between the results of different studies linking attributional style and performance in activity: (1) *Activity type* – According to Seligman (1990), optimistic people are likely to be more successful in activities that require persistence and initiative and that involve high risk of disappointment or rejection by others; at the same time, there are professions in which mild pessimism resulting in prudence and stronger sense of reality could be an advantage. For instance, optimistic explanatory style was shown to be beneficial for salespeople (Corr & Gray, 1996; Seligman & Shulman, 1986), but optimistic explanations of positive events made a negative impact upon academic success and performance of law school students (Satterfield et al., 1997); (2) *Activity difficulty* – One study (Gibb, Zhu, Alloy, & Abramson, 2002) has found the relationship between attributional style for negative events and academic performance in college students to be dependent on their academic ability levels: pessimism was associated with lower GPAs in students with lower ability but was beneficial for high-ability students; (3) *Measurement confusion* – Different studies use different and often incomparable measures of attributional style. Some researchers do not differentiate attributional styles for positive and negative events and only report composite scores, which do not allow to estimate unique contributions of the two attributional styles to observed effects; (4) *Other variables* – The effects of optimism upon performance might be mediated by other variables, such as expectations, goals or anxiety. For instance, Martin-Krumm and Salama-Younes (2007) found that the effect of attributional style upon school grades was mediated by expectations of success (the authors do not clarify the type of attributional style that contributed to performance, using a composite score).

Two studies were undertaken to investigate the relationship between explanatory style for positive and negative events, well-being, and performance in two different academic settings.

Study 1: Attributional Optimism, Well-Being, and Academic Achievement at School

Aim

The aim of the first study was to investigate the relationship of optimistic attributional style to well-being and academic performance in high school students.

Method

Participants

The sample comprised students of several high schools in Russian cities of Moscow, Magadan, and Bijsk ($N = 224$) aged between 14 and 18 (mean age was 15.3 years, standard deviation 0.98); 38% were male.

Instruments

Success and Failure Attributional Style Questionnaire for Adolescents (SFASQ-A, Gordeeva et al., 2009) was used to measure attributional style. A set of 24 positive and negative life situations was developed on the basis of ASQ and its extended versions, Adversity Quotient Questionnaire (Stoltz, 1999), and approximately one-third of the situations were original, formulated in accordance with the ASQ logic for Russian culture. Each situation is rated on two out of three parameters (stability, globality, and controllability) using a response scale with points ranging from 1 to 6, anchored by "This cause will never arise again... will exist always" (stability), "This cause is associated with this specific situation... all situations of my life" (globality), "This cause is outside my control... I can control completely" (controllability). The scale internal consistency (Cronbach's alpha coefficient) was .83 for both positive and negative event scales and ranged between .70 and .82 for the stability, globality, and controllability parameter subscales. No significant gender differences were found on any of the SFASQ scales.

Russian versions of three other questionnaires were used to measure well-being and to control for self-esteem, which could possibly explain the association between optimistic attributional style and achievement. *Subjective Happiness Scale* (Lyubomirsky & Lepper, 1999), a four-item measure with a seven-point response scale and both *Trait Depression Scale* (Ritterband & Spielberger, 1996) and *Self-Esteem Scale* (Rosenberg, 1965), which have ten-item measures using four-point response scales. The internal consistencies (Cronbach's alpha coefficient) of all these scales were adequate, ranging from .75 for the self-esteem scale to .79 for the trait depression scale. Each total score was divided by the number of items in the respective scale.

In addition to completing the questionnaires, students were asked to indicate their last term's grades in four principal school subjects (Algebra, Geometry, Russian language, and Literature). The academic performance in Russia is evaluated on a five-point scale (5 – excellent, 4 – good, 3 – satisfactory, 2 – unsatisfactory; 1 is never used in practice). The grades were averaged, resulting in an academic achievement indicator with a Cronbach's alpha coefficient reliability of .82.

Procedure

The students anonymously completed a battery of tests administered by a psychologist in a group setting during their regular school hours. Individual feedback on personality traits was offered as a reward for participation.

Results

The Association of Optimism with Well-Being and Academic Achievement

The correlations between optimism and other study variables are presented in Table 14.1. Optimistic attributional style for positive events demonstrated modest

Table 14.1 Descriptive statistics and Pearson correlations between optimism and other studied variables

	1	2	3	4	5	6	7	8	9
1. Depression	–								
2. Happiness	–.68**	–							
3. Self-Esteem	–.46**	.48**	–						
4. SFASQ: Stability	–.35**	.28**	.31**	–					
5. SFASQ: Globality	–.26**	.21**	.36**	.61**	–				
6. SFASQ: Controllability	–.14*	.10	.15*	.34**	.27**	–			
7. SFASQ: Positive events	–.19**	.22**	.30**	.44**	.48**	.70**	–		
8. SFASQ: Negative events	–.30**	.17*	.24**	.78**	.69**	.55**	.25**		
9. Grade Average	–.03	.12	.17*	.13	.23**	.05	.26**	.02	
M	1.87	4.87	3.25	4.18	4.39	4.08	4.33	4.14	3.66
SD	0.48	1.09	0.42	0.66	0.61	0.83	0.79	0.62	0.53

*p<.05; **p<.01

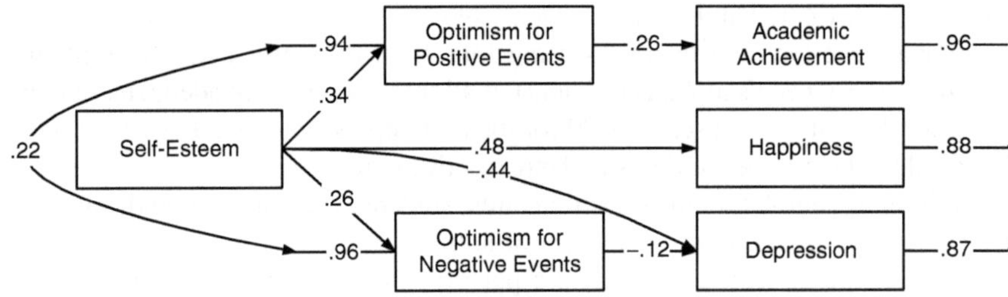

Chi-square = 6.79, df=7, p=.45; RMSEA<.001, CFI>.999, NFI=.98, SRMR=.03
Notes: All path coefficients shown are significant (p < .05)

Fig. 14.1 Path diagram of the associations between optimism, well-being, and academic achievement, controlling for self-esteem

positive association with academic achievement, which was also associated with self-esteem. Both optimistic attributional styles for positive and negative events were associated with measures of subjective well-being and self-esteem.

To clarify these associations, a path model was tested using EQS 6.1 (maximum likelihood estimation method). Optimistic attributional styles for positive and negative events were entered as predictors of well-being and academic achievement, controlling for self-esteem. When five nonsignificant paths were removed, the model still fit the data well (Fig. 14.1). Only the optimistic attributional style for positive events was a significant predictor of academic achievement and only the pessimistic attributional style for negative events predicted depression.

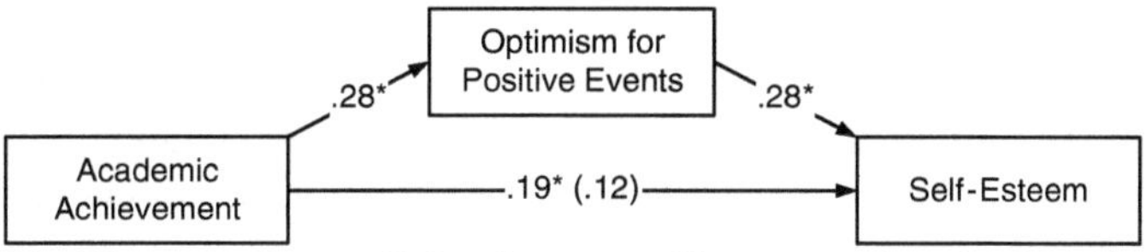

Notes: *p < .01; [a]The regression coefficient between self-esteem and academic achievement controlling for optimism is shown in parentheses; All regression coefficients are standardized.

Fig. 14.2 The relationship between academic achievement and self-esteem mediated by optimism for positive situations

Optimism as Mediator of the Effect of Academic Achievement upon Self-Esteem

It was further hypothesized that optimistic attributional style for positive events might mediate the effect of the students' academic achievement upon their self-esteem. In order to test this hypothesis, Sobel test for mediation was used. Optimistic attributional style for positive events emerged as a full mediator of the association between academic performance and self-esteem (see Fig. 14.2), satisfying all four mediation criteria proposed by Baron and Kenny (1986).

Discussion

The importance of distinction between optimistic attributional style for positive and negative events is confirmed by their specific associations with academic achievement and depression. The relationship between optimism for positive situations and academic performance corresponds well in terms of both magnitude and direction to previous findings obtained in academic (Yates & Yates, 1995) and professional settings (Corr & Gray, 1996; Furnham, et al., 1992).

The causal nature and direction of the associations between attributional style and academic achievement still have to be clarified. On the one hand, optimistic attributional style for positive events may promote goal setting and implementation, persistence, and effective coping within academic activity, resulting in higher grades. On the other hand, optimistic attributional style for positive events may form on the basis of repeated mastery experiences associated with school successes, and, thus, it may simply reflect, rather than motivate, academic achievement. The study limitations (correlational design and use of indicators of past academic performance) did not allow us to distinguish between these associations: the data most likely revealed a mixed picture of both, but further studies should be done to analyze these effects separately.

The associations between optimistic attributional style and well-being are not particularly strong. However, this association might be more intricate, supposing that the way an individual interprets a success or failure situation determines the type of ensuing emotional experience and the effect of this situation upon future motivation and self-image. Thus, attributional style seems to be *the* link between performance and well-being, but the studies needed to reveal the dynamics of these processes need to be longitudinal, rather than cross-sectional.

The results suggest that interventions fostering optimistic explanation of their successes can help students to improve their academic performance, maintain positive self-esteem, and mitigate the detrimental effects of academic failures upon self-esteem, preventing depression.

Study 2: Attributional Optimism, Well-Being, and Entrance Examination Performance

Aim

The aim of the second study was to investigate the relationship of optimistic attributional style for positive and negative events to well-being and academic performance in a realistic competitive setting of university entrance examinations.

Method

Participants

The sample comprised a group of entrants to the Moscow State University Psychology Department ($N = 108$), aged between 15 and 22 (mean age 17.2, standard deviation 1.38); 16% were male. The study participants comprised ~20% of all 2006 applicants and did not differ significantly in age or gender from the rest of applicants. Successful entrants are chosen by the examination board from among those who passed all three written examinations (Math, Essay, and Biology) on the basis of average scores.

Instruments

Success and Failure Attributional Style Questionnaire for Adolescents (SFASQ-A, Gordeeva et al., 2009) was used to measure attributional style. The internal consistency (Cronbach's alpha coefficient) was .80 for the positive events scale, .83 for the negative events scale, and between .70 and .72 for the stability, globality, and controllability parameter subscales. The grades were averaged across the examinations taken by each entrant, giving an overall success indicator with Cronbach's alpha coefficient reliability of .56.

To measure well-being, Russian versions of ten-item *Trait Depression Scale* (Ritterband & Spielberger, 1996) with answer options ranging from 1 to 4, and a .80 reliability, as well as a four-item *Subjective Happiness Scale* (Lyubomirsky & Lepper, 1999) with a 1 to 7 response scale, and a .77 reliability were used. Russian version of the ten-item *General Self-Efficacy Scale* (Schwartzer, 1993) with response scale options ranging from 1 to 4, and a .83 overall reliability was used to assess general self-efficacy beliefs. Each total score was divided by the number of items in the respective scale. To obtain a measure of situational self-efficacy (success expectations), participants were asked to indicate their chances of entering the University on a 0–100% scale.

Procedure

During the initial application period (2 weeks immediately prior to the entrance examinations), entrants who submitted their applications were invited to participate in a psychological study of "personality traits and their relation to achievement in a university entrance situation". To strengthen their motivation, the participants were told that the results would "help the advancement of psychological knowledge", and a popular psychology book was offered in reward for participation. The information leaflet stated that the study was being conducted by a research team independent from the university administration and that individual scores would remain confidential. The university application area and the research room were physically separated by three floors. The tests were administered by undergraduate and graduate students. Participants were asked to indicate their real names, which would be used to match their results to their examination scores as part of the research.

Results

Comparison of the Examination and the No-Attempt Group

Only 87 study participants took at least one examination (after a failed examination, subsequent ones are not taken), the remaining 21 participants (no-attempt group) did not even try one. Two-tailed *t*-test (see Table 14.2) revealed higher levels of depression, lower general and situational self-efficacy, lower happiness and more pessimistic attributional style in the no-attempt group.

Given that the number of available attempts to enter a higher educational institution was practically limited to two or three per year, it is likely that the entrants who had applied but did not actually take any exams were conservative in estimating their chances and decided to avoid potential failure by changing their goal for

Table 14.2 Comparison of the examination and the no-attempt group on all variables

	Examination		No-attempt			
	$N = 87$		$N = 21$			
Scale	*M*	SD	*M*	SD	*t*	Cohen's *d*
Expected success	64.08	19.45	52.62	27.34	2.23*	.55
General self-efficacy	3.24	0.40	2.91	0.45	3.32**	.81
Depression	1.71	0.41	2.05	0.37	3.39**	.83
Happiness	5.42	0.95	4.66	0.81	3.37**	.83
SFASQ: Positive events	4.45	0.68	4.07	0.74	2.21*	.55
SFASQ: Negative events	3.92	0.63	3.57	0.73	2.21*	.55
SFASQ: Total optimism	4.12	0.56	3.76	0.65	2.54*	.64

$^*p < .05$; $^{**}p < .01$

Table 14.3 Comparison of the successful and the unsuccessful group on all variables

	Successful		Unsuccessful			
	$N = 32$		$N = 55$			
Scale	*M*	SD	*M*	SD	*t*	Cohen's *d*
Expected success	71.94	19.13	59.51	18.29	3.00**	.68
General self-efficacy	3.22	0.32	3.25	0.44	0.34	.09
Depression	1.95	0.37	1.93	0.42	0.08	.07
Happiness	5.49	1.00	5.38	0.93	0.51	.11
SFASQ: Positive events	4.22	0.69	4.58	0.64	2.46*	.55
SFASQ: Negative events	3.64	0.64	4.08	0.57	3.36**	.76
SFASQ: Total optimism	3.86	0.51	4.27	0.53	3.53**	.79

$^*p < .05$; $^{**}p < .01$

different universities with lower competition, after it became clear at the end of the application campaign that it would be as high as five applicants per place at the MSU.

Optimism and Examination Outcome

Based on the examination session outcome, the examination group was split into successful (admitted to the university) and unsuccessful (not admitted) entrant subgroups. The unsuccessful group was constituted by entrants who had failed an examination or passed all three but scored below the cut-off average score set by the examination board for full- or part-time studies. When the two groups were compared (see Table 14.3), SFASQ was the only scale to reveal any significant differences: successful entrants showed less optimism across all the parameters of attributional style. This effect was somewhat more pronounced for negative situations than for positive situations. Interestingly, despite lower level of attributional optimism, successful entrants had higher expectations of success.

When the three groups described above with different examination outcomes were compared together using one-way ANOVA (see Fig. 14.3), no significant

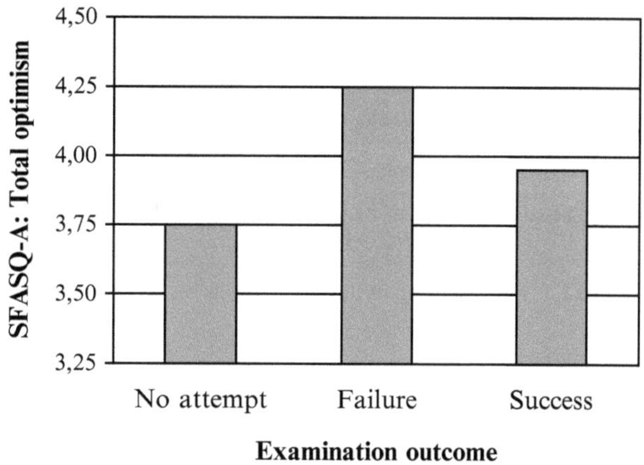

Fig. 14.3 Differences in optimism associated with examination outcome

Table 14.4 Descriptive statistics and Pearson correlations between well-being, optimism, and examination success in the examination group

	1	2	3	4	5	6	7
1. Average exam grade							
2. Expected success	.39**						
3. General self-efficacy	–.07	.27**					
4. Depression	–.01	–.18	–.32**				
5. Happiness	–.05	.26*	.41**	–.72**			
6. SFASQ: Positive events	–.08	.20	.36**	–.31**	.28**		
7. SFASQ: Negative events	–.26*	.10	.42**	–.40**	.30**	.47**	
M	3.06	64.08	3.24	1.71	5.42	4.45	3.92
SD	0.65	19.45	0.40	0.41	0.95	0.68	0.63

$^*p < .05$; $^{**}p < .01$

differences in optimism were found between the successful group and the no-attempt group ($F_{2,\ 104} = 9.23$, $p < .001$, $\eta^2 = .15$). Fisher post-hoc test suggested that the observed differences in optimism between the examination and the no-attempt group were due to the failure subgroup, exhibiting extremely high optimism scores.

The Association of Optimism with Expected and Actual Success

These analyses were carried out in the examination group only ($N = 87$). Only pessimistic attributional style and success expectations were correlated with the average examination grade (see Table 14.4).

A path model (presented on Fig. 14.4) was tested in EQS, revealing that only pessimistic explanatory style for negative events and success expectations predicted actual performance. Success expectations, in turn, were predicted by optimistic attributional style for positive events.

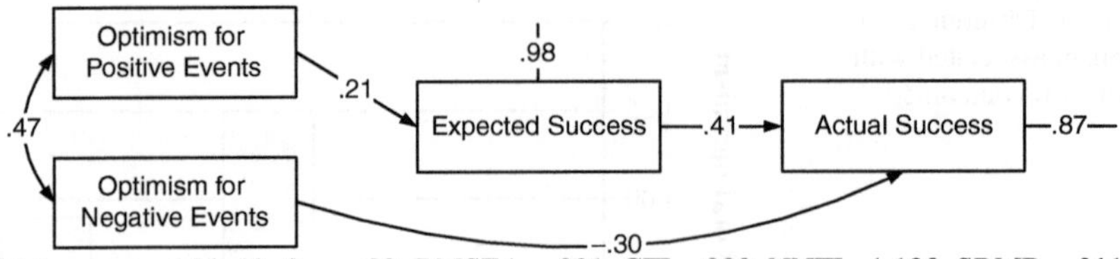

Chi-square = .166, df = 2, p = .92; RMSEA = .001, CFI = .999, NNFI = 1.130, SRMR = .011

Notes: All path coefficients shown are significant (p < .05)

Fig. 14.4 Path diagram of the associations between optimism and examination success

Discussion

The results suggest that moderately pessimistic attributional style for negative events can be beneficial in some academic situations, confirming the previous findings on university students' exam performance (LaForge & Cantrell, 2003; Yee et al., 2003). The probable explanation is that moderately pessimistic students experience more test anxiety and are less confident of success, which motivates them to invest more time and effort into exam preparation. In turn, high optimism exhibited by the unsuccessful entrants may lead to unrealistic success expectations and, thus, undermine performance in complex tasks, which is in line with existing findings on unrealistic optimism (Armor & Taylor, 2002).

The path model revealing that the link between optimistic explanatory style for positive situations and success is mediated by success expectations reproduces the results of Martin-Krumm and Salama-Younes (2007) in the domain of positive life events. Pessimistic explanations of negative events may increase anxiety and motivate a failure-avoidance approach involving additional performance goal setting and preparatory activity. This is associated with higher results, but also higher depression proneness, as the data suggest. Acquired preparedness is likely to be reflected in increased success expectations, but pessimistic attributional style could affect them adversely, which explains the nearly zero association between explanatory style for negative events and success expectations.

In short, the results suggest two different motivational mechanisms behind the relationship of explanatory style to performance. Moderately pessimistic explanations of negative events can elicit anxiety and motivate persistence, concentration on short-term performance goals but can lead to depression and passivity in the long term. In turn, optimistic explanations of positive events may motivate mastery goal setting, persistence and effective coping with difficulties in the long term, but can also result in unrealistically high success expectations, particularly detrimental in difficult activity.

The principal limitation of the study is its modest sample size. However, the study was done in an extremely realistic setting, where school graduates had to make potentially life-changing decisions and take real action by applying to a university. The emerging individual differences were more manifold than it had been expected, and the findings allow drawing meaningful hypotheses for future studies in controlled settings.

General Discussion

The results of the two studies are in line with the existing findings, suggesting that optimistic attributional style is moderately associated with both emotional and cognitive aspects of subjective well-being, predicting higher happiness and lower depression, as well as higher self-esteem and self-efficacy. More importantly, attributional style seems to be the link between well-being and performance. On the one hand, attributional style is the way an individual interprets any given situation in the light of his/her personal dispositions, which results in helplessness or motivated activity, as early studies have shown. On the other hand, attributional style is the way an individual processes feedback from his/her activity, and, therefore, it should moderate the effects of successes and failures upon subjective well-being and future performance.

The findings of the two studies seem to be contradictory at the first glance, but do, in fact, complement each other, demonstrating the relationship of two types of optimism to performance in two academic situations of different types. The Study 1 results reflect the effects of explanatory style for positive life events on long-term, everyday performance in high school learning activity. This activity is continuous, familiar, manageable in terms of difficulty and requires, first of all, motivation for constant persistence, to which optimistic explanations of one's own past successes may contribute. The Study 2 data reflect a short-term positive effect of moderately pessimistic explanatory style for negative events, which is likely to be peculiar to difficult and new situations, such as entering a university. In this case, a realistic prognosis of future difficulties is essential to success, and moderate pessimism may be beneficial, as long as it is not pronounced enough to undermine motivation and activity altogether via the helplessness mechanism.

The findings suggest that optimism is associated with both positive and negative outcomes. It is generally beneficial to both success (via increased self-efficacy) and well-being: in failure situations, optimism may facilitate recovery of positive emotional states, making it easier for one to carry on some difficult activity. However, unrealistically high optimism, particularly concerning negative events, may result in rigid and inaccurate explanations and prognoses of life events. These findings can be seen from different angles: students who have extremely optimistic explanatory style may actually perform worse than those who have a moderate explanatory style *or* who are able to switch and find balance between optimistic and pessimistic explanations. Although attributional style is a stable personality characteristic, it is likely that rigid explanatory style, either pessimistic or optimistic, is less adaptive in terms of resulting performance, than flexible, *realistic* explanatory style, reflecting not only personal dispositions, but also specific features of different situations. Additional studies aimed to test this hypothesis are underway.

The distinction between explanatory style for positive and negative situations, as well as between different types of academic situations, makes it possible to resolve the contradictions between the existing findings concerning the relationship between optimism and performance. The present findings constitute strong evidence in favor of measuring attributional styles for positive and negative events as separate variables. We propose to conclude that attributional style *is* associated with performance in different situations, but the specific pattern of this association depends on the situation type and perspective (whether long-term or short-term performance is considered). In the light of this conclusion, it seems more productive to study the effects of attributional style using longitudinal approach and in concrete settings of specific situations.

Acknowledgement The authors would like to thank Dmitry Leontiev for his useful comments, as well as Oleg Sychev and Valentina Shevyakhova, who assisted in the data collection.

References

Abramson, L. Y., Metalsky, G. I., & Alloy, L. B. (1989). Hopelessness depression: A theory-based subtype of depression. *Psychological Review, 96*, 358–372.

Abramson, L. Y., Seligman, M. E. P., & Teasdale, J. D. (1978). Learned helplessness in humans. *Journal of Abnormal Psychology, 87*, 49–74.

Anderson, C. A., & Arnoult, L. H. (1985). Attributional style and everyday problems of living: Depression, loneliness, and shyness. *Social Cognition, 3*, 16–35.

Anderson, C. A., & Riger, A. L. (1991). A controllability attributional model of problems in living: Dimensional and situational interactions in the prediction of depression and loneliness. *Social Cognition, 9*, 149–181.

Armor, D. A., & Taylor, S. E. (2002). When predictions fail: The dilemma of unrealistic optimism. In T. Gilovich, D. Griffin, & D. Kahneman (Eds.), *Heuristics and biases: The psychology of intuitive judgment*. Cambridge, UK: Cambridge University Press.

Ashforth, B. E., & Fugate, M. (2006). Attributional style in work settings: Development of a measure. *Journal of Leadership and Organizational Studies, 12*(3), 12–29.

Baron, R. M., & Kenny, D. A. (1986). The moderator-mediator variable distinction is social psychological research: Conceptual, strategic and statistical considerations. *Journal of Personality and Social Psychology, 51*, 1173–1182.

Bridges, K. R. (2001). Using attributional style to predict academic performance: How does it compare to traditional methods? *Personality and Individual Differences, 31*(5), 723–730.

Cheng, H., & Furnham, A. (2001). Attributional style and personality as predictors of happiness and mental health. *Journal of Happiness Studies, 2*, 307–323.

Cheng, H., & Furnham, A. (2003). Attributional style and self-esteem as predictors of psychological well being. *Counseling Psychology Quarterly, 16*(2), 121–130.

Corr, P. J., & Gray, J. A. (1996). Attributional style as a personality factor in insurance sales performance in the UK. *Journal of Occupational and Organizational Psychology, 69*, 83–87.

Cutrona, C. E., Russell, D., & Jones, R. D. (1985). Cross-situational consistence in causal attributions: Does attributional style exist? *Journal of Personality and Social Psychology, 47*(5), 1043–1058.

Davis, H., & Zaichkowski, L. (1998). Explanatory style among elite jockey athletes. *Perceptual and Motor Skills, 87*, 1075–1080.

Deuser, W. E., & Anderson, C. A. (1995). Controllability attributions and learned helplessness: Some methodological and conceptual problems. *Basic and Applied Social Psychology, 16*(93), 297–318.

Follette, V. M., & Jacobson, N. S. (1987). Importance of attributions as a predictor of how people cope with failure. *Journal of Personality and Social Psychology, 52*, 1205–1211.

Furnham, A., Sadka, V., & Brewin, C. R. (1992). The development of an occupational attributional style questionnaire. *Journal of Organizational Behavior, 13*(1), 27–39.

Gibb, B. E., Zhu, L., Alloy, L. B., & Abramson, L. Y. (2002). Attributional styles and academic achievement in university students: A longitudinal investigation. *Cognitive Therapy and Research, 26*(3), 309–315.

Gordeeva, T. O., Osin, E. N., & Shevyakhova, V. Y. (2009). *Measurement of optimism as attributional style for negative and positive life events: Success and failure attributional style questionnaire*. Moscow: Smysl.

Hale, B. (1993). Explanatory style as a predictor of academic and athletic achievement in college athletes. *Journal of Sport Behavior, 16*, 63–75.

Johnson, J., Crofton, A., & Feinstein, S. (1996). Enhancing attributional style and positive life events predict increased hopefulness among depressed psychiatric inpatients. *Motivation and Emotion, 20*, 285–296.

Johnson, J. G., Han, Y. S., Douglas, C. J., Johannet, C. M., & Russell, T. (1998). Attributions for positive life events predict recovery from depression among psychiatric inpatients: An investigation of the Needles and Abramson model of recovery from depression. *Journal of Counseling and Clinical Psychology, 66*(2), 369–376.

LaForge, M. C., & Cantrell, S. (2003). Explanatory style and academic performance among college students beginning major course of study. *Psychological Reports, 92*(3), 861.

Lyubomirsky, S., & Lepper, H. (1999). A measure of subjective happiness: Preliminary reliability and construct validation. *Social Indicators Research, 46*, 137–155.

Martin-Krumm, C., & Salama-Younes, M. (2007). Mode explicatif et résultants scolaires chez des enfants préadolescents. *Carrefours de l'Éducation, 24*, 1–12.

Martin-Krumm, C. P., Sarrazin, P., Peterson, C., & Famose, J. P. (2003). Explanatory style and resilience after sport failure. *Personality and Individual Differences, 35*, 1685–1695.

Martinez, R., & Sewell, K. W. (2000). Explanatory style as a predictor of college performance in students with physical disabilities. *Journal of Rehabilitation, 1*, 30–36.

Mezulis, A. H., Abramson, L. Y., Hyde, J. S., & Hankin, B. L. (2004). Is there a universal positivity bias in attributions: A meta-analytic review of individual, developmental, and cultural differences in the self-serving attributional bias. *Psychological Bulletin, 130*(5), 711–747.

Musgrave-Marquart, D., Bromley, S. P., & Dalley, M. B. (1997). Personality, academic attributions, and substance use as predictors of academic achievement in college students. *Journal of Social Behavior and Personality, 12*(2), 501–511.

Needles, D. J., & Abramson, L. Y. (1990). Positive life events, attributional style, and hopefulness: Testing a model of recovery from depression. *Journal of Abnormal Psychology, 99*(2), 156–165.

Peterson, C. (2000). Optimistic explanatory style and health. In J. F. Gillham (Ed.), *The science of optimism and hope: Research essays in honor of Martin E.P. Seligman* (pp. 145–162). Philadelphia: Templeton Foundation.

Peterson, C., & Barrett, L. (1987). Explanatory style and academic performance among university freshmen. *Journal of Personality and Social Psychology, 53*(3), 603–607.

Peterson, C., Bishop, M. P., Fletcher, C. W., Kaplan, M. R., Yesko, E. S., Moon, C. H., et al. (2001). Explanatory style as a risk factor for traumatic mishaps. *Cognitive Therapy and Research, 25*(6), 633–649.

Peterson, C., & Seligman, M. E. P. (1984). Causal explanations as a risk factor for depression: Theory and evidence. *Psychological Review, 91*(3), 347–374.

Peterson, C., & Seligman, M. E. P. (1987). Explanatory style and illness. *Journal of Personality, 55*, 237–265.

Peterson, C., Seligman, M. E. P., & Vaillant, G. E. (1988). Pessimistic explanatory style is a risk factor for physical illness: A thirty-five-year longitudinal study. *Journal of Personality and Social Psychology, 55*, 23–27.

Peterson, C., Semmel, A., von Bayer, C., Abramson, L., Metalsky, G., & Seligman, M. E. P. (1982). The attributional style questionnaire. *Cognitive Therapy and Research, 6*(3), 287–300.

Peterson, C., & Vaidya, R. S. (2001). Explanatory style, expectation, and depressive symptoms. *Personality and Individual Differences, 31*, 1217–1223.

Rigby, B. N., & Huebner, E. S. (2005). Do causal attributions mediate the relationship between personality characteristics and life satisfaction in adolescence? *Psychology in the Schools, 42*(1), 91–99.

Ritterband, L. M., & Spielberger, C. D. (1996). Construct validity of the Beck Depression Inventory as a measure of state and trait depression in non-clinical populations. *Depression and Stress, 2*, 123–145.

Rosenberg, M. (1965). *Society and the adolescent self-image*. Princeton, NJ: Princeton University Press.
Rowe, J. E., & Lockhart, L. K. (2005). Relationship of cognitive attributional style and academic performance among a predominantly Hispanic college student population. *Individual Differences Research, 3*(2), 136–139.
Russel, D. (1982). The causal dimension scale: A measure of how individuals perceive causes. *Journal of Personality and Social Psychology, 42*, 1137–1145.
Sanjuan, P., Perez Garcia, A. M., Rueda, B., & Ruiz, A. (2008). Interactive effects of attributional style for positive and negative events on psychological distress. *Personality and Individual Differences, 45*, 187–190.
Sanjuan, P., & Magallares, A. (2009). Coping strategies as a link between optimistic explanatory styles and well-being. In T. Freire (Ed.), *Understanding positive life: Research and practice on positive psychology* (pp. 167–180). Lisbon: Climepsi Editores.
Satterfield, J. M., Monahan, J., & Seligman, M. E. P. (1997). Law school performance predicted by explanatory style. *Behavioral Sciences and the Law, 15*, 95–105.
Schwartzer, R. (1993). *Measurement of perceived self-efficacy. Psychometric scales for cross cultural research*. Berlin, Germany: Freie Universität Berlin, Institut für Psychologie.
Seligman, M. E. P. (1975). *Helplessness: On depression, development, and death*. San Francisco: Freeman.
Seligman, M. E. P. (1990). *Learned optimism*. New York: Simon & Schuster.
Seligman, M. E. P. (2002). *Authentic happiness*. New York: Free Press.
Seligman, M. E. P., Abramson, L. Y., Semmel, A., & Von Baeyer, C. (1979). Depressive attributional style. *Journal of Abnormal Psychology, 88*, 242–247.
Seligman, M. E. P., Nolen-Hoeksema, S., Thornton, N., & Thornton, K. M. (1990). Explanatory style as a mechanism of disappointing athletic performance. *Psychological Science, 1*(2), 143–146.
Seligman, M. E. P., & Shulman, P. (1986). Explanatory style as a predictor of productivity and quitting among life insurance sales agents. *Journal of Personality and Social Psychology, 50*, 832–838.
Stolz, P. G. (1999). *Adversity quotient: Turning obstacles into opportunities*. New York: Wiley.
Sweeney, P. D., Anderson, K., & Bailey, S. (1986). Attributional style in depression: A meta-analytic review. *Journal of Personality and Social Psychology, 50*(5), 974–991.
Tennen, H., & Herzberger, S. (1985). A review of attributional style questionnaire. In D. J. Keyser & R. S. Herzberger (Eds.), *Test critiques* (Vol. 4, pp. 20–32). Kansas City: Test Corporation of America.
Voelz, Z., Haeffel, G., Joiner, T., & Wagner, K. (2003). Reducing hopelessness: The interaction of enhancing and depressogenic attributional styles for positive and negative life events among youth psychiatric inpatients. *Behavior Research and Therapy, 41*, 1183–1198.
Ward, C. W. (2003). Explanatory style among undergraduate students in Christian higher education. Part 1: A single-institution case study. *Christian Higher Education, 2*(2), 169–185.
Yates, S. M., & Yates, G. C. R. (1995). Explanatory style, ego-orientation and primary school mathematics. *Educational Psychology, 15*, 28–34.
Yee, P. L., Pierce, G. R., Ptacek, J. T., & Modzelesky, K. L. (2003). Learned helplessness attributional style and examination performance: Enhancement effects are not necessarily moderated by prior failure. *Anxiety, Stress, and Coping, 16*(4), 359–373.
Xenikou, A., Furnham, A., & McCarrey, M. (1997). Attributional style for negative events: A proposition for a more reliable and valid measure of attributional style. *British Journal of Psychology, 88*, 53–69.
Zautra, A. J., Guenther, R. T., & Chartier, G. M. (1985). Attributions for real and hypothetical events: Their relation to self-esteem and depression. *Journal of Abnormal Psychology, 94*, 530–540.

Chapter 15
To Flourish, Arm or Fade Away? Proactive, Defensive and Depressive Patterns of Self-Regulated Learning

Darko Lončarić

A self-regulation and strategic approach to every aspect of our lives is becoming increasingly popular. We are constantly reminded by popularized science that taking control of our lives and leaving almost nothing to pure chance or destiny is an impetus for our well-being and success. Although overly exaggerated, this statement reflects a well-established, paradigmatic shift from reactive to proactive perspective on human thought and action. This perspective has been specially promoted by positive psychology theorists and researchers (e.g. Clonan, Chafouleas, McDougal, & Riley-Tillman, 2003; Fung, Rice, & Carstensen, 2005; Greenglass, 2002; Netzel & Eber, 2003). Most prominent ideas about self-regulation can be abstracted in a statement that human beings have the ability to exert control over their inner states, processes and responses, resist their own impulses and adapt and change their current behavior in order to attain relatively distal goals. Self-control is a human strength most relevant to self-regulation. With focus being shifted from positive to some negative influences of self-control, it became obvious that it depends on limited resources and may cause short-term impairments like ego depletion (Baumeister, Vohs, & Tice, 2007). Research has reached high level of methodological rigor and excellence in this field. For example, findings about life-long perspective on cognitive control and efficiency (Eigsti et al., 2006) are strongly supported even on the neurophysiologic level of analysis.

As opposed to ever presence of self-regulation in scientific and lay person's everyday jargon, there is still not enough consensus or conceptual and terminological clarity in self-regulation theory and practice. Most of self-regulation research and self-regulation ideas are fragmented and scattered across different, not always compatible, theoretical frameworks, applied over several different domains resulting in a great number of different terms and labels. That situation hinders an exchange of ideas between scientists who investigate similar or even same real-life phenomena.

D. Lončarić (✉)
Faculty of Teacher Education, University of Rijeka, Rijeka, Croatia
e-mail: darko@ufri.hr; loncaricd@gmail.com

I. Brdar (ed.), *The Human Pursuit of Well-Being: A Cultural Approach*,
DOI 10.1007/978-94-007-1375-8_15,

On the other hand, Boekaerts and colleagues optimistically suggest that self-regulatory constructs could be a cohesive force for integrating different areas of psychology (Boekaerts, Pintrich, & Zeidner, 2005). Therefore, the main goal of this investigation is to contribute to conceptual, theoretical and terminological unity of the self-regulation construct through the investigation of related structures and processes within the domain of self-regulated learning.

To meet the challenges of conceptualization and measurement of self-regulation components, three simple organizing constructs will be proposed and partially tested in this research. I propose that all self-regulated components can be described in terms of two functional patterns labeled as proactive and defensive self-regulation. Furthermore, these patterns can be supplemented with a depressive pattern indicating self-defeating cognitions and strategies, absence of motivation and self-regulation efforts.

Proactive pattern can be related to perseverance and growth as two of three important human strengths elaborated by Carver and Scheier (2003). On the other hand, relatively new perspective in positive psychology describes "giving up" as a third human strength. It can be a valuable and adaptive response when it leads to changing goals to more attainable alternatives. Giving up is related to the depressive self-regulation pattern when a person is committed to unattainable goal, leading to distress, futility and helplessness. When person does not adopt a new/different goal, we can expect problems leading to aimlessness, emptiness and loneliness. Depressive self-regulation could also be related to specific attributional patterns (e.g., stable, internal attributions of failure and unstable, external attributions of success), helplessness, procrastination and apathy. Persons entangled in such processes and interpretations could be described metaphorically as fading away instead of growing and flourishing. They even lack the "rouses thorns" for self-defense, as the main characteristic of depressive pattern is absence of defensive self-regulation efforts. Empirical part of this work is focused on self-regulation efforts, with guidelines for developing and testing a depressive pattern in future research.

Patterns of Self-Efficacy and Outcome Expectations

Bandura's theory proposes that outcome expectations form important construct related to motivational behavior and affect. Outcome expectations are defined as judgments or beliefs regarding the contingency between behavior and the anticipated outcome. Although self-efficacy beliefs are highly correlated with outcome expectations, these two constructs should not be confused. Bandura (1986, p. 391) provides us with an example of these constructs, differentiating them as follows: "The belief that one can high jump six feet is an efficacy judgment; the anticipated social recognition, applause, trophies and self-satisfaction for such a performance constitute the outcome expectations".

Bandura (1982) has suggested that students can be classified into four groups according to their high or low self-efficacy and high or low outcome expectations. The crossing of these dimensions forms a two by two contingency table and four different patterns that might provide some insight into behavioral and affective reactions for individuals who vary in efficacy and outcome expectation beliefs. These patterns can also be related to the proactive, defensive and depressive self-regulation patterns proposed in this paper.

Students who are high in both self-efficacy and outcome expectations are confident and assured in their performance; they invest high levels of effort, are persistent when faced with troubles and obstacles and have a high level of cognitive engagement in academic tasks. This would be characteristic for the proactive self-regulation pattern.

Students who are high in efficacy but low in outcome expectations are most likely to keep investing effort in combination with protest and social activism for problems that led to low expectations. If nothing changes, they are likely to change the environment or become school-dropouts. While these students are focused on their high self-efficacy, they would still exhibit the proactive self-regulation pattern. When their focus shifts on low outcome expectations, the defensive self-regulation pattern is likely to emerge.

Students who are low in both self-efficacy and outcome expectations are prone to resignation, apathy, and might be unwilling or unable to invest high levels of effort. They usually give up on learning efforts and, in most ways, are similar to students with problems related to learned helplessness (Pintrich & Schunk, 2002) and learned hopelessness (Au, Watkins, Hattie, & Alexander, 2009). On the other hand, they still have the opportunity to attribute some of the problems to external factors influencing low outcome expectations. They can perceive other students failing at the same task and conclude that the task is too difficult and that no effort would lead to the wanted outcomes. If these students focus more on their low self-efficacy, they are likely to demonstrate the depressive self-regulation pattern, but if they focus more on external factors leading to low outcome expectations, they might use the defensive self-regulation pattern.

The last group of students is at the highest risk of falling into the depressive self-regulation pattern as they have low self-efficacy but high outcome expectations. These students believe that they are not able to do the required task, but they are aware (by seeing others getting rewarded for performing as required) that if they were able to do the task, the environment would be responsive, and they would be appropriately rewarded. That would lead to negative self-evaluations and students would focus on themselves as the cause of all failure resulting in the depressive self-regulation pattern.

Motivational and Cognitive Components of Knowledge, Beliefs, Strategies and Outcomes

Conceptual six-component framework presented by Garcia and Pintrich (1994) outlines two general domains (motivational and cognitive) and three organizing constructs (knowledge/beliefs, strategies used for regulation and outcomes).

The first component represents the motivational domain of knowledge and beliefs. Knowledge and beliefs can also be considered as cognitions, but this component can be characterized as a list of "hot" cognitions for its motivational relevance. The second component is also comprised of knowledge and beliefs, but it can be characterized as a list of "cold" cognitions. It includes conceptual knowledge (such as content knowledge and disciplinary knowledge) and metacognitive knowledge regarding tasks and strategies. The third component describes various motivational strategies (self-handicapping, defensive pessimism, self-affirmation, disidentification and attributional style) that students may use to accomplish their social and personal goals. Furthermore, motivational strategies, in conjunction with students' motivational beliefs and self-schemas, directly influence motivational learning outcomes described in the fifth component as quantity of effort, task choice and persistence.

Cognitive strategies represent the fourth component of this model. Cognitive learning strategies usually include rehearsal, elaboration and organization. They are an integral part of various academic tasks. Regulatory learning strategies include goal-setting, planning, monitoring and self-testing. They are usually used to improve the students' learning process. Cognitive strategies are supposed to be directly linked to motivational outcomes described in the fifth and sixth components that include the quality of effort (such as deep processing), knowledge activation/restructuring and academic performance.

Promotion and Prevention Focus

The regulatory focus theory (Higgins, 1997) proposes that self-regulation operates differently when serving fundamentally different needs, such as nurturance and security. Nurturance-related regulation is assumed to involve a promotion focus, which is a regulatory state concerned with ideals, advancement, aspiration and accomplishment. A promotion focus is sensitive to presence or absence of positive outcomes. Security-related regulation involves a prevention focus which is a regulatory state concerned with obligations, protection, safety and responsibility. A prevention focus is sensitive to presence or absence of negative outcomes.

Promotion and prevention focus provide incentives for the use of different means and strategies activated to achieve the desired outcomes. Promotion-focused people prefer to use eagerness-related means, most suited to striving for advancement, aspiration and accomplishment, while prevention-focused people prefer to use vigilance-related means, most suited to striving for protection, safety and responsibility (Crowe & Higgins, 1997). This regulatory focus is supposed to explain differences in judgmental processes and goal pursuit above and beyond such fundamental factors as expectancy and value of attainment.

Learning and Well-Being Patterns

Pioneering work on two processing modes in academic settings was done by Diener and Dweck (1978). They examined children's reactions to failure and differentiated two groups of children demonstrating different behavioral patterns: helpless and mastery group. Soon enough, it become obvious that if we want to understand and model such behavior, we have to ask ourselves how students interpret academic situation and what meaning do they construct from such situations.

Boekaerts (1992) assumed that students continuously judge whether a learning situation is being neutral or threatening for their well-being. She defined appraisals as ongoing comparison processes between task or situational demands and personal resources to meet these demands (Boekaerts, 1991, 1993). Appraisals are the central construct of Boekaerts' (1992, 1996) model of adaptable learning. She developed the model as an attempt to integrate and extend the fragmented research and theory within the domains of learning, motivation, anxiety, coping with stress and action control.

Predominantly positive appraisals activate the processing mode, called mastery or learning mode. Students' attention and energy is focused on adaptive payoffs, such as the increase in competence and other resources. Unfavorable appraisals and intense emotions draw a learner's attention away from a learning process which may lead to avoidance behavior. The predominance of negative appraisals activates a processing mode called coping or well-being mode focusing students to protect their ego or restore their well-being. Students are said to be learning in an adaptable way when they have found the balance between the two processing routes and the basic priorities underlying them.

Conceptual Framework for the Study

When investigating numerous interrelated constructs, such as motivation, cognition, self-regulation strategies and their outcomes, an elaborated framework is needed to focus and guide empirical research efforts. Such a framework could help us to select relevant variables to be measured, assume relations between different concepts, model direct and indirect effects and formulate prior hypotheses to be tested.

The conceptual framework displayed in Fig. 15.1 (Lončarić, 2008) has been based predominantly on the previously discussed models of self-regulated learning. The taxonomy developed by Garcia and Pintrich (1994) provides a well-elaborated network of cognitive and motivational knowledge, beliefs and strategies encompassing most relevant components for this study. Boekaerts' model of adaptable learning provides the opportunity to integrate these components into functional self-regulation processes that are hypothesized to reflect proactive and defensive self-regulation patterns. Garcia and Pintrich describe various learning strategies,

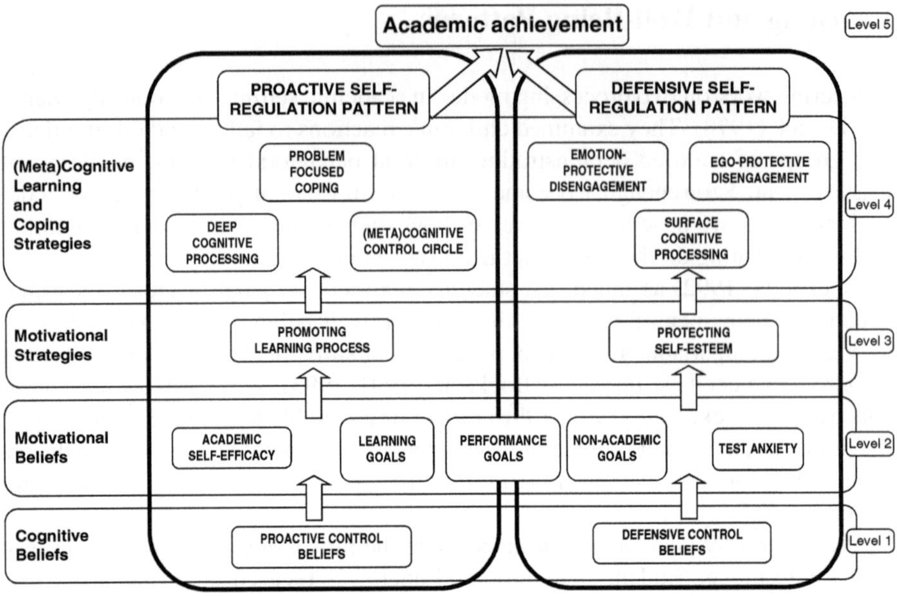

Fig. 15.1 Proactive and defensive patterns of cognitive and motivational beliefs/strategies affecting academic achievement (Lončarić, 2008)

while Boekaerts' model specifically considers coping strategies as a part of the "coping mode". Coping strategies are an important component of self-regulation as they represent volitional processes in postdecisional phases of self-regulation efforts.

Another important element of this conceptual framework is the assumption about direct and indirect effects among the components of self-regulated learning and academic achievement. It is hypothesized that cognitive beliefs (Level 1) have direct effect on motivational beliefs (Level 2). Cognitive beliefs can also exert direct or indirect effects on motivational strategies, cognitive strategies and academic outcomes, but these relations are not explicit in this schematic model. As proposed by Ames (1992) and Garcia and Pintrich (1994), students' motivational beliefs about the tasks and general goal orientation (Level 2) can have direct and strong effect on motivational strategies (Level 3), cognitive strategies (Level 4) and effort. Cognitive strategies together with increased quality and quantity of effort are supposed to directly affect academic achievement (Level 5).

The described conceptual framework provides general guidance for empirical investigation of the self-regulated learning patterns. It represents a theoretically guided sample of variables relevant for self-regulated learning and gives some general predictions about directionality of relations between different components and constructs. It describes relevant independent variables, dependent variables and possible mediated effects. It also provides some affirmative hypotheses about the classification of self-regulation components into proactive and defensive self-regulation patterns.

Primary objective of this research is to investigate the relationships between the cognitive, motivational and strategic components of self-regulated learning. As a preliminary test of the proposed model, we can investigate if there are specific patterns of cognitive beliefs, motivational beliefs, motivational strategies, learning and coping strategies that would result in empirical distinction between the proactive and defensive self-regulation pattern.

Method

Participants

The sample for the study included 461 children and young adolescents (243 girls and 218 boys) and was obtained from two suburban public elementary schools in the northwest part of Croatia. The students ranged from 11 to 14 years of age with a mean of 12.68 years (SD = 1.15) and were attending upper elementary school. The families from the school area were largely middle-class families.

Procedure

The participants were randomly assigned to complete one of the two versions of the survey with different order of the presented material. There were no significant differences between the versions, so they were combined for subsequent analyses. In order to make the procedure less invasive for the students, the questionnaires were administered during two 35-minute sessions, with the second session administered after approximately 1 or 2 weeks.

The questionnaires were administered in the classroom, during the regular teaching periods. The students completed their questionnaires in the regular classroom groups (20–30 students) with a research assistant available to explain the procedure and answer questions. After completing the measures, all the participants were debriefed about the purpose of the study and had the opportunity to express themselves, comment on the survey and ask questions.

Measures

In order to collect a wide range of motivational and cognitive self-regulation components, self-regulated learning component scale[1] (SRLC, Lončarić, 2008) was used. All scales use the five-point Likert-type response format ranging from 1 ("strongly disagree") to 5 ("strongly agree"). As presented in Table 15.1, this scale

[1] Scales are available on request (English and Croatian version).

Table 15.1 Motivational and cognitive components of self-regulated learning

Constructs	Scales	Subscales	M^a	SD	n	α
Cognitive beliefs	Proactive control beliefs	Means-ends beliefs: Effort	4.22	0.83	4	.81
		Generalized control beliefs	4.12	0.92	4	.90
	Defensive control beliefs	Means-ends beliefs: External	2.27	1.13	4	.87
		Means-ends beliefs: Ability	2.27	1.07	4	.80
		Entity theory of intelligence	2.56	1.02	4	.74
Motivational beliefs	Test anxiety	Physiological component	3.50	1.27	2	.79
		Emotional component	3.57	1.14	2	.62
		Cognitive and behavioral component	2.54	1.04	4	.77
	Academic self-efficacy	Self-efficacy in learning process	3.56	0.84	4	.75
		Attribution of success to effort	4.38	0.66	4	.72
	Self-referenced learning goals	Learning approach	4.16	0.78	4	.81
		Avoiding mistakes	3.58	0.97	4	.81
	Other referenced performance goals	Competition approach	3.10	1.13	4	.87
		Competition avoidance	2.32	1.02	3	.78
		Self-protective	2.89	1.13	3	.79
		Self-promoting	2.54	1.10	4	.88
	Nonacademic goals	Work-avoidance	2.84	1.08	4	.80
		Social	2.88	1.12	4	.80
Motivational strategies	Promoting learning process	Setting up goals	2.94	0.68	5	.76
		Effort regulation	3.45	0.90	5	.81
		Work, place, and time management	4.52	0.93	6	.79
	Protecting self-esteem	Self-handicapping	2.42	1.04	5	.85
		Defensive pessimism	2.85	0.95	4	.70
		Self-affirmative attributions	2.58	1.17	4	.86
Learning strategies	(Meta)cognitive control circle	Repetition and exercise	3.74	0.88	4	.81
		Controlling learning process and outcome	3.97	0.78	7	.87
	Deep cognitive processing	Elaboration	3.64	0.91	4	.84
		Organization	3.72	0.82	7	.84
		Application	3.55	0.84	4	.70
		Critical thinking	3.41	0.86	5	.81
	Surface cognitive processing	Focusing on minimal requirements	2.27	1.14	4	.85
		Unrelated memorizing	2.58	1.08	4	.85
Academic coping strategies	Problem-focused coping	Problem solving behaviors	4.26	0.75	4	.82
		Problem solving cognitions	3.97	0.85	4	.78
	Emotion-protective disengagement	Avoidance	2.23	1.12	5	.88
		Wishful thinking	3.04	1.11	4	.75
		Distraction	2.62	1.16	5	.89
	Ego-protective disengagement	Giving up and reinterpretation	2.54	0.91	8	.81
		Ignoring the problem	2.86	1.09	4	.79
		Using humour	2.65	1.26	4	.90

[a] Mean score is computed as the sum of the items divided by the number of items

includes several motivational and cognitive components of self-regulated learning: cognitive beliefs, motivational beliefs, motivational strategies, learning strategies and academic coping strategies.

Cognitive Beliefs

Cognitive beliefs are measured with the control beliefs scales based on an action theoretical approach as formulated by Skinner, Chapman and Baltes (1988), and on students' implicit theories of intelligence (Dweck, 2000). Cognitive beliefs include proactive control beliefs (belief that effort leads to success and belief that most situations are controllable) and defensive control beliefs (belief that external agents or intelligence leads to success).

Motivational Beliefs

The motivational beliefs scales are based on the expectancy-value model as described by Pintrich and his colleagues (Pintrich, 1988; Pintrich & De Groot, 1990; Pintrich & Schunk, 2002). The test anxiety scales represent the affective component of motivational beliefs and include physiological, emotional, cognitive and behavioral components of anxiety. The academic self-efficacy scales were constructed to represent the expectancy component of motivational beliefs and measure self-efficacy in the learning process and reliance on effort. The goal orientation scales were constructed to represent the value component of motivational beliefs and they included self-referenced learning goals, other referenced performance goals and nonacademic (work avoidance and social) goals.

Motivational Strategies

The motivational strategies scales are in line with various learning strategies measures that differentiate motivational strategies and management of external resources from other, more (meta)cognitively oriented learning strategies: MSLQ (Pintrich, Smith, Garcia, & McKeachie, 1991), LASSY (Weinstein, Zimmerman, & Palmer, 1988), CSRL (Niemivirta, 1996) and LIST (Wild & Schiefele, 1994). The motivational strategies scales include strategies for promoting learning process such as setting up goals and effort/work/place/time management and strategies for protecting self-esteem that include self-handicapping, defensive pessimism and external attribution of failure.

Cognitive Strategies

The learning strategies scales are constructed with the respect to two conceptually different models. One model makes the principal distinctions between students who adopt a deep approach versus those who adopt a surface approach to learning (Marton & Saljo, 1976a, 1976b; Tait, Entwistle, & McCune, 1998), while the other model defines learning strategies mostly in terms of cognitive vs. metacognitive components (MSLQ; Pintrich et al., 1991).

The preliminary results gathered in the early stages of the scale development showed more support for the deep vs. surface processing distinction than for the cognitive vs. metacognitive distinction of learning strategies. It also showed that repetition and exercise as predominantly cognitive strategies (sometimes considered as surface cognitive strategies) were strongly related to metacognitive self-monitoring strategies (learning acquisition and outcome control), suggesting the functional unity of the cognitive–metacognitive circle. This finding also indicates that cognitive and metacognitive distinctions are less empirically supported when compared to other, more functionally organized constructs. The learning strategies scales include (meta)cognitive control circle (measuring functionally related constructs such as repetition and exercise, controlling learning process and outcome), deep cognitive processing and surface cognitive processing.

The academic coping strategies scales is a self-report measure of students' efforts to cope with academic failure. The initial scale construction was in line with the transactional perspective (Lazarus & Folkman, 1984). As the scales were further developed, modifications were made to make them more in line with proposed model of proactive and defensive self-regulation. The academic coping strategies scales include problem-focused coping, emotion-protective disengagement and ego-protective disengagement.

Results

The objective of this research was to investigate the possibility that relationships between cognition, motivation and self-regulated strategies suggest empirical evidence for proactive and defensive self-regulation patterns. There is no previous research that would relate the used measures with the proactive or defensive self-regulation pattern. This attempt to integrate all these measures and account for some of the findings provided in previous models is exploratory in nature, so exploratory factor analysis is used.

The factor analysis with the maximum likelihood (ML) extraction method and oblimin rotation using the scree plot criteria suggested two significant factors explaining 44.37% of the total variance. Eigen values for the two extracted factors were 4.90 and 2.84, respectively (eigenvalues for the third and fourth factor were 1.15 and 1.05, respectively). The correlation between the extracted factors was 0.02, indicating independent constructs.

The factor loadings presented in the pattern matrix (Table 15.2) indicate that the first factor can be labeled as the *proactive self-regulation pattern* as it includes proactive learning (metacognitive control circle and deep cognitive processing), proactive coping (problem-focused coping), proactive motivational components (self-efficacy,

Table 15.2 Common factor analysis (ML) of cognitive, motivational and strategic components of self-regulated learning: Pattern matrix

	Factors	
	Proactive SR pattern	Defensive SR pattern
Promoting learning process	**.87**	.07
Learning goals	**.81**	−.10
(Meta)Cognitive control circle	**.71**	.05
Deep cognitive processing	**.68**	.32
Problem-focused coping	**.61**	−.04
Self-efficacy	**.61**	−.24
Proactive control beliefs	**.39**	−.18
Nonacademic goals	**−.57**	**.46**
Protecting self-esteem	**−.40**	**.55**
Performance goals	.21	**.64**
Defensive control beliefs	−.18	**.63**
Emotion-protective disengagement	.06	**.60**
Surface cognitive processing	−.12	**.59**
Ego-protective disengagement	−.16	**.48**
Test anxiety	.18	**.43**

Note: Values in bold face denote factor loadings greater than 0.32 (indicating more than 10% of overlapping variance)

motivation for promoting learning process, learning goals), and proactive control beliefs. The second factor could be labeled as the *defensive self-regulation pattern* as it includes defensive learning (surface cognitive processing), defensive coping (emotion-protective disengagement and ego-protective disengagement), defensive motivational components (test anxiety, protecting self-esteem, performance goals, nonacademic goals) and the defensive cognitive beliefs.

The nonacademic goals and motivation to protect self-esteem demonstrated considerable cross-loadings. These components had negative loadings on the proactive and positive loadings on the defensive self-regulation pattern indicating that nonacademic goals, self-handicapping, defensive pessimism and self-affirmative attribution of failure intensify defensive and suppress proactive self-regulation.

Discussion

Several self-regulation models (e.g., Boekaerts, 1993; Higgins, 1997; Higgins & Spiegel, 2004) suggest that self-regulation operates differently when serving two fundamentally different needs or basic priorities. In different models, these dichotomised processes were given different names and have somewhat different features, but, basically, they represent a combination of self-regulation processes and components that can be labeled as proactive and defensive self-regulation patterns.

The main goal of this research was to determine whether proactive and defensive self-regulation patterns can be empirically differentiated. The exploratory investigation of the relationships between cognitive, motivational and strategic components of self-regulated learning revealed two different factors that were in accordance with the proposed proactive and defensive self-regulation patterns. The proactive self-regulation pattern is characterized by proactive control beliefs, self-efficacy and learning approach goals and also avoiding nonacademic goals. As for strategic behavior, it is indicated by motivational strategies for promoting learning process and less reliance on motivational strategies for protecting self-esteem, proactive use of the (meta)cognitive control circle, deep cognitive processing learning strategies and problem-focused coping. The defensive self-regulation pattern is characterized by defensive control beliefs, test anxiety and adopting performance and nonacademic goals. It is also related to increased use of protecting self-esteem strategies, surface cognitive processing learning strategies and emotion- and ego-protective disengagement coping strategies.

Extending sufficient amount of effort in learning is a predominant characteristic of the proactive self-regulation factor as indicated with highest factor loadings onto motivation strategies that promote a learning process (e.g., effort regulation and work-place-time management), learning goals and metacognitive and cognitive control processes (e.g., repetition and exercise). Therefore, it is not surprising that nonacademic goals (e.g., work avoidance) and motivation to protect self-esteem (e.g., self-handicapping) had relatively high negative loadings onto the proactive factor in addition to relatively high positive loadings onto the defensive factor. These cross-loadings suggest that nonacademic goals and motivation to protect self-esteem could easily be used to differentiate proactive and defensive self-regulation patterns. Regarding future research, it remains to be seen whether nonacademic goals and motivation to protect self-esteem actively defer students from extending effort when learning. Alternatively, proactive students might consider these self-regulation components as particularly detrimental and avoid them actively. These processes and interpretations might both have synergic effect on producing such cross-loadings onto different factors.

In this and some previous research (Končarić, 2008), I have formulated the model of proactive and defensive self-regulation patterns integrating numerous findings from different fields of psychology. Several authors proposed a deep vs. surface approach to learning (Marton & Saljo, 1976a, 1976b; Tait et al., 1998) reinforcing my belief that even cognitive strategies might have two distinctive proactive and defensive functions. Boekaerts (1993) made further distinction between different information processing modes, called mastery or learning mode and coping or well-being mode. Similar constructs were proposed by Diener and Dweck (1978) as they differentiated two groups of children demonstrating different behavioral patterns and called them helpless and mastery group. Higgins (1997) has come to similar conclusions formulated in the regulatory focus theory describing promotion and prevention regulatory focus. Finally, it may be said that the strongest support for proactive and defensive self-regulation patterns was given by the patterns of self-efficacy and outcome expectations (Bandura, 1982). Students who are high in both self-efficacy and outcome expectations are most likely to engage in proactive self-regulation, while students who are low in outcome expectations are most likely to engage in defensive self-regulation.

Proactive and defensive patterns cover most but not all of the students' behavior in different academic situations. There are students who do not extend effort to increase their knowledge or skills and to protect their self-esteem when faced with failure. From the perspective of functional analysis, it seems very difficult to explain such behavior. So far, they are best described by one of self-efficacy and outcome expectations patterns (Bandura, 1982). They probably have low self-efficacy but high outcome expectations. These students believe that they are not able to do a required task (no proactive self-regulation pattern) but they are aware that if they were able to do the task, the environment would be responsive, and they would be appropriately rewarded. This way, they cannot have positive reinterpretation of the problem and attribute failure to the lack of environmental responsiveness, and they cannot lower the value of academic activities, leaving them with no opportunity to use the defensive self-regulation pattern. These children might be at highest risk because they are inclined to the depressive self-regulation pattern and learned helplessness. Instead of flourishing and developing their potential in academic context, they might vain and fade away, usually unnoticed and isolated by peers and relevant adults who are more concerned with defensive children who have antiacademic goals. Further research needs to address this question of specific self-regulation failures described as the depressive self-regulation pattern in samples that include larger proportion of poorly adapted and under-achieving students.

Self regulation in learning is just a part of general self-regulation processes that are important for understanding why some children prevail when going through adverse situations while others fail to adapt to problems and stressful situations. Adaptive self-regulation is related to resilience. Resilience is usually described as a trait that renders people invulnerable to harsh, extreme and impoverished child-rearing circumstances, but, recently, it has been conceptualized as a self-regulation process (Dishion & Connell, 2006). Longitudinal research has showed that self-regulation-based resilience buffers adverse effects of peer deviance and stress on an adolescent's antisocial behavior and internalizing symptoms like depression. Resilience was also considered as an outcome of self-regulation strategies and research findings indicated that motivational strategies were strong predictors of academic resilience defined as students' inclination to pursue long and demanding learning experiences (Nota, Soresi, & Zimmerman, 2004).

Further research should improve investigation into self-regulation patterns in several ways. Academic and motivational outcomes like GPA, school drop-out, truancy, students' choice of activities, task value and persistence should also be considered. Methodology should be extended to cover microanalytic (investigating self-regulation on specific academic tasks within a specific academic subject and relating it to specific, immediate outcomes) and longitudinal perspective (self-regulation is usually considered as a process that unfolds over time).

Regardless of these limitations presented, results give additional support for the reconceptualization of self-regulation components into distinctive proactive and defensive patterns. These findings, in collaboration with some previous research, present us with an opportunity to develop a new network of self-regulation concepts in learning and academic achievement.

References

Ames, C. (1992). Classrooms: Goals, structures and student motivation. *Journal of Educational Psychology, 84*(3), 261–271.
Au, R. C. P., Watkins, D., Hattie, J., & Alexander, P. (2009). Reformulating the depression model of learned hopelessness for academic outcomes. *Educational Research Review, 4*, 103–117.
Bandura, A. (1982). Self-efficacy mechanism in human agency. *The American Psychologist, 37*, 122–147.
Bandura, A. (1986). *Social foundations of thought and action: A social cognitive theory*. Englewood Cliffs, NJ: Prentice-Hall.
Baumeister, R. F., Vohs, K. D., & Tice, D. M. (2007). The strength model of self-control. *Current Directions in Psychological Science, 16*, 396–403.
Boekaerts, M. (1991). Subjective competence, appraisals and self-assessment. *Learning and Instruction, 1*(1), 1–17.
Boekaerts, M. (1992). The adaptable learning process: Initiating and maintaining behavioural change. *Journal of Applied Psychology: An International Review, 41*, 377–397.
Boekaerts, M. (1993). Being concerned with well-being and with learning. *Educational Psychologist, 28*(2), 149–167.
Boekaerts, M. (1996). Coping with stress in childhood and adolescence. In M. Zeidner & N. S. Endler (Eds.), *Handbook of coping: Theories, research, applications* (pp. 452–484). New York: Wiley.
Boekaerts, M., Pintrich, P. R., & Zeidner, M. (2005). Self-regulation: An introductory overview. In M. Boekaerts, P. R. Pintrich, & M. Zeidner (Eds.), *Handbook of self-regulation* (pp. 1–9). San Diego, CA: Academic.
Carver, C. S., & Scheier, M. F. (2003). Three human strengths. In L. G. Aspinwall & U. M. Staudinger (Eds.), *A psychology of human strengths: Fundamental questions and future directions for a positive psychology* (pp. 87–102). Washington, DC: American Psychological Association.
Clonan, S. M., Chafouleas, S. M., McDougal, J. L., & Riley-Tillman, T. C. (2003). Positive psychology goes to school: Are we there yet? *Psychology in the Schools, 41*, 101–110.
Crowe, E., & Higgins, E. T. (1997). Regulatory focus and strategic inclinations: Promotion and prevention in decision-making. *Organizational Behavior and Human Decision Processes, 69*, 117–132.
Diener, C. I., & Dweck, C. S. (1978). An analysis of learned helplessness: Continuous changes in performance, strategy and achievement cognitions following failure. *Journal of Personality and Social Psychology, 36*, 451–462.
Dishion, T. J., & Connell, A. (2006). Adolescents' resilience as a self-regulatory process: Promising themes for linking intervention with developmental science. *Annals of the New York Academy of Sciences, 1094*, 125–138.
Dweck, C. S. (2000). *Self-theories: Their role in motivation, personality, and development*. Philadelphia: Psychology press.
Eigsti, I.-M., Zayas, V., Mischel, V., Shoda, Y., Ayduk, O., Dadlani, M. B., et al. (2006). Predicting cognitive control from preschool to late adolescence and young adulthood. *Psychological Science, 17*, 478–484.
Fung, H. L., Rice, C., & Carstensen, L. L. (2005). Reactive and proactive motivational changes across adulthood. In W. Greve, K. Rothermund, & D. Wentura (Eds.), *The adaptive self: Personal continuity and intentional self-development* (pp. 171–184). New York: Hogrefe/Huber Publisher.
Garcia, T., & Pintrich, P. R. (1994). Regulating motivation and cognition in the classroom: The role of self-schemas and self-regulatory strategies. In D. H. Schunk & B. J. Zimmerman (Eds.), *Self-regulation of learning and performance: Issues and educational applications* (pp. 127–153). Hillsdale, NJ: Erlbaum.
Greenglass, E. R. (2002). Proactive coping. In E. Frydenberg (Ed.), *Beyond coping: Meeting goals, vision, and challenges* (pp. 37–62). London: Oxford University Press.

Higgins, E. T. (1997). Beyond pleasure and pain. *The American Psychologist, 52*, 1280–1300.
Higgins, E. T., & Spiegel, S. (2004). Promotion and prevention strategies for self-regulation: A motivated cognition perspective. In R. F. Baumeister & K. D. Vohs (Eds.), *Handbook of self-regulation: Research, theory and applications* (pp. 171–187). New York: Guilford Press.
Lazarus, R. S., & Folkman, S. (1984). *Stress, appraisal, and coping*. New York: Springer.
Lončarić, D. (2008). Kognitivni in motivacijski dejavniki procesov samoregulacije pri ucenju in soocanju s solskim neuspehom [Cognitive and motivational factors in self-regulation of learning and coping with school failure]. Unpublished doctoral dissertation, Department of Psychology, University of Ljubljana, Slovenia.
Marton, F., & Saljo, R. (1976a). On qualitative differences in learning: I. Outcome and process. *The British Journal of Educational Psychology, 46*, 4–11.
Marton, F., & Saljo, R. (1976b). On qualitative differences in learning: II. Outcome as a function of the learner's conception of the task. *The British Journal of Educational Psychology, 46*, 115–127.
Netzel, D. M., & Eber, L. (2003). Shifting from reactive to proactive discipline in an urban school district: A change of focus through PBIS implementation. *Journal of Positive Behavior Interventions, 5*, 71–79.
Niemivirta, M. (1996). *Motivational-cognitive components in self-regulated learning*. Paper presented in 5th Workshop on Achievement and Task Motivation, 26–29 March, Landau.
Nota, L., Soresi, S., & Zimmerman, B. J. (2004). Self-regulation and academic achievement and resilience: A longitudinal study. *International Journal of Educational Research, 41*, 198–215.
Pintrich, P. R. (1988). A process-oriented view of student and motivation. In J. Stark & L. Mets (Eds.), *Improving teaching and learning through research: New Directions for institutional research* (Vol. 57, pp. 65–79). San Francisco: Jossey-Bass.
Pintrich, P. R., & De Groot, E. V. (1990). Motivational and self-regulated learning components of classroom academic performance. *Journal of Educational Psychology, 82*, 33–40.
Pintrich, P. R., & Schunk, D. H. (2002). *Motivation in education: Theory, research, and applications* (2nd ed.). Englewood Cliffs, NJ: Prentice Hall Merrill.
Pintrich, P. R., Smith, D. A. F., Garcia, T., & McKeachie, W. J. (1991). *A manual for the use of the Motivational Strategies for Learning Questionnaire (MSLQ)* (Tech. Rep. No. 91-B-004). Ann Arbor: University of Michigan, School of Education.
Skinner, E. A., Chapman, M., & Baltes, P. B. (1988). Control, means-ends, and agency beliefs: A new conceptualization and its measurement during childhood. *Journal of Personality and Social Psychology, 54*, 117–133.
Tait, H., Entwistle, N. J., & McCune, V. (1998). ASSIST: A reconceptualisation of the approaches to studying inventory. In C. Rust (Ed.), *Improving students as learners* (pp. 112–141). Oxford: Oxford Brookes University, The Oxford Centre for Staff and Learning Development.
Weinstein, C. E., Zimmerman, S. A., & Palmer, D. R. (1988). Assessing learning strategies: The design and development of the LASSI. In C. E. Weinstein, P. A. Alexander, & E. T. Goetz (Eds.), *Learning and study strategies: Issues in assessment, instruction, and evaluation* (pp. 25–40). New York: Academic.
Wild, K. P., & Schiefele, U. (1994). Lernstrategien im studium: ergebnisse zur faktorenstruktur und reliabilität eines neuen fragebogens, [Learning strategies at the university level: Testing the factor structure and reliability of a new questionnaire]. *Zeitschrift für Differentielle und Diagnostische Psychologie, 15*, 185–200.

Chapter 16
Moderator Effect of Burnout in Secondary School Context

Charles Martin-Krumm, Marie Oger, Philippe Sarrazin, and Patrick Pelayo

Burnout has been studied according to a physiological point of view (e.g., Berthoin, Pelayo, Baquet, Marais, & Robin, 1999; Pelayo, Mujika, Sidney, & Chatard, 1996). It has also been studied according to a psychological approach, and the first conceptualization has been made by Freudenberger (1974) in the workplace. He used the term *burnout* to describe the workers' incapacity to effectively carry out their roles. At the same time, Maslach (1982a, 1982b) described burnout as a gradual process of exhaustion, cynicism and reduced commitment among poverty lawyers. She has proposed burnout to have three central characteristics: emotional and physical exhaustion, the feeling of reduced sense of accomplishment and depersonalization (Raedeke, 1997).

Although many studies have examined burnout in human service, coaching settings (e.g., Kelley, Eklund, & Ritter-Taylor, 1999; Schaufeli, Maslach, & Marek, 1993), athletes (e.g., Cresswell & Eklund, 2005a, 2005b, 2005c, 2006a, 2006b, 2006c; Gustafsson Hassmén, Kenttä, & Johansson, 2008; Raedeke & Smith, 2001), competitive adolescent athletes (e.g., Gustafsson, Kenttä, Hassmén, & Lundqvist, 2007) elementary school or college teachers (e.g., Laugaa, Rascle, & Bruchon-Schweitzer, 2005; Lowenstein, 1991; Steffgen & Recchia, 2008; Unterbrink et al., 2008),

C. Martin-Krumm (✉)
CREAD EA 3875, IUFM de Bretagne, Ecole Interne UBO, Rennes, France

IFEPSA, Les Ponts de Cé, France
e-mail: charles.martin-krumm@wanadoo.fr

M. Oger • P. Pelayo
Université Lille Nord de France, Faculté des Sciences du Sport et de l'Education Physique, EA 4488, F-59000 Lille, France

P. Sarrazin
SENS, University Joseph Fourier, Grenoble 1, Grenoble, France

I. Brdar (ed.), *The Human Pursuit of Well-Being: A Cultural Approach*,
DOI 10.1007/978-94-007-1375-8_16,

university teachers (Azeem & Nazir, 2008), performance improvement at school (Walker & Stott 2000), PE teaching (Fejgin, Talmor, & Erlich, 2005; Koustelios & Tsigilis, 2005) and studies showing that it may be involved in teachers training according to the promotion of health in schools (Jourdan, Samdal, Diagne, & Carvalho, 2008); we have found only a very few studies focused on pupils (Oger, Martin-Krumm, & Sarrazin, 2006; 2007; Martin-Krumm, Oger, & Sarrazin, 2009).

These researches were focused on the validation of a questionnaire devoted to: its measurement in the secondary school context, the evolution of the burnout during a school year and the links with motivation. However, the links between the pupils' burnout and their performances at school, particularly during PE classes, have not been studied. The target of this chapter is to fill that gap. How does burnout influence performance at school during PE classes? Is there a direct link or is it possible to identify a process by which burnout has an impact on performance?

Answering these questions could lead to a better comprehension of this possible phenomenon in the domain of school, and, furthermore, it could lead to reduced occurrence of these dysfunctional schemata in case of overtiredness, which may happen in the French school context. Indeed, it is one of the most exhausting in Europe. Pupils have four to seven 50-min lessons per day, during 5–6 school days per week. The school year is organized with 5–7 weeks' periods between each holiday separated by 1–2 weeks' holiday periods. At the end of the school year, there is an 8-week holiday period in summer. Altogether, it is a 34-week school year. This organization is balanced neither for the teachers nor for the pupils, and it may generate burnout for them. It may affect their performances, especially the pupils'.

The link between burnout and performance has been established in different domains, and according to Smith (1986), its behavioral consequences involve a decreased level of efficiency and a psychological, if not physical, withdrawal from the activity. Burnout was originally conceived in human care settings to describe the inability of workers to effectively carry out their roles (Freudenberger, 1975). In this particular domain, burnout was identified as an important factor altering performance of the workers. Shutte, Toppinen, Kalimo, and Schaufeli (2000) identified its impact on performance in general work settings. In sports, athlete burnout is a concern because of its consequences include performance decrements and negative welfare outcomes (Cresswell & Eklund, 2006a). Burnout has consequences on motivation (Cresswell & Eklund, 2005a, 2005b, 2005c, 2006a). It may be involved in injury, perception of the team environment and training loads (Cresswell & Eklund, 2006b), overtraining (Lemyre, Roberts, & Stray-Gundersen, 2007; Teeple, Shalvoy, & Feller, 2006), dropout (see Cresswell & Eklund, 2006c, for a review) or anxiety (Wiggins, Crenades, Lai, Lee, & Erdmann, 2006; Wiggins, Lai, & Deiters, 2005). It may be considered as an endpoint of excessive physical training (Silva, 1990). It is possible to study the symptoms and consequences associated with its three dimensions (Goodger, Wolfenden, & Lavallee, 2007). All these variables have potential effect on performances. But, as questioned previously, will burnout affect pupils' performances during PE? Are there any effects on pupils' motivation, especially their motivation at school?

Eccles and her colleagues' model is particularly useful in predicting behavior at school (Eccles et al., 1983; Eccles & Wigfield, 2002). According to it, success expectancies and subjective task value are the two most immediate predictors of achievement behavior like task choices, persistence in an activity, strength involvement and performance (see Wigfield & Eccles, 2000, for a review). Expectancies for success are defined as individuals' beliefs about how well they will do on upcoming tasks (see Eccles & Wigfield, 2002). According to Eccles et al.'s model (1983), they are influenced by goals and more general self-schemata. In this study, we focused only on self-views in discrete and specific areas, namely the self-concept of one's ability in a subject because particular beliefs are generally better predictors of behavior than general beliefs (e.g., Pajares & Schunk, 2001). Self-concept of one's ability, or perceived ability, can be defined as an individual perception of the actual competence in a particular subject (e.g., Eccles & Wigfield, 2002). Thus, the concepts of success expectancies and perceived ability can be distinguished insofar as the latter corresponds to the ability at a given moment in a general domain (e.g., the "sport" or a particular kind of sport), whereas the formers are "projections" (thus focused on future) onto someone's capacity to succeed in a particular task or activity. Eccles and her colleagues (1983) defined task value in terms of four major components: (a) intrinsic value (enjoyment of the activity), (b) utility value (usefulness of the task in terms of current and future goals), (c) attainment value (personal importance of doing well at the task), and (d) cost (perceived negative aspects of engaging in the task). Among the different antecedents of subjective task value, Eccles et al. again underlined the importance of goals and the more general self-schemata. For example, McIver, Stipek, and Daniels (1991) showed that changes in students' (aged 12–15 years) perceived ability over one semester predicted changes in their interest for subject matter, much more than the reverse. In short, according to Eccles et al.'s model, the student who perceives high ability will develop high success expectancies and high subjective task value, which in turn will positively influence his/her grade point average. Conversely, the dynamics will be negative for a student who perceives low ability in this subject. But in every case, the perceived ability remains a direct predictor of performance. For example, Martin-Krumm, Sarrazin, and Peterson (2005) have shown a process by which a variable (i.e., explanatory style) may influence the relationship between perceived ability, success expectancies, subjective task value, and performance, but their results showed a partial mediation of success expectancies and subjective task value in the link between perceived ability and performance. The direct link between perceived ability and performance do persist.

In this study, we focused only on this direct link between perceived ability and performances. We were especially interested in the nature and the role played by the burnout in this relationship. Is a high perceived ability student expected to have only high performances or does burnout moderate the link between these two variables? We think this process may be more complex, and that perceived ability interacts with burnout to predict performances at school during PE classes as shown by the dotted arrows on Fig. 16.1, which summarizes the theoretical model of this study. If a high perceived ability is associated with a low level of burnout, the effect of

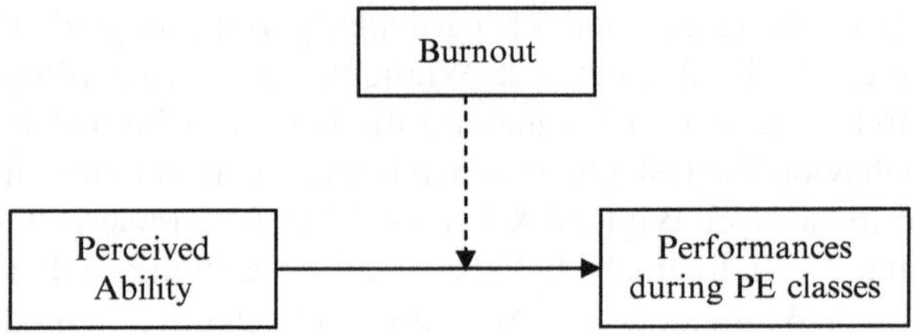

Fig. 16.1 Study conceptual model. The *arrow* expresses the direct links whereas the *dotted one* shows the moderating effects

perceived ability will be in keeping with Eccles and Wigfield models, and if it is associated with a high level of burnout, the links may be modified. Burnout may moderate the relationship between perceived ability and performance. A low perceived ability will be associated with low performances, both in case of low or high levels of burnout.

Indeed, we think that students who feel competent in PE, but who do not feel overtired, will attend to have high performances, whereas if they feel overtired, their performance will decrease. For those who feel incompetent, the burnout will confirm the relationship with performances, lower in both cases than those who feel competent. Moreover, a high perceived ability may not preserve pupils from the deleterious effects of burnout on performance.

In summary, the present research was conducted in PE classes and had one primary aim, to test the moderating effects of burnout on the relationships between students' perceived ability and their performances in PE. More precisely, we expected that burnout would interact with perceived ability to predict performances in PE in the following ways: (a) a high level of burnout inhibits the effect of a high perceived ability on performance, (b) a high level of burnout exacerbates the effects of a low perceived ability on performance, (c) a low level of burnout does not affect the Eccles and Wigfield motivation model. To resume, the aim was to test the possibility that burnout has only indirect effects on outcomes. It may be a distal variable (indirect effects) and not a proximal one (direct effects).

Method

In order to test these hypotheses, 143 college students have been followed during the first term of a school year (84 girls and 59 boys; $M = 12.6$ years, $SD = 0.86$, sixth and seventh grade). At the beginning of it, perceived ability in PE was assessed. Three months later, the participants filled questionnaires out to measure their level of burnout. Lastly, the average of the marks in PE class at the end of the first term, before the Christmas vacation, was used as an indicator of achievement during PE classes.

Measures

Burnout During PE Classes

Burnout level has been assessed with a 12-item questionnaire (EMB, Oger et al., 2006; Gautheur, Oger, Guillet, & Martin-Krumm, 2010). It is made of four items for each component of burnout, (emotional/physical exhaustion [e.g., *I feel so tired from my PE classes that I have trouble finding energy to do other things*], reduced sense of accomplishment [e.g., *I'm not achieving much during PE classes*], and devaluation [e.g., *The effort I spend during PE classes would be better spent doing other things*], ["almost never"... "almost always"]). It is a five-point scale. Internal consistency was comprised between α = .61 and .80. A global score has been computed.

Perceived Ability in PE

To assess perceived ability in PE, a three-item questionnaire similar to the one developed by Nicholls and colleagues (Nicholls, Patashnick, & Nolen, 1985) was used (e.g., "When you practice sports and you compare yourself to most friends of your age, you feel..."). The answers are indicated on a seven-point scale anchored by "very bad" (1) and "very good" (7). In previous research conducted on teenagers (Sarrazin, Roberts, Cury, Biddle, & Famose, 2002), the questionnaire has shown good construct validity, internal consistency (alpha coefficient greater than .78), test–retest stability over 10 weeks (r = .77) and predictive validity. In the present study, the internal consistency was high (α = .77); consequently, the average was computed and used in subsequent analyses.

Results

Means, standard deviations and correlations between each variable of the study are presented in Table 16.1. All the variables were significantly intercorrelated. Particularly, pupils' marks were correlated with perceived ability in PE and burnout. Perceived ability was negatively and significantly correlated with burnout (see Table 16.1).

Hierarchical regression model was used to test the moderating effects of the burnout on the links between perceived ability and performances in PE. The hierarchical regression model was constructed as follows: the burnout and perceived ability were entered at Step 1, and burnout by perceived ability interaction was entered at Step 2. Following Aiken and West (1991), all the measured predictor variables were standardized.

The overall model was significant (Table 16.2). Simple effect analyses showed a nonsignificant effect of the interaction for (a) high (β = .09) or (b) medium level of

Table 16.1 Means, standard deviation, and correlations

Variables	Burnout	Perceived ability	Marks in physical education
Burnout	–		
Perceived ability	–.55**	–	
Marks in physical education	–.30**	.35**	–
Means	1.83	4.62	14.01
SD	0.73	1.48	2.21

** $p<.01$

Table 16.2 Estimated parameters in multiple regression predicting performances in physical education

	$F_{1,139}$	β
Perceived ability	8.63	.40**
Burnout	4.40	–.59*
Perceived ability x Burnout	7.64	–.43**
$R^2 = .18$	$F_{3,139} = 10.46$***	

* $p < .05$; ** $p < .01$; ***$p < .001$

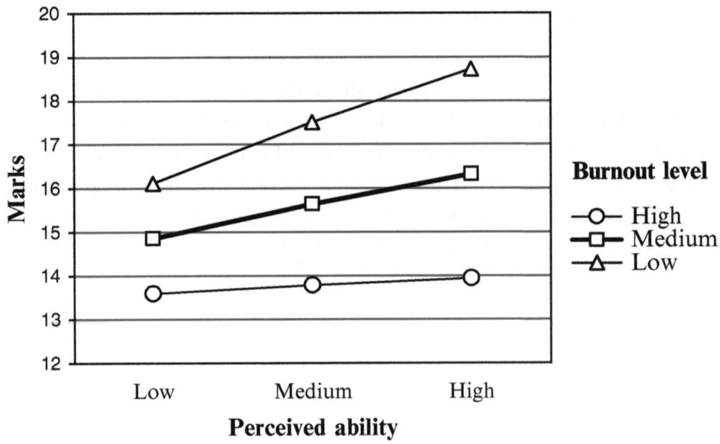

Fig. 16.2 Moderating effect of burnout on the relationships between perceived ability and marks in physical education

burnout ($\beta = .40$). On the other hand, results revealed a significant effect at a low level of burnout ($\beta = .71$, $p < .02$, Fig. 16.2). The interaction terms accounted for a small but statistically significant portion of the variance in predicting performances in PE ($\Delta R^2 = .04$, $p < .01$).

Figure 16.2 shows the slope of perceived ability at low (1 SD below the mean), at medium (the mean) and high (1 SD above the mean) levels of burnout. Perceived ability predicted performances strongly when burnout level was low, but not anymore at medium or high levels of burnout.

More specifically, a high level of burnout inhibits the positive effects of a high perceived ability on performance, whereas a low level of burnout increased its effects. In other words, in the case of a high level of burnout, the Eccles and Wigfield's model does not predict the performances anymore; high perceived ability is not associated with greater performances than low perceived ability. To complete the analyses and according to Aiken and West (1991), a *t*-test was computed to test whether the two slopes, at a high and at a low level of burnout, were significantly different or not. Results revealed significant differences [t (139) = 17.70; $p < .001$].

Discussion

This study was designed to explore whether burnout moderates the effect of perceived ability on school pupils' performances in PE classes. First, in accordance with former studies in the field of deleterious effect of burnout on performance, results showed that burnout was negatively associated with performances. Second, the results confirmed the role played by the perceived ability, according to Eccles and Wigfield's motivation model, but only in the case of a low level of burnout. Indeed, burnout interacted with perceived ability to predict subsequent performances in PE classes. More specifically, in the case of a low or medium level of burnout, the motivation model was confirmed, but in the case of a high level of burnout, it was not possible to observe the positive effect of a high level of perceived ability on performance ($\beta = .09$). A low level of perceived ability is not associated with lower performances in PE classes in the case of a high level of burnout, but neither is a high level of perceived ability. In contrast with these results, at a low level of burnout, perceived ability had a significant impact on performance in PE ($\beta = .71$). The lower the level of perceived ability is, the lower the performances are, and the higher it is, the better they are. Consequently, in concerns with performances during PE classes, it is possible to conclude that the association of high perceived ability and high-level performances, which has been ascertained in previous researches (see Eccles, Wigfield, & Schiefele, 1998; Wigfield & Eccles, 2000 for a review) is not systematic: a high burnout level may inhibit the positive effect of a high perceived ability on performances.

Although the present results provided support for the suggested model, some limitations should be acknowledged and kept in mind when interpreting findings. First of all, as with all correlational data, these results must be interpreted cautiously insofar as predictor variables (e.g., burnout) were not manipulated. Although a reciprocal causal link is not plausible given the longitudinal data (e.g., final students' marks cannot have caused perceived ability or burnout at the beginning of the school year), it is difficult to make sure that all relevant variables have been taken into account. Thus, the ascertained links between the variables can be due to other variables, which have not been measured (see Judd & McClelland, 1989). Among the omitted potential variables, it would have been interesting to have, at our disposal, an objective indicator of the students' real ability in PE and other personality variables like self-esteem, anxiety or negative affectivity. Thus, future researches should probably control such variables. Along these lines, the marks given by the teacher for the students' performances may not be the correct reflection of the students' achievement in PE. As emphasized by Jussim (1991), marks can be biased by the teacher's beliefs or his a priori opinion. In other words, the performance measure used in this study may have underestimated the model variables' effects. Future studies should have recourse to another performance indicator to reduce this possible bias. According to self-concept models (e.g., Harter, 1990; Marsh, 1990; Skaalvik, 1997), our study confirmed the links between the self-concept of one's ability and performances in specific conditions. A high level of burnout may buffer the positive effect of a high perceived ability, whereas a low level one tends to confirm the motivation model previously described; high perceived ability is linked with good performances. However, more studies are necessary to confirm this link and the interaction with burnout in connection with the other subjects at school (i.e., mathematics, foreign language) and with the general school context.

Thus, from an applied perspective, it seems important to enhance, at the same time, the self-concept of pupils' ability and to balance their work load at school to decrease the possible occurrence of burnout. Because it may be possible to identify possible early signs in the domain of sport (Cresswell & Eklund, 2004), it is likely that it is also possible in the school context. Thus, teachers should be trained both, at the same time, to prevent the occurrence of burnout and to identify its early signs.

References

Aiken, L., & West, S. (1991). *Multiple regression: Testing and interpreting interactions*. Newbury Park, CA: Sage.

Azeem, S. M., & Nazir, N. A. (2008). A study of job burnout among university teachers. *Psychology Developing Societies, 20*, 51–64.

Berthoin, S., Pelayo, P., Baquet, G., Marais, G., & Robin, H. (1999). *Variations du volume plasmatique et des concentrations de lactate lors de la récupération après des exercices maximal et supramaximal*. Communications affichées, 8ème Congrès de l'ACAPS, Macolin, 1999.

Cresswell, S. L., & Eklund, R. C. (2004). The athlete burnout syndrome: Possible early signs. *Journal of Science and Medicine in Sport, 7*(4), 481–487.

Cresswell, S. L., & Eklund, R. C. (2005a). Motivation and burnout in professionnal rugby players. *Research Quarterly for Exercise and Sport, 76*(3), 370–376.

Cresswell, S. L., & Eklund, R. C. (2005b). Motivation and burnout among top amateur rugby players. *Medicine and Science in Sport and Exercise, 37*(3), 469–477.

Cresswell, S. L., & Eklund, R. C. (2005c). Changes in athlete burnout and motivation over a 12-week league tournament. *Medicine and Science in Sport and Exercise, 37*(11), 1957–1966.

Cresswell, S. L., & Eklund, R. C. (2006a). Changes in athlete burnout over a thirty-week "rugby year". *Journal of Science and Medicine in Sport, 9*, 125–134.

Cresswell, S. L., & Eklund, R. C. (2006b). The nature of player burnout in rugby: Key characteristics and attributions. *Journal of Applied Sport Psychology, 18*, 219–239.

Cresswell, S. L., & Eklund, R. C. (2006c). Athlete burnout: Conceptual confusion, current research and future research directions. In S. Hanton & D. Mellalieu (Eds.), *Literature reviews in sport psychology* (pp. 91–126). Hauppauge, NY: Nova Science.

Eccles, J. S., & Wigfield, A. (2002). Motivational beliefs, values, and goals. *Annual Review of Psychology, 53*, 109–132.

Eccles, J. S., Adler, T. F., Futterman, R., Goff, S. B., Kaczala, C. M., Meece, J. L., et al. (1983). Expectancies, values, and academic behaviors. In T. J. Spence (Ed.), *Achievement and achievement motivation* (pp. 75–146). San Francisco, CA: W. H. Freeman.

Eccles, J. S., Wigfield, A., & Schiefele, U. (1998). Motivation to succeed. In W. Damon (Series Ed.) & N. Eisenberg (Vol. Ed.), *Handbook of child psychology* (5th ed., Vol. III, pp. 1017–1095). New York: Wiley.

Fejgin, N., Talmor, R., & Erlich, I. (2005). Inclusion and burnout in physical education. *European Physical Education Review, 11*, 29–50.

Freudenberger, H. J. (1974). Staff burnout. *Journal of Social Issues, 30*, 159–165.

Freudenberger, H. J. (1975). The staff burnout syndrome in alternative institutions. *Psychotherapy: Theory, Research and Practice, 12*, 73–82.

Gautheur, S., Oger, M., Guillet, E., & Martin-Krumm, C. (2010). Validation of a French version of the Athlete Burnout Questionnaire. *European Journal of Psychological Assessment, 26*(3), 203–211.

Goodger, K., Wolfenden, L., & Lavallee, D. (2007). Symptoms and consequences associated with three dimensions of burnout in junior tennis players. *International Journal of Sport Psychology, 38*, 342–364.

Gustafsson, H., Hassmén, P., Kenttä, G., & Johansson, M. (2008). A qualitative analysis of burnout in elite Swedish athletes. *Psychology of Sport and Exercise, 9*, 800–816.

Gustafsson, H., Kenttä, G., Hassmén, P., & Lundqvist, C. (2007). Prevalence of burnout in competitive adolescent athletes. *The Sport Psychologist, 21*, 21–37.

Harter, S. (1990). Causes, correlates and the functional role of global self-worth: A life span perspective. In J. Kolligian & R. Stenberg (Eds.), *Perceptions of competence and incompetence across the life span* (pp. 67–98). New Haven, CT: Yale University Press.

Jourdan, D., Samdal, O., Diagne, F., & Carvalho, G. S. (2008). The future of health promotion in schools goes through the strengthening of teacher training at a global level. *Promotion & Education, 15*, 36–38.

Judd, C. M., & McClelland, G. H. (1989). *Data analysis: A model-comparison approach*. Orlando, FL: Harcourt Brace Jovanovitch.

Jussim, L. (1991). Social perception and social reality: A reflection-construction model. *Psychological Review, 98*, 54–73.

Kelley, B. C., Eklund, R. C., & Ritter Taylor, M. (1999). Stress and burnout among collegiate tennis coaches. *Journal of Sport and Exercise Psychology, 21*, 113–130.

Koustelios, K., & Tsigilis, N. (2005). Teachers: A multivariate approach. The relationship between burnout and job satisfaction among physical education. *European Physical Education Review, 11*, 189–203.

Laugaa, R., Rascle, N., & Bruchon-Schweitzer, M. (2005). Construction et validation d'une échelle de stress spécifique pour les enseignants en école primaire. *Psychologie et Education, 1*, 13–32.

Lemyre, P.-N., Roberts, G. C., & Stray-Gundersen, J. (2007). Motivation, overtraining, and burnout: Can self-determinated motivation predict overtraining and burnout in elite athletes? *European Journal of Sport Science, 7*(2), 115–126.

Lowenstein, L. (1991). Teacher stress leading to burnout – Its prevention and cure. *Education Today, 41*, 12–16.

Marsh, H. W. (1990). The causal ordering of academic self-concept and academic achievement: A multiwave, longitudinal path analysis. *Journal of Educational Psychology, 82*, 646–656.

Martin-Krumm, C., Oger, M., & Sarrazin, P. (2009). College pupils' burnout in France: Links to motivation and evolution during a school year. In T. Freire (Ed.), *Understanding positive life. Research and practice on positive psychology* (pp. 251–269). Lisboa: Climepsi Editores.

Martin-Krumm, C., Sarrazin, P., & Peterson, C. (2005). The moderating effects of explanatory style in physical education performance: A prospective study. *Personality and Individual Differences, 38*, 1645–1656.

Maslach, C. (1982a). *Burnout: The cost of caring*. London: Prentice Hall.

Maslach, C. (1982b). Understanding burn-out: Definitional issues in analyzing a complex phenomenon. In W. S. Paine (Ed.), *Job stress and burnout*. Beverly Hills, CA: Sage.

McIver, D. J., Stipek, D. J., & Daniels, D. H. (1991). Explaining within-semester changes in student effort in junior high school and senior high school courses. *Journal of Educational Psychology, 83*, 201–211.

Nicholls, J. G., Patashnick, M., & Nolen, S. B. (1985). Adolescents' theories of education. *Journal of Educational Psychology, 77*, 683–692.

Oger, M., Martin-Krumm, C., & Sarrazin, P. (2006). *Burnout among French college pupils: Preliminary studies*. Abstract of the 3rd European Conference on Positive Psychology, Braga, Portugal, p. 72

Oger, M., Martin-Krumm, C., & Sarrazin, P. (2007). Le burnout en milieu scolaire: évolution et processus engagés. In Y. Dufour, *Contribution de l'E.P.S. à l'éducation au bien-être*. Collection Journées Debeyre n°2.

Pajares, J., & Schunk, D. H. (2001). Self-efficacy, self-concept, and academic achievement. In J. Aronson & D. Cordova (Eds.), *Psychology of education: Personal and interpersonal forces*. New York: Academic.

Pelayo, P., Mujika, I., Sidney, M., & Chatard, J. C. (1996). Blood lactate recovery measurements, training, and performance during a 23-week period of competitive swimming. *European Journal of Applied Physiology, 74*, 107–113.

Raedeke, T. D. (1997). Is athlete burnout more than just stress? A sport commitment perspective. *Journal of Sport and Exercise Psychology, 19*, 396–417.

Raedeke, T. D., & Smith, A. L. (2001). Development and preliminary validation of an athlete burnout measure. *Journal of Sport and Exercise Psychology, 23*, 281–306.

Sarrazin, P., Roberts, G., Cury, F., Biddle, S., & Famose, J. P. (2002). Exerted effort and performance in climbing among boys: The influence of achievement goals, perceived ability, and task difficulty. *Research Quarterly for Exercise and Sport, 73*(4), 425–436.

Schaufeli, W. B., Maslach, C., & Marek, T. (Eds.). (1993). *Professional burnout: Recent developments in theory and research*. Washington, DC: Taylor & Francis.

Schutte, N., Toppinen, S., Kalimo, R., & Schaufeli, W. (2000). The factorial validity of the Maslach Burnout Inventory-General Survey (MBI-GS) across occupational groups and nations. *Journal of Occupational and Organizational Psychology, 73*, 53–65.

Silva, J. M. (1990). An analysis of the training stress syndrome in competitive athletics. *Applied Sport Psychology, 2*, 5–20.

Skaalvik, E. (1997). Issues in research on self-concept. In M. Maehr & P. Pintrich (Eds.), *Advances in motivation and achievement* (Vol. 10, pp. 51–97). London: JAI Press.

Smith, R. E. (1986). Toward a cognitive-affective model of athletic burnout. *Journal of Sport Psychology, 8*, 36–50.

Steffgen, G., & Recchia, S. (2008). Les problèmes psychosociaux, un défi en promotion de la santé. *Promotion & Education, 15*, 60–63.

Teeple, E., Shalvoy, R. M., & Feller, E. R. (2006). Overtraining in young athletes. *Medicine and Health, 89*(7), 236–238.

Unterbrink, T., Zimmermann, L., Pfeifer, R., Wirsching, M., Brähler, E., & Bauer, J. (2008). Parameters infuencing health variables in a sample of 949 German teachers. *International Archive of Occupational and Environmental Health, 82*, 117–123.

Walker, A., & Stott, K. (2000). Performance improvement in schools: A case of overdose? *Educational Management Administration Leadership, 28*, 63–76.

Wigfield, A., & Eccles, J. S. (2000). Expectancy-value theory of achievement motivation. *Contemporary Educational Psychology, 25*, 68–81.

Wiggins, M. S., Crenades, J. G., Lai, C., Lee, J., & Erdmann, J. B. (2006). Multidimensional comparison of anxiety direction and burnout over time. *Perceptual and Motor Skills, 102*(3), 788–790.

Wiggins, M. S., Lai, C., & Deiters, J. A. (2005). Anxiety and burnout in female collegiate ice hockey and soccer athletes. *Perceptual and Motor Skills, 101*(2), 519–524.

Part V
Measurement

Chapter 17
Factor Structure of the French Ryff's Psychological Well-Being Scales for Active Older Adults

Mareï Salama-Younes, Amany Ismaïl, Ali Montazeri, and Charles Roncin

People have always been interested in answering the question: What is a good life? Frequently, good life is directly connected to well-being and happiness. Research into the good life has been encouraged by the seminal work of Ryff (1989a, 1989b). She, on the basis of an extensive literature review, developed an integrated theoretical framework of well-being. She found that the most important perspectives of well-being were life span theories (Erikson, 1959), clinical theories on personal growth (Allport, 1961; Maslow, 1968; Rogers, 1961) and the criteria of positive mental health formulated by Jahoda (1958). In addition, she incorporated insights from her own research on development during the course of life (Ryff & Keyes, 1995) and on an elaborated overview of philosophical attempts to define the good life (Becker, 1992). She argued that all these perspectives contain similar and complementing criteria of positive psychological functioning. An important similarity is that the criteria are all formulated in terms of well-being instead of illness. In fact, this perspective has generated a new model of health based in the conception of health as "not only the absence of illness but the presence of something positive" (Ryff & Singer, 1998; WHO, 1948).

In her model, Ryff distinguished six core dimensions and also developed an instrument that is now widely used by researchers interested in well-being. The theoretically derived dimensions of positive psychological health include self-acceptance, positive relations with others, autonomy, environmental mastery, purpose in life and personal growth (Ryff, 1989a). Recently, this model has been criticized. Using data

M. Salama-Younes (✉)
Psychology Department, European University of Brittany, Rennes, France

Sport Psychology Department, Helwan University, Helwan, Egypt
e-mail: marei.salama@uhb.fr; msalamayounes@hotmail.com

A. Ismaïl • C. Roncin
Laboratory of Sociology and Anthropology, Department of Sociology, Rennes II University, Rennes, France

A. Montazeri
Iranian Institute for Health Sciences Research, ACECR, Tehran, Iran

I. Brdar (ed.), *The Human Pursuit of Well-Being: A Cultural Approach*,
DOI 10.1007/978-94-007-1375-8_17,

from three major surveys, Springer and Hauser (2006) raised serious doubts on the validity of the six-factor model. Their results showed that four of the six dimensions (i.e., personal growth, purpose in life, self-acceptance and environmental mastery) empirically might be one dimension only.

This article builds on the recent discussion in the literature (Ryff & Singer, 2006; Springer & Hauser, 2006; Springer, Hauser & Freese, 2006; Van Dierendonck, 2004) on the measurement of well-being with the Ryff's scales of psychological well-being. The discussion raised the need for further testing of the six-dimensional nature of the model. A recent study by Abbott et al. (2006) added to this discussion by testing an additional second order dimension underlying the four above-mentioned dimensions (inspired by the model suggested by Springer & Hauser, 2006). It should be noted, however, that Abbott et al. (2006) kept the six original well-being dimensions intact. They argued that given the problems with the psychometric quality of this measure, more research is certainly needed to help researchers interested in using the Ryff's six-factor model and instrument with additional information to make an informed decision on what to use in future research.

A limitation of all the above-mentioned studies and accompanying analysis is that, in all instances, different versions of the Ryff's measurement instrument were used and these have been criticized for their lack of factorial validity or internal consistency. It is very well possible that part of the overlap between the four dimensions is due to problems with the factorial validity of the original measure. In a previous construct of validity of the instrument, an alternative short version was suggested that combines reasonable factorial validity with good internal consistency (see Van Dierendonck, 2004, for a review). More specifically, in the short version that came out of the latter study, several of the items, whose content overlapped dimensions, were eliminated. Other studies also emphasized the necessity to remove items with too much content overlap between dimensions (Abbott et al., 2006; Cheng & Chan, 2005). Another limitation refers to the ordinal nature of the Ryff's measure. Springer & Hauser (2006) argued that all studies applying this measure analyzed it using continuous factor statistical procedures that produce biased estimates and inaccurate results if the variables are ordinal or non-normal. Therefore, to accurately analyze the measure, researchers need to take that into consideration.

In the present article, we used the French version of the Ryff's instrument (Labelle et al., 2001). This study aimed to (1) have a consistent version of the instrument and (2) test the factorial structure of the Ryff's psychological well-being scales using the consistent well-being version.

Method

Participants and Procedure

The sample consisted of a group of French adults. In all, 427 individuals, age ranging from 55 to 74 years ($M = 61.85$, $SD = 7.11$), participated in the study. They were 297 females (69%) and 130 males (31%). This entire sample was regularly practicing physical activities (e.g., walking, swimming, cycling, running). They filled in the questionnaire just after they finished their sport training in groups. The investigation was presented as a research on quality of life and health perception for physically active adults. Participation was voluntary and anonymous, and no incentives were offered to participants.

Measure

The Ryff's psychological well-being scales. The Ryff inventory consists of either 84 questions (long form) or 54 questions (medium form). There is also a short form, but it is statistically unreliable and, therefore, should not be used for assessment. Both the long and medium forms consist of a series of statements reflecting the six areas of psychological well-being: autonomy, environmental mastery, personal growth, positive relations with others, purpose in life and self-acceptance. Respondents rate statements on a scale of 1–6, with 1 indicating strong disagreement and 6 indicating strong agreement (Ryff & Keyes, 1995; Ryff & Singer, 2006). In this study, we used the medium form consisting of six dimensions of 14 items each. A six-point response category was used for all scales, ranging from 1 (*strongly disagree*) to 6 (*strongly agree*).

Results

Exploratory Factor Analysis

The factorial structure of the Ryff's psychological well-being scales was firstly tested by explanatory factor analysis. Using principal axis factoring as an extraction method and promax with Kaiser Normalization as a rotation method, only five, not six, factors have been well loaded in pattern matrix. Items composing the purpose of life loaded in more than one factor (two, three, or four factors), or they are saturated a low of .30. For example, items 29, 35 and 77 loaded in three different factors. However, item 11 and 23 saturated at .18 and .21. The analysis indicated that the five-factor model jointly accounted for 47.32% of the variance, and only 20 items have been conserved with at least .30 (see Table 17.1). The subscale length of this shortened version varied between three items (environmental mastery and personal growth), four items (positive relation with others) and five items (autonomy and self-acceptance). The eigenvalues were 2.75, 2.23, 2.20, 1.63 and 1.34, respectively.

Internal Consistency

Cronbach's alpha coefficient has then been calculated. The five factors have an acceptable consistency. The Cronbach's alpha coefficients of the five well-being

Table 17.1 Exploratory factor analyses of the Ryff's psychological well-being (shortened version)

Item	Autonomy	Environmental mastery	Personal growth	Positive relations	Self-acceptance
1	.77				
7	.83				
43	.86				
49	.74				
73	.32				
2		.58			
14		.61			
44		.69			
3			.69		
45			.94		
57			.57		
4				.54	
10				.40	
32				.76	
38				.62	
12					.78
18					.58
24					.59
30					.54
54					.54
% of var.	12.85	8.02	6.18	5.85	14.42
Cronbach's α	.84	.74	.86	.88	.72

Only loadings >.30 are presented

dimensions were as follows: autonomy .84, self-acceptance .74, positive relations with others .86, environmental mastery .88 and personal growth .72.

Confirmatory Factor Analysis

We performed confirmatory factor analyses (CFA) to assess the Ryff's psychological well-being scales structure. The intention was to indicate which model better fits the data. There are varying suggestions in the literature about the number, type and cut-off values for goodness-of-fit required to be reported for CFA (Byrne, 1998). A popular recommendation is to present three of four indices from different areas. Accordingly, we report several goodness-of-fit indicators including: goodness of fit index (GFI), adjusted goodness of fit index (AGFI), root mean square error of approximation (RMSEA) and relative chi-square (χ^2/df). The GFI and AGFI are chi-square- based calculations independent of degrees of freedom. The recommended cut-off values for acceptable values are ≥.90. The RMSEA tests the fit of the model to the covariance matrix. As a guideline, values of <.05 indicate a close fit and values below .11 are an acceptable fit. The value of 2 alone may be used as an index, but 2 divided by the degrees of freedom (2/*df*) reduces its sensitivity to sample size (cut-off values: <2–5). It should be noted that, in this evolving area of research, there is not a definitive set of criteria to define the best-fitting model (French & Tait, 2004; Hu & Bentler, 1999).

Using the consistent and shortened version, confirmatory factor analysis by Lisrel 8.50 also has been performed (Jöreskog & Sörbom, 1996). The items were indicated as categorical variables following the recommendations of Springer & Hauser (2006). They argued that due to the specific nature of the Ryff' variables, the items should be treated as ordinal and not as continuous variables for a more accurate estimation of the models. Estimation was done using the weighted least squares mean and variance (WLSMV)-adjusted procedure. This provides for asymptotically unbiased, consistent and efficient parameter estimates and correct goodness of fit indices for variables that have a non-normal distribution. The following factor analytic models were specified: (1) one-factor model, which assumes that all items load on a general composite well-being factor, (2) two-factor model, in which all negatively formulated items load on one factor and all positively formulated items load on a second factor, (3) a three-factor model, in which self-acceptance, environmental mastery and purpose in life load on one factor, autonomy on the second factor and personal relations with others on the third factor, (4) the original six-factor structure as described by Ryff (with exception of purpose in life).

In the present study, the single factor model was used as the starting point and provided a poor fit for the data as shown by the fit indices. The indices were: GFI= .69, AGFI = .61, the RMSEA = .16 and the χ^2/df= 12.45. (Table 17.2). The CFA indicated that a 20-item uni-dimensional model was not well fitted in the data. Results indicated that either two-dimensional or three-dimensional model did not fit the data well (see Table 17.2). However, CAF indicated that a five-dimensional model well fitted the data. We found the following figures: GFI = .92, AGFI = .90, RMSEA = .06 and the χ^2/df=4.31. The analysis showed a well-fitting model with our data only for five factors.

Table 17.2 Confirmatory factor analyses, scales of psychological well-being (shortened version)

Models	χ^2	*df*	GFI/AGFI	RMESA	χ^2/df
One factor	2119.28	170	.69/.61	.16	12.45
Two factors[a]	1662.84	167	.77/.72	.14	9.93
Three factors[b]	791.43	130	.88/.84	.11	6.08
Five factors[c]	473.96	110	.92/.90	.06	4.31**

GFI goodness of fit index, *AGFI* adjusted goodness of fit index, *RMSEA* root mean square error of approximation

$**p<.01$

[a]Positive and negative items with correlated factors

[b](1) autonomy, (2) positive relationships (3) self-acceptance, personal growth and environmental mastery

[c]The goodness-of-fit of the consistence five factors model as loaded using the explanatory factor analysis

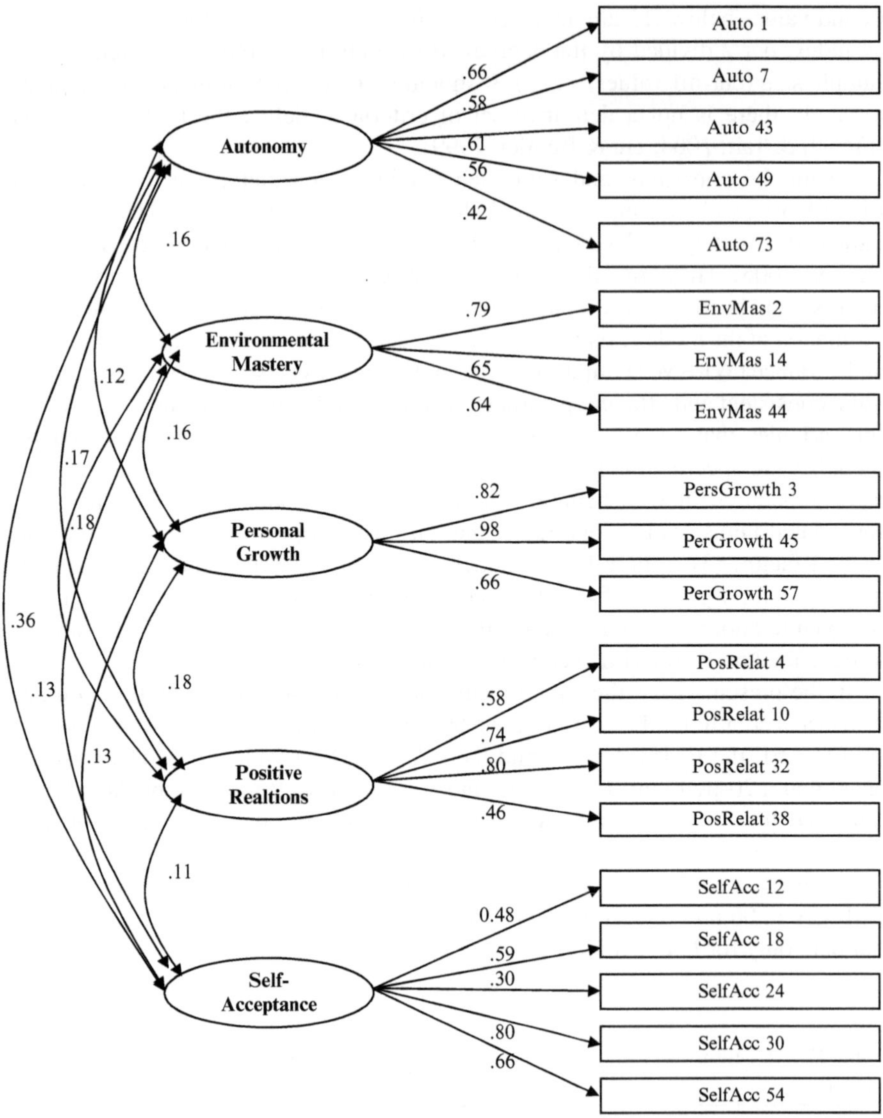

Fig. 17.1 Confirmatory factor analysis for the five factor model

Figure 17.1 shows that the best-fitting model was the five-factor model with a single first order factor. This confirms the Ryff's underlying model for the Spanish language sample using a shortened version. Therefore, her results suggest one well-being dimension underlying all six dimensions, not underlying only four out the six dimensions, as was previously suggested by Abbott et al. (2006). Van Dierendonck (2004), for Spanish population, indicated that the factor loading of one item of the personal growth scale

("I don't want to try new ways of doing things, my life is fine the way it is") was not significant. After removing that item from the model, the resulting fit became even better with relative fit indices of .84 for comparative fit index (CFI) .94 for Tucker-Lewis index (TLI) and .06 for the root mean square residual (RSMR). These scores were very good, given the previously noted problems with the factorial validity of this measure. Threshold values were reached for the RSMR and almost reached for the TLI. Last author indicated also that the exception is purpose in life that showed very high inter-correlations with self-acceptance and with environmental mastery. Noteworthy, however, is the relative lower correlations for personal growth with the other three scales (self-acceptance, purpose in life and environmental mastery) that Springer and Hauser (2006) proposed to collapse as one, which could explain why in this Spanish language sample, the six-factor model had the best fit indices. In our study, the purpose of life has low consistence and has not even been loaded as an independent factor. This might be due to culture differences or population age (older adults).

Discussion

The factor structure and internal consistency of Ryff's SPWB have been studied with different ages and countries. Clark, Marshall, Ryff, and Wheaton (2001) tested from one-factor to six-factor models with Canadian older adults. They found a low internal consistency and reliability for all models. Kafka and Kozma (2002) showed that unrestricted model extracted 15 factors; a model restricted to six-factor did not correspond to a priori Ryff dimensions. Results failed to support the hypothesis that performing factor analytic procedures on the items of the SPWB should produce a six-factor solution. They tested a range of models with Chinese sample (including one factor, six factors with second order). Six-factor a priori model with correlated negative method factor, correlated errors for adjacent questions and three error correlations had lowest BIC (Springer & Hauser, 2006). However, with Dutch sample, a priori six-factor with second order returned lower AIC than other models (e.g., 1 F, two-factor negative and positive, five-factor and six-factor) but CFI was unacceptably low: .65 (84 item), .73 (54 item), .88 (18 item). Factorial validity was only acceptable for the 18-item version, but internal consistency was below acceptable limits for the 84-, 54- and 18-item versions. (Van Dierendonck, 2004). Last author confirmed that the internal consistencies of these 3-item scales were unacceptably low, suggesting that these scales should not be used. The selection of items on the basis of theoretical arguments is, of course, legitimate. However, for the SPWB, the internal consistency of the resulting scales is so low that its use in correlational research is questionable. A low reliability will lead to an underestimation of the correlation between constructs (Hunter & Schmidt, 1990). In Van Dierendock's publication, alternative short scales are, therefore, suggested that showed good internal consistency and reasonable factorial fit indices. In the present study, we also tried to have short scales having good internal consistency and acceptable fit indices for the French active older adults.

This article described preliminary tests of the internal consistency and factorial structure of the Ryff's six-factor model for eudaimonic well-being in a French language sample. A recently published handbook on positive psychological assessment (Lopez & Snyder, 2003) emphasized the importance of valid and reliable instruments for this research field. With the growing interest for studying well-being in cross-cultural settings (Salama-Younes & Delle Fave, in press), it is vital to collect more information on the validity of the Ryff's measure in different countries and, especially, in different languages. A strong element of this instrument is the theoretical base that underlies its development. The results allow for the following conclusions.

The factorial validity of the shortened French version developed from the Ryff's SPWB was better than the longer version preliminarily used for older adult samples. The reliability in terms of internal consistency was good. This confirms the previous findings that this version is a good compromise between the importance of factorial validity and good reliability, something that were missing in the original versions of the SPWB (see, van Dierendonck, 2004). The last author mentioned that one personal growth item was removed due to a nonsignificant factor loading. In our study, purpose of life had a very low coefficient for the item 14 (.13). Using exploratory factor analysis, this factor has not been loaded. Therefore, since this factor, in terms of Cronbach's alpha coefficient, also showed very low coefficient (.38), we recommend that for French older adults, it is better that we use only five- and not six-factor model.

Although different shortened versions were used, other studies in countries with languages different from English also pointed toward a confirmation of the Ryff's model, e.g., Chinese (Cheng & Chan, 2005) and Swedish (Lindfors, Berntsson, & Lundberg, 2006). We found no confirmation for Springer and Hauser's (2006) position that there may be not six, but only three dimensions, while following their recommendations for statistical analyses. Furthermore, the results did not replicate Abbott et al.'s (2006) suggestion of a second order factor underlying only four of the six dimensions. Our results caution researchers regarding lumping dimensions within this model together because there is a risk of losing valuable information when deleting the purpose in life factor from the original measure.

There are some limitations of this study that need to be highlighted. The first limitation pertains to the fact that the measuring instruments used in the study were developed neither for non-French populations nor for older physically active. Although an attempt was made to analyze the characteristics of the scale through the use of factor analyses, one cannot be certain about the validity of the scale. Secondly, the SPWB were a self-report measure, and, thus, it provides no potential for assessing whether respondents were faking good or faking bad or neither. It also relied on their self-knowledge and subjective experience of situations, and this may impact the accuracy of the results. Thirdly, the measuring instruments were administrated to about 20 physically active older adult populations. These groups were different in their educational and socio-demographical levels and age. This might result in more frequently practicing leisure activities in older adults, such as social, spiritual or cultural activities. In this study, we did not study any socio-demographic factors that probably could affect the perception of well-being. Nevertheless, the most important contribution of our study is that the model was tested in older adults, in a non-Anglo-Saxon culture. Also, we used a shortened version of the Ryff's scales, in which some items with too much overlap between dimensions removed. Of course, factor analysis is only the first step in validating an instrument. As a next step, we suggest to examine the extent to which five dimensions differently predict different behaviors.

In conclusion, when using the Ryff's SPWB for French older adults, it is recommended to keep the five dimensions intact so that insight into the full breath of the well-being construct can be gained.

Acknowledgment The first author thanks Prof. Dirk, van Dierendonck, RSM Erasmus University, Netherlands, for his permanent help, Prof. Sylvie Lapierre for her permission to use the French version established for Canadian adults and Charles Roncin for his cooperation in the early version.

References

Abbott, R. A., Ploubidis, G. B., Huppert, F. A., Kuh, D., Wadsworth, M. E. J., & Croudace, T. J. (2006). Psychometric evaluation and predictive validity of Ryff's psychological well-being items in a UK cohort sample of women. *Health and Quality of Life Outcomes, 76*.

Allport, G. W. (1961). *Pattern and growth in personality*. New York: Holt, Rinehart & Winstom.

Becker, L. C. (1992). Good lives: Prolegomena. *Social Philosophy and Policy, 9*, 15–37.

Byrne, B. M. (1998). *Structural equation modelling*. Mahwah, NJ: Lawrence Erlbaum Associates Publishers.

Cheng, S.-T., & Chan, A. C. M. (2005). Measuring psychological well-being in the Chinese. *Personality and Individual Differences, 38*, 1307–1316.

Clark, P., Marshall, V., Ryff, C., & Wheaton, B. (2001). Measuring psychological well-being in the Canadian study of health and aging. *International Psychogeriatrics, 13*, 79–90.

Erikson, E. (1959). Identity and the life cycle. *Psychological Issues, 1*, 18–164.

French, D. J., & Tait, R. J. (2004). Measurement invariance in the General Health Questionnaire-12 in young Australian adolescents. *European Child & Adolescents Psychiatry, 13*, 1–7.

Hu, L., & Bentler, P. M. (1999). Cutoff criteria for fit indexes in covariance structure analysis: Conventional criteria versus new alternatives. *Structural Equation Modeling, 6*(1), 1–55.

Hunter, J. E., & Schmidt, H. L. (1990). *Methods of meta-analysis: Correcting for sources of error and bias in research findings*. Newbury Park, CA: Sage.

Jahoda, M. (1958). *Current concepts of positive mental health*. New York: Basic Books.

Jöreskog, K. G., & Sörbom, D. (1996). *LISREL 8: Structural equation modeling with the SIMPLIS command language*. Chicago: Scientific Software International.

Kafka, G. J., & Kozma, A. (2002). The construct validity of Ryff's scales of psychological well-being (SPWB) and their relationship to measures of subjective well-being. *Social Indicators Research, 57*, 171–190.

Labelle, R., Alain, M., Bastin, É., Bouffard, L., Dubé, M., & Lapierre, S. (2001). Bien-être et détresse psychologique: vers un modèle hiérarchique cognitivo-affectif [Welfare and psychological distress: Towards a hierarchical cognitive-affective model]. *Québécoise de Psychologie, 22*(1), 71–87.

Lindfors, P., Berntsson, L., & Lundberg, U. (2006). Factor structure of Ryff's psychological well-being scales in Swedish female and male white-collar workers. *Personality and Individual Differences, 40*, 1213–1222.

Lopez, S. J., & Snyder, C. R. (2003). *Positive psychological assessment: A handbook of models and measures*. Washington, DC: American Psychological Association.
Maslow, A. (1968). *Toward a psychology of being* (2nd ed.). New York: Van Nostrand.
Rogers, C. R. (1961). *On becoming a person*. Boston: Houghton Mifflin.
Ryff, C. D. (1989a). Beyond Ponce de Leon and life satisfaction: New directions in quest of successful aging. *International Journal of Behavioral Development, 12*, 35–55.
Ryff, C. D. (1989b). Happiness is everything, or is it? Explorations on the meaning of psychological well-being. *Journal of Personality and Social Psychology, 57*, 1069–1081.
Ryff, C. D., & Keyes, C. L. M. (1995). The structure of psychological well-being revisited. *Journal of Personality and Social Psychology, 69*, 719–727.
Ryff, C. D., & Singer, B. H. (1998). The contours of positive human health. *Psychological Inquiry, 9*, 1–28.
Ryff, C. D., & Singer, B. H. (2006). Best news yet on the six-factor model of well-being. *Social Science Research, 35*, 1103–1119.
Salama-Younes, M., & Delle Fave, A. (in press). *Positive psychology for all: Introduction, concepts and applications in school age*.
Springer, K. W., & Hauser, R. M. (2006). An assessment of the construct validity of Ryff's scales of psychological well-being: Method, mode, and measurement effects. *Social Science Research, 35*, 1080–1102.
Springer, K. W., Hauser, R. M., & Freese, J. (2006). Bad news indeed for Ryff's six-factor model of well-being. *Social Science Research, 35*, 1120–1131.
Van Dierendonck, D. (2004). The construct validity of Ryff's scales of psychological well-being and its extension with spiritual well-being. *Personality and Individual Differences, 36*, 629–643.
World Health Organization (1948). *Preamble to the Constitution of the World Health Organization*. Adopted by the International Health Conference, New York, 19–22 June, 1946; signed on 22 July 1946 by the representatives of 61 States (Official records of the World Health Organization, no. 2, p. 100) and entered into force on 7 April 1948.

Chapter 18
Further Evaluation of the Test-Retest Reliability of the Children Hope Scale and Students' Life Satisfaction Scale

Susana C. Marques, José Pais-Ribeiro, and Shane J. Lopez

Psychologists have placed an increased emphasis on the study and identification of psychological variables that promote a positive human development. Hope and satisfaction with life are two of the most well-established indicators associated with general wellness and, additionally, positive functioning. These variables are linked with a variety of adaptive outcomes and viewed as potential contributors to the development of other positive behaviors and attitudes.

Snyder and colleagues have developed a detailed theory and definition of hope as goal-directed thinking in which the person has the perceived capacity to find routes to goals (pathways thinking) and the motivation to use those routes (agency thinking). Snyder's theory incorporates three distinct components of hope – goals, pathways and agency. Goals, whether short-term or long-term, provide the targets of mental action sequences and vary in the degree to which they are specified, but all goals must be of sufficient value to warrant sustained conscious thought about them (Snyder, 2002). Pathways represent a person's perceived ability to generate workable routes to desired goals (Snyder, Rand, & Sigmon, 2002) and the production of several pathways is important when encountering impediments. It is illustrated by internal speech, such as "I'll find a way to get this done!" Agency thinking is the motivational component in hope theory that reflects a person's cognitions about his or her ability to begin and sustain goal-directed behavior (Snyder, Lopez, Shorey, Rand, & Feldman, 2003). Mobilizing agency thoughts is a prerequisite to motivate the movement along pathways to desired goals. These self-referential thoughts can be seen in internal speech, such as "I can do this" and "I am not going to be stopped" (Snyder, LaPointe, Crowen, & Early, 1998). Agency and pathways components of

S.C. Marques (✉) • J. Pais-Ribeiro
Faculty of Psychology and Educational Sciences, University of Porto, Porto, Portugal
e-mail: dscmarques@mail.telepac.pt

S.J. Lopez
The Clifton Strengths School and Gallup, Omaha, USA

I. Brdar (ed.), *The Human Pursuit of Well-Being: A Cultural Approach*,
DOI 10.1007/978-94-007-1375-8_18,

hope are reciprocal, additive, or both, necessary for hopeful thinking and positively related; however, they are not synonymous (Snyder et al., 1991). Hope reflects relative enduring, cross-situational subjective appraisals of goal-related capabilities (Snyder, 2000).

Hope has been found to play a significant role in a large number of successful goal pursuits (e.g., academics, athletics, psychological adjustment, health, coping) (see Snyder, 2002, for a summary review). For example, scores on the CHS are significantly correlated with global life satisfaction, extraversion, perceived social support (Valle, Huebner, & Suldo, 2004), personal adjustment (Gilman, Dooley, & Florell, 2006), psychological well-being (Snyder, Feldman, Taylor, Schroeder, & Adams, 2000), greater parental support (Hodgkins, 2001), secure attachments (Shorey, Snyder, Yang, & Lewin, 2003), greater satisfaction with interpersonal relationships (Snyder, 2002) and self-worth and perceived physical competence (Snyder, Hoza et al., 1997). Studies consistently revealed that the CHS provides predictive power with regard to academic achievement (Gilman et al., 2006; Snyder et al., 1997) and recent research has shown that hope reports of adolescents moderate the relationship between their global life satisfaction and their later internalizing behaviors (Valle, Huebner, & Suldo, 2006), providing preliminary evidence that hope reflects a psychological strength that can buffer against the effects of acute negative life events.

Global life satisfaction has been defined as individuals' cognitive evaluations of the positivity of their lives as a whole, based on their own standards (Shin & Johnson, 1978). Life satisfaction is the subjective evaluation of the quality of a person's life that can include global life satisfaction judgments or specific domains of life, as it underlies an overall or a multidimensional evaluation, respectively. Child and adolescent life satisfaction reports demonstrate moderate levels of stability, reflecting somewhat enduring trait-like components, but also sensitivity to changing life circumstances (Huebner, 2004; Suldo & Huebner, 2004a).

Life satisfaction has been linked with several adaptive outcomes and receives special interest related to their importance of building on human positive development, both as a by-product of various life events and as an important determinant of many life outcomes, such as successful interpersonal, intrapersonal, educational and health outcomes (Huebner, 2004; Suldo, Riley, & Shaffer, 2006). Life satisfaction has been studied first and extensively in adults (Diener, Suh, Lucas, & Smith, 1999) and more recently and lesser extensively in children and adolescents (Huebner, 1997; Huebner, Suldo, Smith, & McKnight, 2004; Suldo & Huebner, 2004b). Specifically, children and adolescents with high levels of life satisfaction have, in general, extraverted temperament, internal locus of control, active coping, positive self-concept and purpose in life and participation in meaningful, prosocial activities. On the other hand, low levels of life satisfaction have been linked with negative outcomes, such as aggressive behavior (Valois, Zullig, Huebner, & Drane, 2001), chemical abuse (Zullig, Valois, Huebner, Oeltmann, & Drane 2001), neuroticism (Fogle, Huebner, & Laughlin, 2002), depression, anxiety, social stress (Huebner, Funk, & Gilman, 2000), stressful life events, and externalizing and internalizing behavior (McKnight, Huebner, & Suldo, 2002). Recent research has shown that life satisfaction reports of adolescents moderate the relationship between their experiences of stressful life events and their later externalizing behavior (Suldo & Huebner 2004a). Finally, other studies have revealed that global life satisfaction mediates the impact of stressful life events (McKnight et al., 2002) and parenting behavior (Suldo & Huebner, 2004b).

The special attention to hope and satisfaction with life constructs is in line with the importance of promoting positive youth development; they are associated with a large number of adaptive outcomes and viewed as potential contributors to the development of other positive behaviors and attitudes. Moreover, hope and satisfaction with life in children and youth act as true strength, mitigating against the development of psychopathological behavior in the face of adverse life circumstances (Suldo & Huebner, 2004b; Valle et al., 2006). In this later regard, having as foundation the characteristics and potentialities of hope and satisfaction with life, we consider, is relevant to evaluate the stability of these variables across time. The goal of the present study is to examine and report the students' hope and satisfaction with life scores over a 6 months and 1 year period.

Method

Participants

At Time 1 (Fall 2006), the scales were administered to a sample of 367 sixth and eighth grade students with a mean age of 11.78 years, range 10–15 years and 53.1% female. This sample is similar to the sample in the original scale development study (Snyder et al., 1991). Participants were from seven schools in the north of Portugal.

At Time 2 (Spring 2007) and Time 3 (Fall 2007), participation was sought from all original participants. A total of 62 students at Time 2 (mean age 10.95 years, range 10–12 years and 73.5% female) and 215 students at Time 3 (mean age 12.57 years, range 11–16 years and 53% female) were retested on the CHS and SLSS.

Instruments

Children's hope scale (*CHS*). The CHS is a dispositional scale developed by Snyder, Hoza et al. (1997) to measure goal-related hopeful thinking in children and adolescents aged 8–16. The measure contains six items (each item is presented as an affirmation) responded to on a six-point scale ranging from 1=*none of the time* to 6=*all of the time*. This self-report measure contains three questions to evaluate pathways thinking and three questions to examine agency thinking. The pathways and agency items are alternated within the scale. Possible scores range from 6 to 36, with higher scores denoting higher levels of hope. Previous studies with CHS revealed adequate psychometric properties, including internal consistencies ranging between .72 and .86 for the total score (see Snyder et al., 2003 for a review). The CHS has been validated for Portuguese children (Marques, Pais-Ribeiro, & Lopez, 2009a) with a Cronbach's alpha coefficient of 0.81 for the total score.

Students' life satisfaction scale (*SLSS*). The SLSS is a self-report measure to evaluate the satisfaction with life as a whole in individuals ranging in age from 8to18 years. Respondents are asked to answer the questions based on the thoughts that they had in the last few weeks. For each of the seven items of the scale, presented as an affirmation, there are six response choices ranging from 1 = *strongly disagree* to 6 = *strongly agree*. Items are summed to produce a global index of life satisfaction. The scale scores range from 7 to 42, with higher scores denoting higher levels of global satisfaction with life. The internal consistency of the SLSS has been reported as .82 (Huebner, 1991) and .86 in a subsequent exploratory study (Dew & Huebner, 1994). The SLSS has been validated for Portuguese children (Marques, Pais-Ribeiro, & Lopez 2007) and reported a Cronbach's alpha coefficient of .89.

Procedure

Approval to collect data was secured through the administrator from each school. A letter describing the study and requesting permission for student participation was sent home to parents of potential participants. Approximately 31% of the students returned the signed parental permission forms. The motives and potential difference in these motives of the 31% of the parents who enrolled their children in the study and those that declined are unknown. However, this rate is comparable to that reported in similar studies (Valle et al., 2004, 2006). Students then were asked to assent to the research process. Each student who obtained parental consent and gave assent to participate in the study was administered each of the measures described above in groups of 15–30 students. The size of the group was dependent upon the space available within each school, as well as the amount of adult assistance present to promote the full understanding of instructions and the confidential completion of all measures. The measures completed by all participants were presented in a counter-balanced order. The students were first asked to complete the demographic survey and then the psychological scales. They were then thanked for their participation and dismissed. Research assistants were available during all administration sessions to answer questions and ensure confidentiality. At Time 2 and Time 3, student assent was re-obtained from all participants and survey administration procedures were the same as described at Time 1.

Results

Table 18.1 presents the means, standard deviations and internal consistency coefficients of all variables assessed at Time 1, 6 months later at Time 2 and 1 year later at Time 3.

Table 18.1 Descriptive statistics and internal consistency estimates for hope and life satisfaction at Time 1, Time 2, and Time 3

	Time 1			Time 2			Time 3		
Variable	*M*	SD	α	*M*	SD	α	*M*	SD	α
Hope	24.10	5.01	.81	23.79	4.62	.76	25.41	5.12	.79
Life satisfaction	29.32	6.69	.89	30.16	5.85	.81	29.48	6.86	.86

Table 18.2 Intercorrelations between hope and satisfaction with life at Time 1 and Time 2

	Variable	1	2	3
Time 1	1. Hope	–		
N=367	2. Life satisfaction	.63**	–	
Time 2	3. Hope	.60**	.42**	–
N=62	4. Life satisfaction	.49**	.69**	.61**

** $p<.01$

Table 18.3 Intercorrelations between hope and satisfaction with life at Time 1 and Time 3

	Variable	1	2	3
Time 1	1. T1 Hope	–		
N=367	2. T1 Life satisfaction	.63**	–	
Time 3	3. T3 Hope	.51**	.41**	–
N=215	4. T3 Life satisfaction	.43**	.56**	.53**

** $p<.01$

Means and standard deviations for CHS scores at Times 1, 2 and 3 of the current study were lower than the samples reported in studies with the English language version ($M=25.41$–28.86; SD from 3.01 to 6.11; Snyder, Cheavens et al., 1997; Snyder, Hoza et al., 1997; Valle et al., 2006). Related to satisfaction with life, means and standard deviations for SLSS, scores of the current study are similar to the scores reported in studies with the English language version (Gilman & Huebner, 1997; Huebner, 1991; Huebner, Suldo, & Valois, 2003; Valle et al., 2006). The internal consistency of each scale, represented by Cronbach's alpha coefficient, is adequate and comparable to Cronbach's alpha coeffients ranged from .72 to .86 for the English language version of CHS (Snyder, Hoza et al., 1997) and .80 for the English language version of SLSS (Dew & Huebner, 1994).

Tables 18.2 and 18.3 presents the intercorrelations among the variables at each time point, as well as correlations between hope and life satisfaction at Time 1 and Time 2 and Time 1 and Time 3.

Relationships between CHS and SLSS scores and demographic variables (gender, age) were considered. Correlations with age ($r=.02$; $r=-.002$) were non-significant for CHS and SLSS, respectively. Gender was unrelated to CHS and SLSS scores; there were no significant differences between males and females on the CHS, $t\,(367)=.70$, $p>.05$ and on the SLSS, $t\,(367)=.84$, $p>.05$.

All correlations between hope and life satisfaction were significant at the .01 level. Correlations between the variables are consistent with other studies using the English language versions (Huebner et al., 2003).

The test-retest reliability coefficient is .60 and .51 for the CHS and .69 and .56 for the SLSS, after 6 months and 1 year, respectively.

The studies examining test-retest reliability with the English language version found scores of .73 (Snyder, Hoza et al., 1997) and .76 (Terry & Huebner, 1995) for 1–2 weeks' test-retest correlation; .71 (Snyder, Hoza et al., 1997) and .64 (Gilman & Huebner, 1997) for 1 month; and .47 and .61 (Valle et al., 2006) for 1 year for CHS and SLSS, respectively.

Discussion

This study represents one of the first efforts to examine the test-retest reliability of the Portuguese versions of the CHS and the SLSS. Students' CHS and SLSS scores showed moderate test-retest reliability over a 6-month and 1-year period. This finding implies that, similar to the case for adults (Diener et al., 1999; Snyder et al., 1991), hope and satisfaction with life represent a moderately stable characteristic of children and adolescents, including some trait-like properties. Taken together with previous studies of shorter time frames, the data provides some support for the theoretical premise. However, the moderate magnitude of the coefficients also suggests that hope and satisfaction with life reports are sensitive to changing life circumstances.

Further, the moderate test-retest reliability of the Portuguese versions of the CHS and SLSS are consistent with the results from the English language version (Gilman & Huebner, 1997; Huebner, Funk, & Gilman, 2000; Snyder, Cheavens et al., 1997; Snyder, Hoza et al., 1997; Terry & Huebner, 1995; Valle et al., 2006); both versions demonstrate that hope and satisfaction with life reflect relative enduring variables across time.

The longitudinal design of this study, in which hope and satisfaction with life scores were reassessed after a 6 month and 1-year period, goes beyond previous studies that have assessed test-retest reliability after a 1-, 2-week or 1-month interval (e.g., Gilman & Huebner, 1997; Snyder, Hoza et al., 1997) and introduce a reliability indicator to the validation studies of the Portuguese versions of the CHS (Marques et al., 2009a) and SLSS (Marques et al., 2007).

We suggest continuity of work with different time intervals and transition times of human development to increase our understanding regarding the properties, strengths and vulnerabilities of hope and satisfaction with life.

As the positive psychology initiative continues, studies are needed in different countries to explore the influence of cultural and societal factors on positive constructs and positive functioning. Currently, Portuguese research regarding hope and life satisfaction in middle schoolers is limited. Finally, the present study should be analyzed in the elaboration and implementation of interventions oriented to the promotion of hope and satisfaction with life in middle school children. Future studies are underway to examine the effectiveness of a hope-based intervention with regard to hope, life satisfaction, self-worth, mental health and academic achievement

(Marques, Lopez, & Pais-Ribeiro, 2009b) and to examine the role of positive psychology constructs in predicting mental health and academic achievement in Portuguese students (Marques, Pais-Ribeiro, & Lopez, 2011).

Acknowledgments This research was funded via a Foundation for the Science and Technology (FCT) grant obtained by the first author.

References

Dew, T., & Huebner, E. S. (1994). Adolescents' perceived quality of life: An exploratory investigation. *Journal of School Psychology, 33*, 185–199.

Diener, E., Suh, E. M., Lucas, R. E., & Smith, H. L. (1999). Subjective well-being: Three decades of progress. *Psychological Bulletin, 125*(2), 276–302.

Fogle, L. M., Huebner, E. S., & Laughlin, J. E. (2002). The relationship between temperament and life satisfaction in adolescence: Cognitive and behavioural mediation models. *Journal of Happiness Studies, 3*, 373–392.

Gilman, R., Dooley, J., & Florell, D. (2006). Relative levels of hope and their relationship with academic and psychological indicators among adolescents. *Journal of Social and Clinical Psychology, 25*, 166–178.

Gilman, R., & Huebner, E. S. (1997). Children's reports of their life satisfaction. *School Psychology International, 18*, 229–243.

Hodgkins, N. M. (2001). The relationship of parental acceptance/rejection to hope and shame in adolescents. *Dissertation-Abstracts-International: Section B: The Sciences-and-Engineering, 62*, 550.

Huebner, E. S. (1991). Initial development of the student' life satisfaction scale. *School Psychology International, 12*, 231–240.

Huebner, E. S. (1997). Happiness and life satisfaction. In G. Bear, K. Minke, & A. Thomas (Eds.), *Children's needs II* (pp. 271–278). Bethesda, MD: National Association of School Psychologists.

Huebner, E. S. (2004). Research on assessment of life satisfaction of children and adolescents. *Social Indicators Research, 66*, 3–33.

Huebner, E. S., Funk, B. A., & Gilman, R. (2000). Cross-sectional and longitudinal psychosocial correlates of adolescent life satisfaction reports. *Canadian Journal of School Psychology, 16*, 53–64.

Huebner, E. S., Suldo, S. M., Smith, L. C., & McKnight, C. G. (2004). Life satisfaction in children and youth: Empirical foundations and implications for school psychologists. *Psychology in the Schools, 41*, 81–93.

Huebner, E. S., Suldo, S. M., & Valois, R. F. (2003). *Psychometric properties of two brief measures of children's life satisfaction: The students' life satisfaction scale and the brief multidimensional students' life satisfaction scale*. Paper presented at the Indicators of Positive Development Conference, Washington, DC

Marques, S. C., Lopez, S. J., & Pais-Ribeiro, J. L. (2009). Building hope for the future – A program to foster strengths in middle-school students. *Journal of Happiness Studies*. doi: 10.1007/s10902-009-9180-3.

Marques, S. C., Pais-Ribeiro, J. L., & Lopez, S. J. (2007). Validation of a Portuguese version of the students' life satisfaction scale. *Applied Research in Quality of Life, 2*, 83–94.

Marques, S. C., Pais-Ribeiro, J. L., & Lopez, S. J. (2009). Validation of a Portuguese version of the children hope scale. *School Psychology International, 30*, 538–551.

Marques, S. C., Pais-Ribeiro, J. L., & Lopez, S. J. (2011). The role of positive psychology constructs in predicting mental health and academic achievement in children and adolescents: A two-year longitudinal study. *Journal of Happiness Studies*. doi: 10.1007/s10902-010-9244-4.

McKnight, C. G., Huebner, E. S., & Suldo, S. M. (2002). Relationships among stressful life events, temperament, problem behavior, and global life satisfaction in adolescents. *Psychology in the Schools, 39*, 677–687.

Shin, D. C., & Johnson, D. M. (1978). Avowed happiness as an overall assessment of the quality of life. *Social Indicators Research, 5*, 475–492.

Shorey, H. S., Snyder, C. R., Yang, X., & Lewin, M. R. (2003). The role of hope as a mediator in recollected parenting, adult attachment, and mental health. *Journal of Social and Clinical Psychology, 22*, 685–715.

Snyder, C. R. (2000). The past and the future of hope. *Journal of Social and Clinical Psychology, 19*, 11–28.

Snyder, C. R. (2002). Hope theory: Rainbows in the mind. *Psychological Inquiry, 13*, 249–275.

Snyder, C. R., Cheavens, J., & Sympson, S. C. (1997). Hope: An individual motive for social commerce. *Group Dynamics: Theory, Research, and Practice, 1*, 107–118.

Snyder, C. R., Feldman, D. B., Taylor, J. D., Schroeder, L. L., & Adams III, V. (2000). The roles of hopeful thinking in preventing problems and enhancing strengths. *Applied and Preventive Psychology, 15*, 262–295.

Snyder, C. R., Harris, C., Anderson, J. R., Holleran, S. A., Irving, L. M., Sigmon, S. T., et al. (1991). The will and the ways: Development and validation of an individual-differences measure of hope. *Journal of Personality and Social Psychology, 60*, 570–585.

Snyder, C. R., Hoza, B., Pelham, W. E., Rapoff, M., Ware, L., Danovsky, M., et al. (1997). The development and validation of the children's hope scale. *Journal of Pediatric Psychology, 22*, 399–421.

Snyder, C. R., LaPointe, A. B., Crowson, J. J., Jr., & Early, S. (1998). Preferences of high- and low-hope people for self-referential input. *Cognition and Emotion, 12*, 807–823.

Snyder, C. R., Lopez, S. J., Shorey, H. S., Rand, K. L., & Feldman, D. B. (2003). Hope theory, measurements, and applications to school psychology. *School Psychology Quarterly, 18*, 122–139.

Snyder, C. R., Rand, K. L., & Sigmon, D. R. (2002). Hope theory: A member of the positive psychology family. In C. R. Snyder & S. J. Lopez (Eds.), *Handbook of positive psychology* (pp. 257–266). New York: Oxford University Press.

Suldo, S. M., & Huebner, E. S. (2004a). Does life satisfaction moderate effects of stressful life events on psychopathological behaviour during adolescence? *School Psychology Quarterly, 19*, 93–105.

Suldo, S. M., & Huebner, E. S. (2004b). The role of life satisfaction in the relationship between authoritative parenting dimension and adolescent problem behavior. *Social Indicators Research, 66*, 165–195.

Suldo, S. M., Riley, K. N., & Shaffer, E. J. (2006). Academic correlates of children and adolescents' life satisfaction. *School Psychology International, 27*, 567–582.

Terry, T., & Huebner, E. S. (1995). The relationship between self-concept and life satisfaction in children. *Social Indicators Research, 35*, 39–52.

Valle, M. F., Huebner, E. S., & Suldo, S. M. (2004). Further evaluation of the children's hope scale. *Journal of Psychoeducational Assessment, 22*, 320–337.

Valle, M. F., Huebner, E. S., & Suldo, S. M. (2006). An analysis of hope as a psychological strength. *Journal of School Psychology, 44*, 393–406.

Valois, R. E., Zullig, K. J., Huebner, E. S., & Drane, J. W. (2001). Relationship between life satisfaction and violent behaviours among adolescents. *American Journal of Health Behavior, 25*, 353–366.

Zullig, K. J., Valois, R. F., Huebner, E. S., Oeltmann, J. E., & Drane, W. J. (2001). Relationship between perceived life satisfaction and adolescent substance abuse. *The Journal of Adolescent Health, 29*, 279–288.

Chapter 19
Validation of the Mental Health Continuum Short Form and Subjective Vitality Scale with Egyptian Adolescent Athletes

Mareï Salama-Younes

The multidimensional model of positive mental health proposed by Keyes and his colleagues (Keyes, 2003, 2007; Keyes, Shmotkin, & Ryff, 2002; Keyes & Waterman, 2003) includes both emotional and functional well-being as important domains of mental health. These two domains reflect concepts identified by many writers (e.g., Ryan & Deci, 2001; Waterman, 1990). More specifically, emotional well-being reflects the Greek concept of *hedonic* well-being (i.e., happiness or pleasure in life). It is comprised of avowed quality of life (i.e., happiness and satisfaction with life) and positive affect, which parallel Diener's construction of subjective well-being (Diener, Lucas, & Oishi, 2002). Functional well-being reflects the Greek concept of eudaimonic well-being, i.e., feelings experienced when engaging in behaviors aimed at reaching one's potential (Ryff, 1989).

Three scales served as indicators of positive mental health (Keyes, 1998, 2007): the summed scale of emotional well-being (EWB) (i.e., single item of happiness, single item of life satisfaction and single item of positive affect), the summed scale of psychological well-being (PWB) (i.e., single item of the six subscales added together) and the summed scale of social well-being (SWB) (i.e., single item of the five subscales added together). Thus, Keyes' model of mental health consists of three broad domains: EWB, PWB and SWB, which can be further subdivided into 14 specific dimensions. Each measure of subjective well-being is considered a symptom or characteristic of mental health insofar as it represents an outward sign of an otherwise unobservable state of mental health. Using these multiple dimensions of mental health, Keyes (2002, 2003, 2005a, 2007) conceptualized a mental health continuum that included three levels: flourishing, moderately mentally healthy and languishing. This continuum can be measured either categorically through a diagnosis or continuously as a summary measure (Keyes, 2005a, 2007).

M. Salama-Younes (✉)
Sport Psychology Department, Helwan University, Helwan, Egypt

Psychology Department, European University of Brittany, Rennes, France
e-mail: marei.salama@uhb.fr; msalamayounes@hotmail.com

I. Brdar (ed.), *The Human Pursuit of Well-Being: A Cultural Approach*,
DOI 10.1007/978-94-007-1375-8_19, © Springer Science+Business Media B.V. 2011

According to the 1996 US Surgeon Generals' Report on Physical Activity and Health, physically active people tend to have better mental health when compared to inactive people (Benedetti, Borges, & Petroski, 2008). Mental health benefits have been observed with minimal levels of physical activity (Hamer, Stamatakis, & Steptoe, 2008). Thus, compared to general or inactive samples, it may be expected that a sample of physically active individuals would tend to score toward the flourishing end of the mental health continuum as measured by the MHC-SF. While there are ample indicators that physical activity can have both a preventative and curative role in various forms of mental ill-health (Landers & Arent, 2007; Faulkner & Taylor, 2005), research on the relationship between flourishing and physical activity is still very limited. In a recent study, Salama-Younes, Montazeri, Ismaïl, and Roncin (2009) focused on a related concept, subjective vitality, and found a positive relationship with physical activity.

As a subjective feeling, vitality has been variously defined as a sense of feeling really alive, invigorated or full of energy and enthusiasm for life. Subjective vitality scale, when used as a trait measure, has been correlated with both physical and mental health variables (Ryan & Bernstein, 2004). Kasser and Ryan (1999) and Ryan and Frederick (1997) mentioned that these results are available in college age, adult and elderly populations.

In this paper, we present the results of two studies using the MHC-SF with Egyptian adolescents. We had three aims for these two studies. First, in the absence of specific diagnostic tests such as the MHC-SF for Egyptian youth, we wanted to test the factor structure and internal consistency of the Arabic version of MHC-SF for adolescents, using exploratory and confirmatory factor analyses. Second, using MCA[1], we aimed to test if this sample could be divided along Keyes' three classifications – flourishing, moderately mentally healthy and languishing – and what the percentage of these three categories might be for adolescents. Finally, we wanted to explore the relationship between mental health, as reflected in the total score of the MHC-SF, and subjective vitality.

Study 1: Method

Participants and Procedure

Data were collected from January to March 2007. Participants were Egyptian adolescents, aged from 12 to 18 years ($M = 14.8$; SD = 3.6). The sample consisted of 339 adolescents from Cairo, 123 girls and 216 boys. The athletes represented both team

[1] Multiple correspondence analyses (MCA) is a statistical technique used to highlight correspondences between variables describing a population. The aim of MCA is, on one hand, to study the links between several variables defined on a given population, and, on the other hand, to study the structure induced by this set of variables on the population (Escofier, 2003).

and individual sports (e.g., handball, football, judo, swimming and cycling), and participated regularly, usually at least three times per week, for a total of 6–8 h each week. Most competed in national level competitions. The athletes completed the MHC-SF in groups, immediately after a training session.

Measure

The Mental Health Continuum-Short Form (MHC–SF, Keyes, 2005b) consists of 14 items. It measures the degree of (1) EWB (items 1–3) as defined in terms of positive affect/satisfaction with life; (2) SWB (items 4–8) as described in Keyes' (1998) model of SWB (one item on each of the facets of social acceptance, social actualization, social contribution, social coherence and social integration); (3) PWB (items 9–14) as described in Ryff's (1989) model (including one item on each of the dimensions of autonomy, environmental mastery, personal growth, positive relations with others, purpose in life and self-acceptance). The MHC–SF has been used in the child development supplement in 2002 (Keyes, 2006), where it had been completed by a random sample of youth between the ages of 12 and 18 years. Adolescents confirmed the three factor structure of subjective well-being (Keyes, 2005b). Confirmatory factor analysis (CFA) results have supported the structure of the MHC-SF in both adults and adolescents (Keyes, 2005b; Keyes et al., 2008; Keyes & Waterman, 2003; Robitschek & Keyes, 2009).

The response option for the short form was changed to measure the frequency with which respondents experienced each symptom of positive mental health and, thereby, provided a clear standard for the assessment and a categorization of levels of positive mental health that was similar to the standard used to assess and diagnose a major depressive episode (see Keyes, 2002, 2005a, 2007). Each item ranged from 1 (never) to 6 (everyday). Using forward and reverse translation by four bilingual individuals, an experimental Arabic version equivalent to the original MHC-SF was created. Two independent psychological professionals translated the items and two others translated the response categories and a provisional version was provided. Subsequently, it was back translated into English, and following a careful cultural adaptation, the final version was provided, pilot tested and used in this study. There were no major changes to the original instrument. Egyptian adolescents have replied the translated 14 items in Arabic language.

Results

Exploratory factor analyses, using principal axis factoring with promax rotation (with Kaiser Normalization), revealed that the three factors have eigenvalue greater than 1 as proposed by Keyes' model (Keyes, 2005a). The three-factor structure jointly accounted for 41.60% of the variance. However, only 9 out of the 14 items

Table 19.1 Exploratory factor analysis for the Arabic version of MHC-SF (14 items)

Items	Factor 1	Factor 2	Factor 3
1	.88		
2	.63		
3	.42		
4		.48	
5		.40	
6		(.09)	
7		.59	
8		(.18)	
9			(.13)
10			(.18)
11			.79
12			.61
13			.47
14			(.22)
Eigen value	2.59	2.64	2.29
% of variance	22.09	10.88	8.63

Only items loaded greater than .40 are reported

Table 19.2 Goodness-of-fit of three confirmatory factor analysis models

Latent Model	χ^2	*df*	GFI/AGFI	CN	RMSEA	NFI /IFI	χ^2/df
Single factor	126.74	27	.91/.86	132.41	.11	.73/.79	4.68*
Two factors[a]	71.09	26	.92/.88	224.13	.09	.84/.86	2.74*
Three factors	41.06	24	.97/.95	336.40	.04	.91/.96	1.71*

GFI goodness of fit index, *AGFI* adjusted goodness of fit index, *CN* critical N, *RMSEA* root mean square error of approximation

*$p<.001$

[a] Measure of emotional well–being load on one factor, and measure of psychological and social well–being load on the second factor

proposed in the model were correctly saturated (.40). The items that loaded on the three distinct factors (emotional, social and psychological) were 1, 2, 3, 4, 5, 7, 11, 12, and 13, respectively (see Table 19.1).

CFA was computed to ascertain the factor structure of this version. Results confirmed the factor structure as proposed by Keyes (2002, 2005a)—namely, EWB, SWB, and PWB (see Table 19.2 and Fig. 19.1). This was ascertained on the basis of a comparison with both a single and a two-factor model. The latter two models indicated poor fit in general, yielding a root mean square error of approximation (RMSEA) equal or above the threshold of .10 suggested by MacCullum, Brown, and Sugarawa (1996). The RMSEA measure of fit indicated a good fit of the three-factor model as suggested by the criteria.

The popularity of this particular measure of fit is partly based on the fact that it does not require comparison with a null model and, thus, does not require one to

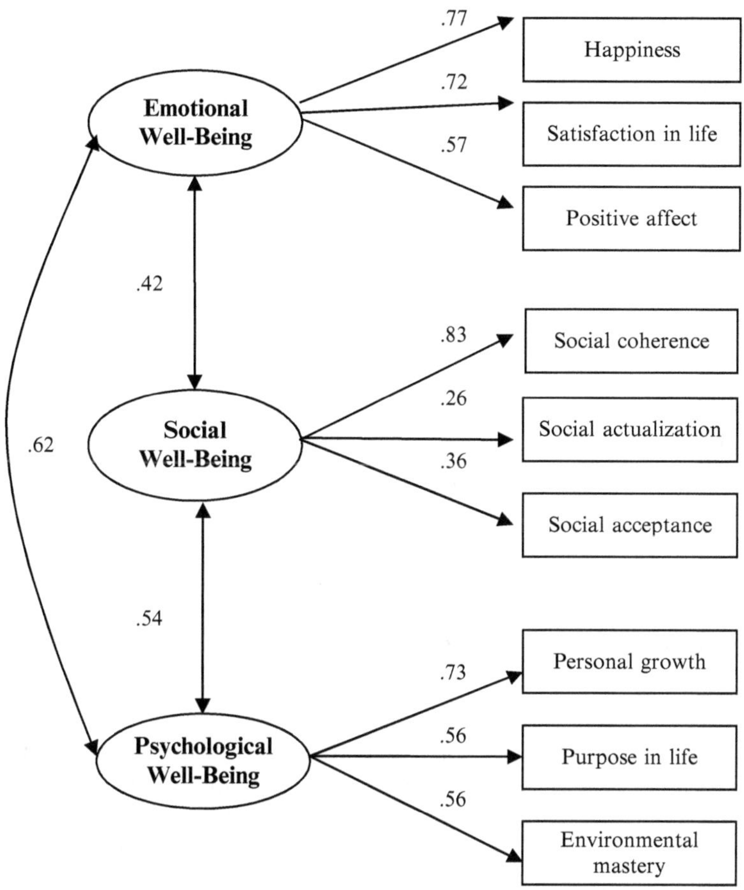

Fig. 19.1 CAF of Keyes' three factor model of mental health, reporting standardized parameters for the nine items

posit, as plausible, a model in which there is complete independence of the latent variables (Arbuckle, 2005). The goodness of fit index (GFI) for the three-factor model also indicated good fit. The GFI varied between 0 and 1 and the closer to 1 it is, the better the fit (Hu & Bentler, 1999). To further attest the good fit of the data, Hoelter's Critical N for the three-factor model was almost twice the recommended cut-off point of 200 (Hoelter, 1983). The chi-square statistics of both the single and two-factor models were significantly higher than the one yielded from the fit of the three-factor model. Thus, the three-factor model is the best-fitting model to these data; its descriptive fit indices suggest it is an excellent fit to the data.

Table 19.3 summarizes the descriptive statistics of each item and the total MHC-SF scale and its three subscales. Table 19.3 shows that the total MHC-SF scale yielded a correctly internal consistency (.72). Nunnally and Bernstein (1994) suggested that Cronbach's alpha coefficient should normally be not less than .70.

Table 19.3 Descriptive statistics of the Arabic MHC-SF subscales and total MHC–SF

			Correlations			
Mental health dimensions	Mean	SD	1	2	3	4
1. Emotional well–being	4.48	1.38	–	.11	.39*	.77*
2. Social well–being	4.67	1.25		–	.09	.21*
3. Psychological well–being	4.61	1.21			–	.75*
4. Total MHC–SF	4.62	1.22				–
Cronbach alpha			.74	.49	.66	.72

* $p < .01$

The EWB subscale had the next highest measure of internal consistency (.74) followed by the PWB subscale (.66), which fell just below the recommended .70. The SWB scale had relatively low internal consistency (.49), although the inclusion of these items in the total MHC-SF scale did not lower its internal consistency. The internal consistency result obtained with Arabic people is similar to that obtained with Setswana speaking South Africans (Keyes et al., 2008).

Assessment of the Mental Health Continuum

The categorical diagnosis using the MHC–SF by Keyes (2006) was applied to the data to obtain estimates of the population prevalence of the mental health categories. To be flourishing, individuals must report that they experience "everyday" or "almost everyday" at least seven of the symptoms, where one of the symptoms is from the hedonic (i.e., EWB) cluster (i.e., happy, interested in life or satisfied). To be languishing, individuals must report that they "never" or "once or twice" experienced at least seven of the symptoms, where one of the symptoms is from the hedonic cluster. Individuals who do not fit the criteria for flourishing or languishing are categorized as moderately mentally healthy.

In order to map both variables and individuals for constructing a complex visual map whose structuring can be interpreted, we used the MCA. The analysis showed the same categories for the Egyptian adolescents (see Table 19.4) as have been found with younger adults in America (Keyes, 2005b). In this study, 23.48% of the participants reported that they experienced "everyday" or "almost everyday" items 3, 4, 5, 10 and 11, which qualified them as flourishing. The second category, languishing, applied to 11.56% of sample who reported that they "never" or "once" experienced the symptoms in items 3, 4, 10, 11 and 12. Finally, the third category is the moderately mentally healthy. People are diagnosed as moderately mentally healthy if their scores are not extreme enough to be diagnosed as either flourishing or languishing. In this study, it was represented by 64.96% of the participants. They reported experiencing the symptoms cited in items 3, 4, 5, 11 and 12 two or three times in a week. In sum, these results support the categorical diagnosis used by Keyes (2006, 2007, 2009).

Table 19.4 Characteristics of the most significant items for the three classes (categories)

Category	Variable	Characteristic modality	% of modality in category	% of modality in sample	% of category in modality
Category 1	Q4	5	37.31	30.68	96.15
23.48%	Q4	6	44.03	37.17	93.65
	Q3	5	36.94	31.27	93.40
	Q1	5	46.27	40.41	90.51
	Q10	5	34.70	29.50	93.00
	Q5	5	28.36	24.48	91.57
	Q11	5	25.75	22.12	92.00
Category 2	Q5	2	56.82	12.09	60.98
64.96%	Q4	3	29.55	4.13	92.86
	Q3	2	38.64	8.85	56.67
	Q11	2	27.27	5.31	66.67
	Q13	3	22.73	4.72	62.50
	Q4	2	29.55	7.96	48.15
	Q12	2	27.27	7.37	48.00
	Q7	2	31.82	10.03	4.25
Category 3	Q2	1	77.78	7.67	80.77
11.56%	Q3	1	77.78	8.55	72.41
	Q1	1	62.96	5.90	85.00
	Q10	1	70.37	9.44	59.38
	Q4	1	70.37	10.03	55.88
	Q11	1	55.56	6.78	65.22
	Q12	1	66.67	14.45	80.77
	Q13	1	77.78	7.67	72.41

Each scale ranged from 1–6. Characteristic modality = score of variable in each category from 1–6. Category 1 is the flourishing people; category 2 is the moderately health and category 3 is languishing people. Characteristic of modality means the score of item from 1–6; % of modality in category and in sample

Discussion

The mental health continuum long form (MHC-LF; Keyes, 2002) represents a clinical approach to the continuous assessment and categorical diagnosis of states of positive mental health. MHC–SF asks individuals how much of the time they functioned in a specific manner: from "none of the time" to "all of the time." This response format was modeled after the approach used in the Composite International Diagnostic Interview, which operationalizes the Diagnostic and Statistical Manual of mental disorder criteria (e.g., for major depressive episode). We believe the results from this paper are encouraging in terms of the potential applicability of the MHC-SF to various cultures. Although that only nine items have been correctly loaded from the explanatory factor analysis, the Arabic short form well replicated the three-factor structure found in the South African (Keyes, et al., 2008) and USA (Keyes, 2005a, 2005b, 2007) studies, and the overall of the Arabic MHC–SF scale had acceptable internal consistency (i.e., above .70). On the other hand, the internal consistency of the PWB subscale and, especially, the SWB subscale were low (i.e., below .70). While inclusion of the PWB and SWB items into the overall scale did not reduce the MHC-SF's internal consistency, future research will need to focus on improving the item content for these respective subscales, at least in terms of physically active adults.

Although the same three categories were found, our results are slightly similar to those of South African and US adult samples, with 23.48% of our sample identified as flourishing. For example, the South African results revealed that 20% of the sample was flourishing, 12.2% were languishing and 67.8% were moderately mentally healthy (Keyes, 2006, 2007; Keyes et al., 2008). The US results revealed that 18% were flourishing, about 17% were languishing and 65% were moderately mentally healthy (Keyes, 2005a). This difference was probably due to the age of the sample or the physical activities in which they engaged. Sample of this study was regularly participated in group physical activities. They responded to the Arabic version of the MHC-SF just after their favorite activity, and they were in a good humor. The mean of age of Egyptian participants was lower than the South African and US samples. The differences between samples could also be due to culture, physical activity levels or age. Now that the psychometrics of the Arabic version of the MHC-SC have been established, future research can begin to investigate these previously confounded variables.

Study 2: Method

Participants and Procedure

Data were collected from July to August 2007. Participants were Egyptian adolescents aged from 12 to 18 years ($M=15.2$; SD$=3.00$). The sample consisted of 127 adolescents from Sadat City,[2] 53 girls and 74 boys. All participants had not participated in Study 1. The athletes represented team sports (i.e., handball, volleyball, and football). Sample completed the MHC-SF in groups, immediately after a training session.

Measures

The Arabic version of the MHC–SF is described in Study 1.

The subjective vitality scale (SVS) is a short instrument that was developed by Ryan and Frederick to measure vitality (Ryan & Frederick, 1997). The original version had seven items derived from an original pool of 19 items. The scale has two

[2]It is about 78 km north of Cairo.

versions: an individual difference level version and the state level version. We used in this study the state level version. Egyptian adolescents have replied the individual difference level version (seven items) translated and adapted in Arabic language by Salama-Younes (2009). The same "forward-backward" procedure as described above was employed to translate the questionnaire from English into Arabic. In general, there were no major changes to the original instrument.

Results

The correlation between the MHC-SF and the SVS scores was investigated and a significant positive correlation emerged (r=.54, p<.01) indicating that those who were more mentally healthy showed higher levels of subjective vitality (Table 19.5). In this study, to test the reliability, the internal consistency of the questionnaire was measured using Cronbach's alpha coefficient and was found to be .83, well above a satisfactory value.

Discussion

There were few studies which have been published to explore the relationships between subjective well-being or positive mental health and subjective vitality. Ryan and Frederick (1997) concluded that subjective vitality is a function of a number of conditions regarding personal agency and growth. As they summarize, it was shown that subjective vitality is, in varied samples, associated with self-actualization, self-determination, mental health, and self-esteem. Conversely, indexes of intrapsychic distress were associated with less vitality. Also, participants reported greater vitality when they felt more self-motivated, and less vitality when they perceived themselves as controlled by external forces, as revealed by measures of treatment motivation in two settings. Ryan and Frederick concluded that vitality has been shown to be strongly associated with a variety of physical and mental health measures (Kasser & Ryan, 1999; Ryan & Frederick, 1997).

Table 19.5 Correlations between the Arabic MHC-SF and subjective vitality

	2	3	4	5
1. Emotional well-being	.14	.16	.62*	.38*
2. Social well-being	–	.15	.72*	.48*
3. Psychological well-being		–	.62*	.19*
4. Total MHC-SF			–	.54*
5. Subjective vitality				–

* p<.05; Each scale ranged from 1–6

Ryan and Frederick (1997) showed that subjective vitality is hypothesized to reflect organismic well-being and thus should co-vary with both psychological and somatic factors that impact the energy available to the self. Associations are shown between subjective vitality and several indexes of PWB, somatic factors such as physical symptoms and perceived body functioning and basic personality traits and affective dispositions. Subsequently, vitality is shown to be lower in people with chronic pain compared to matched controls, especially those who perceive their pain to be disabling or frightening. Subjective vitality is further associated with self-motivation and maintained weight loss among patients treated for obesity. Finally, subjective vitality is assessed in a diary study for its covariation with physical symptoms. Discussion focuses on the phenomenological salience of personal energy and its relations to physical well-being and PWB. In our study, the overall of both of MHC-SF and subjective vitality is positively and significantly correlated. These results are in keeping with those reported by Ryan and Frederick.

General Discussion

MHC-SF is derived from MHC-LF, which consisted of seven items measuring EWB, six 3-item scales (18 items in total) that measured the six dimensions of Ryff's (1989) model of PWB and five 3-item scales (15 items in total) that measure the five dimensions of Keyes' (1998) model of SWB. The measure of EWB in the MHC-LF included six items measuring the frequency of positive affect that was derived, in part, from Bradburn's (1969) affect balance scale and a single item of the quality of life overall based on Cantril's (1967) self-anchoring items. The estimates of internal consistency reliability for each of the three sets of measures—EWB, PWB, and SWB—in the MHC short and long forms have all been high (>.80; see e.g., Keyes, 2005a). The MHC-LF measures of SWB and PWB have been validated (see Keyes, 1998; Ryff, 1989; Ryff & Keyes, 1995) and used in hundreds of studies over the past two decades, and their use as a measure of overall positive mental health was first introduced by Keyes (2002) and recently summarized in Keyes (2007).

While the MHC-LF consisted of 40 items, the MHC-SF consists of 14 items that were chosen as the most prototypical items representing the construct definition for each facet of well-being. Three items (happy, interested in life, and satisfied) were chosen to represent EWB, six items (one item from each of the six dimensions) were chosen to represent PWB and five items (one item from each of the five dimensions) were chosen to represent SWB. The response option for the short form was changed to measure the frequency with which respondents experienced each symptom of positive mental health and, thereby, provided a clear standard for the assessment and a categorization of levels of positive mental health that was similar to the standard used to assess and diagnose major depressive episodes (see Keyes, 2002, 2005a, 2007). To be diagnosed with flourishing mental health, individuals must experience "everyday" or "almost everyday" at least one of the three signs of hedonic well-being and at least six of the eleven signs of positive functioning during the past

2 weeks. Individuals who exhibit low levels (i.e., "never" or "once or twice" during the past 2 weeks) on at least one measure of hedonic well-being and low levels on at least six measures of positive functioning are diagnosed with languishing mental health. Individuals who are neither flourishing nor languishing are diagnosed with moderate mental health.

Keyes (2009) is encouraging in terms of the potential applicability of the MHC–SF in various cultures. Among the black Setswana-speaking population in South Africa, MHC-SF replicated the three-factor structure found in the US studies, the overall MHC-SF scale had acceptable internal consistency (i.e., above .70), and the subscales and overall score of the MHC-SF showed good construct validity with existing measures of subjective well-being. On the other hand, the internal consistency of the PWB subscale and, especially, the SWB subscale were low (i.e., below .70). While inclusion of the PWB and SWB items into the overall scale did not reduce the MHC-SF's internal consistency, future research will need to focus on improving the item content for these respective subscales in this particular South African population (Keyes et al., 2008).

Results from many studies suggest two important findings. First, persons who were completely mentally healthy had the lowest number of chronic physical conditions at all ages. Second, the youngest adults who were languishing had the same number of chronic physical conditions as older flourishing adults. Younger languishing adults who also had major depressive episode (MDE) had 1.5 times more chronic conditions than older flourishing adults. In other words, the absence of mental health – whether it is languishing or languishing combined with a mental illness – appears to compound the risk of chronic physical disease with age (Keyes, in press). Last author noted also that healthcare utilization to be lowest among adults who are flourishing. Rates of overnight hospitalizations over the past year, outpatient medical visits over the past year and number of prescription drugs were lowest among adults who were flourishing and physically healthy, followed by adults who were either flourishing but had physical illness conditions or adults who were not flourishing but were physically healthy. In short, complete mental health (i.e., flourishing and the absence of mental illness) – should be central to any national debate about healthcare coverage and costs (Keyes, 2007). Rather than focusing all discussions around healthcare delivery and insurance, our nation must increase and protect the number of individuals who are healthy, driving down the need for healthcare.

There is a broad-based, self-report measure originally developed in USA. It could be important to test the validity of different models in various cultures. Until now, there are few studies which have been published to explore the relationships between subjective vitality and positive mental health. Neither MHC-SF nor SVS have been used in Arabic culture. In Arabic countries, the construct validity of MHC-SF has never been tested. This study illustrates several issues highlighted in the literature regarding the use of assessment measures in cross-cultural settings (Salama-Younes, 2009). In this paper, we tested the exploratory and confirmatory factor analysis for the Arabic version. In general, results of our study supported its construct validity in the Egyptian country. However, several items in this measure seem to lack reliability and validity. These items were deleted (i.e., 6, 8, 9, 10 and 14).

Only nine items have been correctly loaded. The Arabic short form well replicated the three-factor structure found in the South Africa (Keyes et al., 2008), Germany (Lamers, Westerhof, Bohlmeijer, ten Klooster, & Keyes 2011) and USA (Keyes, 2005a, 2005b, 2007) studies, and the overall of the Arabic version had acceptable internal consistency (i.e., above .70). Moreover, the same three categories (i.e., flourishing, languishing and moderately mentally health) were found. Percentage is slightly similar to those of the South African and US samples. Secondly, the overall of Arabic version was positively and significantly correlated with the subjective vitality.

The first limitation of this study pertains to the fact that the continuum used was developed for American, not for Egyptian populations. Cultural differences have a considerable effect on the two cultures. Secondly, the MHC-SF was a self-report measure, and, thus, it has no potential to assess whether respondents were faking good, faking bad or neither. It also relied on their self-knowledge and subjective experience of situations, and this may impact the accuracy of the results. Thirdly, one of the most important strong points should not be overlooked – we tested only the positive mental health model without the negative part. It would probably be more suitable to test the factor structure of both positive and negative patterns at the same time. This will be done in our current study.

Acknowledgment Author thanks professors Mohamed E. Ali for his help in preparing the Arabic versions. He also thanks professors Mohamed Salama and Mohamed Gebreel for collecting data of Egyptian athletes. Author thanks both Profs. Ineke Vergeer and Stephanie Hanrahan for their help in the early manuscript. Finally, he thanks Professor Corey Keyes for his collaboration.

References

Arbuckle, J. L. (2005). *Amos 6.0 user's guide*. Chicago, IL: SPSS.

Benedetti, T. R. B., Borges, L. J., & Petroski, E. L. (2008). Physical activity and mental health status among elderly people. *Revista de Sade Publica, 42*(2), 302–307.

Bradburn, N. M. (1969). *The structure of psychological well-being*. Chicago: Aldine.

Cantril, H. (1967). *The pattern of human concerns*. New Brunswick, NJ: Rutgers University Press.

Diener, E., Lucas, R. E., & Oishi, S. (2002). Subjective well-being: The science of happiness and life satisfaction. In C. R. Snyder & S. J. Lopez (Eds.), *Handbook of positive psychology* (pp. 63–73). New York: Oxford University Press.

Escofier, B. (2003). *Analyse des Correspondances, Recherches au cœur de l'analyse de données. [Correspondence analysis: Research at the heart of data analysis]*. Campus de la Harpe: Presses Universitaires de Rennes.

Faulkner, G. E. J., & Taylor, A. H. (2005). *Exercise, health and mental health: Emerging relationships*. London: Routledge.

Hamer, M., Stamatakis, E., & Steptoe, A. (2008). Dose response relationship between physical activity and mental health: The Scottish health survey. *British Journal of Sports Medicine, 43*, 1111–1114.

Hoelter, J. W. (1983). The analysis of covariance structures: Goodness of fit indices. *Sociological Methods and Research, 11*, 325–344.

Hu, L. T., & Bentler, P. M. (1999). Fit indices in covariance structure modeling: Sensitivity to under parameterized model misspecification. *Psychological Methods, 3*, 424–453.

Kasser, T., & Ryan, R. M. (1999). The relation of psychological needs for autonomy and relatedness to health, vitality, well-being and mortality in nursing home. *Journal of Applied Social Psychology, 29*, 935–954.

Keyes, C. L. M. (1998). Social well–being. *Social Psychology Quarterly, 61*, 121–140.

Keyes, C. L. M. (2002). The mental health continuum: From languishing to flourishing in life. *Journal of Health and Social Research, 43*, 207–222.

Keyes, C. L. M. (2003). Complete mental health: An agenda for the 21st century. In C. L. M. Keyes & J. Haidt (Eds.), *Flourishing: Positive psychology and the life well–lived* (pp. 293–312). Washington, DC: American Psychological Association Press.

Keyes, C. L. M. (2005a). Mental illness and/or mental health? Investigating axioms of the complete state model of health. *Journal of Consulting and Clinical Psychology, 73*, 539–548.

Keyes, C. L. M. (2005b). The subjective well–being of America's youth: Toward a comprehensive assessment. *Adolescent and Family Health, 4*, 3–11.

Keyes, C. L. M. (2006). Mental health in adolescence: Is America's youth flourishing? *The American Journal of Orthopsychiatry, 76*, 395–402.

Keyes, C. L. M. (2007). Promoting and protecting mental health as flourishing: A complementary strategy for improving national mental health. *The American Psychologist, 62*, 95–108.

Keyes, C. L. M. (2009). The nature and importance of mental health in youth. In R. Gilman, M. Furlong, & E. S. Heubner (Eds.), *Promoting wellness in children and youth: A handbook of positive psychology in the schools* (pp. 9–23). New York: Routledge.

Keyes, C. L. Mental health is a complete state and not merely the absence of mental illness. In M. Salama-Younes & A. Delle Fave (Eds.), Positive psychology for all: Introduction, concepts and application in school age (in press).

Keyes, C. L. M., Shmotkin, D., & Ryff, C. D. (2002). Optimizing well–being: The empirical encounter of two traditions. *Journal of Personality and Social Psychology, 82*, 1007–1022.

Keyes, C. L. M., & Waterman, M. B. (2003). Dimensions of well-being and mental health in adulthood. In M. Bornstein, L. Davidson, C. L. M. Keyes, & K. Moore (Eds.), *Well-being: Positive development throughout the life course* (pp. 477–497). Mahwah, NJ: Erlbaum.

Keyes, C., Wissing, M., Potgieter, J., Temane, M., Kruger, A., & van Rooy, S. (2008). Evaluation of the mental health continuum-short form (MHC–SF) in Setswana speaking South Africans. *Clinical Psychology & Psychotherapy, 15*, 181–192.

Lamers, S. M. A., Westerhof, G. J., Bohlmeijer, E. T., ten Klooster, P. M., & Keyes, C. L. M. (2011). Evaluating the psychometric properties of the Dutch version of the mental health continuum-short form (MHC-SF). *European Journal of Clinical Psychology, 67*(1), 99–110.

Landers, D. M., & Arent, S. M. (2007). Physical activity and mental health. In G. Tenenbaum & R. C. Eklund (Eds.), *Handbook of sport psychology* (3rd ed., pp. 469–491). Hoboken, NJ: Wiley.

MacCallum, R. C., Browne, M. W., & Sugawara, H. M. (1996). Power analysis and determination of sample size for covariance structure modeling. *Psychological Methods, 1*, 130–149.

Nunnally, J. C., & Bernstein, I. H. (1994). *Psychometric theory* (3rd ed.). New York: McGraw–Hill.

Robitschek, C., & Keyes, C. L. M. (2009). The structure of Keyes' model of mental health and the role of personal growth initiative as a parsimonious predictor. *Journal of Counseling Psychology, 56*, 321–329.

Ryan, R. M., & Bernstein, J. (2004). Vitality/Zest/Enthusiasm/Vigor/Energy. In C. Petersen & M. E. P. Seligman (Eds.), *Character strengths and virtues: A handbook and classification* (pp. 273–289). New York: Oxford University Press.

Ryan, R. M., & Deci, E. L. (2001). On happiness and human potentials: A review of research on hedonic and eudaimonic well-being. *Annual Review of Psychology, 52*, 141–166.

Ryan, R. M., & Frederick, C. M. (1997). On energy, personality, and health: Subjective vitality as a dynamic reflection of well-being. *Journal of Personality, 65*, 529–564.

Ryff, C. D. (1989). Happiness is everything, or is it? Explorations on the meaning of psychological well-being. *Journal of Personality and Social Psychology, 57*, 1069–1081.

Ryff, C., & Keyes, C. (1995). The structure of psychological well-being revisited. *Journal of Personality and Social Psychology, 69*, 719–727.

Salama-Younes, M. (2009). Subjective well-being for Arabic athletes: Comparative study. In: 1st World congress on positive psychology, International Positive Psychology Association (IPPA), Philadelphia, PA, 18–21 June 2009.

Salama-Younes, M., Montazeri, A., Ismaïl, A., & Roncin, C. (2009). Factor structure and internal consistency of the 12-item general health questionnaire (GHQ-12) and the subjective vitality scale (VS), and the relationship between them: A study from France. *Health and Quality of Life Outcomes, 22*, 1477–7525.

Waterman, A. S. (1990). The relevance of Aristotle's conception of eudaimonia for the psychological study of happiness. *Theoretical and Philosophical Psychology, 10*, 39–44.

Part VI
Interventions

Chapter 20
School Interventions for Promoting Psychological Well-Being in Adolescence

Chiara Ruini, Fedra Ottolini, Elena Tomba, Carlotta Belaise, Elisa Albieri, Dalila Visani, Ernesto Caffo, and Giovanni A. Fava

Recently, the interest on the positive aspects of adolescence, such as positive development, quality of life, happiness, and social functioning is growing (Kelley, 2003). Also the increasing episodes of bullyism in high schools, behavioral and learning problems, and early leaving of school underline the importance of specific approaches to adolescents' difficulties (Friedman, 2003).

In this scenario, schools represent an ideal setting for promoting interpersonal relationships and human development.

Many school interventions have been proposed and validated: the Paths curriculum (Kam, Greenberg, & Walls, 2003) for the promotion of social competence and the prevention of aggressive behavior; the Gatehouse project (Patton, Bond, Butler, & Glover, 2003) for increasing the attachment and the sense of belonging to a school in students, the Bounce Back program (McGrath & Noble, 2003) and the Bright Ideas (Brandon & Cunningham, 1999) for promoting resilience and coping skills, the Penn Resiliency program (Gillham, Reivich, Jaycox, & Seligman, 1995; Gillham et al., 2007) for promoting optimism and preventing depression, the Stress Inoculation training (Meichenbaum & Deffenbacher, 1998) or the Coping Cat (Kendall, 1994) for preventing anxiety in children and adolescents. However, these programs are focused only on damage repairing, without addressing specifically issues such as the features of well-being in adolescence, which factors are related to its promotion and whether these factors can affect also the individual vulnerability to stress, psychological disturbances, and social maladjustment in adolescence.

C. Ruini (✉) • F. Ottolini • E. Tomba • C. Belaise • E. Albieri • D. Visani • G.A. Fava
Department of Psychology, University of Bologna, Bologna, Italy
e-mail: chiara.ruini@unibo.it

E. Caffo
Mother-Infant Department, University of Modena and Reggio Emilia, Modena, Italy

I. Brdar (ed.), *The Human Pursuit of Well-Being: A Cultural Approach*,
DOI 10.1007/978-94-007-1375-8_20, © Springer Science+Business Media B.V. 2011

This study aims to test the efficacy of a new school program for the promotion of psychological well-being (PWB) and optimal human functioning in adolescence according to the eudaimonic perspective (Ryan & Deci, 2001). This approach appears particularly relevant in developmental settings because it underlines the realization of human potential and individual strengths (Ryan & Deci, 2001; Ryff, 1989). Particularly, Ryff's model of PWB (Ryff, 1989) represents this perspective, assessing different dimensions such as autonomy, environmental mastery, personal growth, positive relations with others, and self-acceptance.

In clinical settings, a specific strategy well-being therapy (WBT) for enhancing PWB according to Ryff's model (Ryff, 1989) has been developed (Fava & Ruini, 2003) and tested in controlled trials, both alone (Fava, Rafanelli, Cazzaro, Conti, & Grandi, 1998a) and in addition to cognitive-behavioral packages (Fava, Rafanelli, Grandi, Conti, & Belluardo, 1998b; Fava, Ruini, Rafanelli & Grandi, 2002; Fava, Ruini, Rafanelli, Finos, Conti, & Grandi, 2004; Fava et al., 2005). These studies have documented the importance of increasing PWB in anxiety and depressive disorders. Further, a modified school protocol of WBT has been tested in a preliminary investigation (Ruini, Belaise, Brombin, Caffo, & Fava, 2006). The results have shown a decrease in anxiety symptoms and an increased well-being in a population of junior high-school students. In the current investigation, the preliminary school program has been improved further and adapted for adolescents, improving specific aspects which need to be achieved during this important crossing age.

Method

Participants

Nine classes of one high school in Northern Italy volunteered to participate to the project, and school interventions were performed in a sample of 227 students (139 females, 88 males; mean age = 14.40 year; SD=0.67).

129 students were assigned to the WBT intervention group. 42 (32.3%) were males and 87 (67.7%) females. Their mean age was 14.47 (SD=07.69). 98 students were assigned to the attention-placebo intervention group. 46 (46.9%) were males and 52 (53.1%) females. Their mean age was 14.32 (SD=0.54).

Procedure

The classes were randomly assigned to: (a) a protocol derived from WBT (five classes) and (b) attention-placebo protocol (four classes). Both school-based interventions consisted of six 2-h sessions, which were held once a week in the class, where role playing and group discussions were performed.

The questionnaires were administered three times: during the first (test) and the last (retest) session of both school interventions and 6 months later (follow-up).

WBT and attention-placebo school interventions were performed by two clinical psychologists, involved in both interventions. Written informed consent was obtained after the procedures were explained to the students and teachers. No student declined to participate.

A 6-month follow-up was performed in the following school year, and students were re-assessed with the same psychometric instruments. The follow-up was not feasible in one WBT class because the class was split and students were no longer available. These students were excluded from follow-up analyses. The number of students in the follow-up was thus 202 instead of 227.

Measures

During the first and last sessions of both school interventions, and in one other school day 6 months later, students were assessed using three questionnaires.

Kellner's symptom questionnaire (SQ, Kellner, 1987). SQ is a 92-item, self-rating scale that yields four scales of distress (anxiety, depression, somatization and hostility-irritability), and four scales of well-being (relaxation, contentment, physical well-being, and friendliness). Each symptom scale score may range from 0 to 17; each well-being scale score from 0 to 6. In the present study, SQ well-being subscales were computed to represent the lack of these well-being dimensions (Kellner, 1987). Test-retest Pearson's coefficients were satisfactory for all SQ scales. They ranged from .44 to .60.

The *psychological well-being scales* (PWB, brief form, Ryff, 1989; Ruini, Ottolini, Rafanelli, Ryff & Fava, 2003) is a self-rating, 18-item inventory that covers the six areas of PWB according to Ryff's model (Ryff, 1989). Each scale score may range from 0 to 18. PWB has been previously validated in an Italian population (Ruini et al., 2003a). In this study, an adapted version of this questionnaire has been used, where items were selected according to their relevance for an adolescent population. Test-retest Pearson's coefficients ranged from .47 (personal growth) to .77 for all six scales. In this investigation, we have also calculated a total PWB score by adding together the scores of the six dimensions.

The *revised children's manifest anxiety scale* (RCMAS, Reynolds & Richmond, 1978) is a self-rating, 37-item inventory for assessing anxiety in children (age range from 6 to 19 years). It has three subscales which represent different aspects of anxiety (i.e., physiological anxiety, worry/oversensitivity, social concerns/concentration), and their scores are added together to form the total anxiety score and one subscale (lie scale) for measuring social desirability in children (Reynolds & Richmond, 1978). The answer scale format is yes/no or true/false.

Interventions

WBT Protocol

In the first session, students were trained to identify, recognize, and express a wide range of emotions (positive and negative), and they were asked to relate different colors or different animals to different emotions to help them realize the variety of emotions they can feel and how all these emotions can influence their behavior.

The second session of the WBT protocol was focused on the relationship between thoughts and emotions, according to the cognitive model (Beck, Rush, Shaw, & Emery, 1979; Muris, Vermeer, & Horselenberg, 2008). Students were trained for self-observation in a diary and were asked to report their daily situations (at school, with friends, with parents) to help them realize that the way they interpret situations can influence their emotions. The third session was based on cognitive restructuring according to cognitive-behavior therapy (CBT) model (Beck, Rush, Shaw & Emery, 1979; Muris, Vermeer, & Horselenberg, 2008) and was performed through role-playing and games in the class.

The last three sessions of the WBT school protocol were based on Ryff's model of well-being (Ryff, 1989), encompassing six dimensions: autonomy, environmental mastery, positive interpersonal relationships, personal growth, purpose in life, and self-acceptance. Particular emphasis has been given to positive interpersonal relationships, purpose in life, and self-acceptance, which are extremely important in adolescence. Also, students were invited to recognize some positive characteristics of their schoolmates and then they were asked to pay each other a compliment. This allowed students to reflect on how it can be difficult to be nice with a schoolmate, but also how it could be gratifying to receive an unexpected compliment.

The fifth session was focused on self-acceptance (awareness of one's good and bad qualities), autonomy (perception of one's skills and abilities) and purpose in life (objectives to be reached in the future). For example, students were asked to write for themselves a personal horoscope concerning their social activities, school, sports, and leisure time for the following year.

The last session was based on happiness and emotional well-being (Ryan & Deci, 2001) and the protocol concluded with some practical advices on how to improve and make one's life happier.

Attention-Placebo Protocol

In the attention-placebo protocol, group discussions, games and role playing were employed as well. Students were taught also some relaxation techniques, but the self-observation diary, cognitive restructuring, emphasis on positive emotions and Ryff's dimensions of PWB were not present. In particular, the second session was focused on the recognition of the physical components of different emotions, and the subsequent session (third) was focused on structured relaxation to help students deal with these physical symptoms. Finally, the last three sessions addressed how to improve communication and conflicts in the class. Students were invited to share their favorite songs or poems with schoolmates explaining the emotions they felt relatively to that song/poem. Students were then also asked to discuss their most feared situations to demonstrate that these fears were common inside the class (i.e., fear to be unpopular in the class, fear of exams and test) (Muris, Hoeve, Meesters, & Mayer, 2004). Finally, in the last session, students were invited to discuss the opinions they have about their schoolmates and about their school, with a particular emphasis on their future expectations.

Data Analysis

The efficacy of the two interventions was compared using a repeated measure analysis of variance (ANOVA). The "group allocation" (WBT school intervention vs. attention-placebo protocol) represented the "between subject factors" while the "test", "retest," and "follow-up" times represented the "within subject factor". PWB, SQ, and RCMAS scale scores were the dependent variables. The efficacy of the two interventions was tested by examining the interaction effect between "group allocation" and "times", using contrast analysis between baseline score – postintervention and follow-up scores.

Results

At baseline, WBT group was larger (five classes vs. four classes attention-placebo) and presented significantly higher levels of SQ somatization, SQ physical well-being (i.e., the higher the score, the higher the distress), and RCMAS physiological anxiety compared to attention-placebo group. Seven students in the WBT group and three in the attention-placebo group were not present at the first assessment. Thirteen students in the WBT group and six in the attention-placebo group were not present at the second assessment. At follow-up, WBT group consisted of 104 students, instead of 129 (one class was missing).

ANOVA for repeated measures, considering time x group allocation interaction (Table 20.1) shows the significant effect of WBT in the PWB total score and in the scale of personal growth (PWB) at retest. WBT, school-based intervention resulted also in a significant improvement in physical well-being (SQ), in physiological anxiety (RCMAS) at retest, in anxiety (SQ) at follow-up and in somatization (SQ) both at retest and at follow-up. All these symptom dimensions display an opposite pattern in the attention-placebo group, i.e., they tend to get worse at follow-up.

Table 20.1 Changes in psychological well-being, anxiety, and somatizations for the intervention and the control group

		Intervention group			Control group			$F_{1,225}$		
									Time × group	
		Test	Retest	Follow-up	Test	Retest	Follow-up	Time	Retest[a]	Follow-up[a]
Psychological well-being	M	79.47	80.63	80.06	80.41	79.10	79.94	1.92	3.95*	0.59
	SD	12.13	11.11	12.20	12.45	13.60	13.31			
Physiological anxiety	M	3.16	2.86	2.91	2.49	2.66	2.53	3.45*	4.15*	1.29
	SD	2.01	2.04	2.01	1.68	1.91	2.01	3.50*		
SQ anxiety	M	4.19	4.20	3.95	3.30	3.59	4.13		0.48	5.00*
	SD	3.73	3.89	3.92	3.18	3.58	3.74			
SQ somatization	M	3.80	3.36	3.34	2.81	3.51	3.16	4.63*	8.46**	3.88
	SD	3.50	3.52	3.58	2.63	3.56	3.30			

* $p<.05$; ** $p<.01$

[a]Time × group within subject contrast

Discussion

This preliminary study has different limitations: the limited number of sessions in each intervention (six sessions, once a week), the sample characteristics (self-selected school students of only one high school in Northern Italy, with no particular physical or mental problems) and the fact that assessment was based on self-rating scales only.

Nevertheless, this investigation has important clinical and preventive implications. The main purpose was to test the efficacy and the feasibility of a school intervention based on the promotion of PWB in adolescence and to compare it to an attention-placebo school protocol. The results of this study show that this intervention, based on promoting positive emotions and well-being, could be effective also in decreasing distress, in particular anxiety and somatization. This is in line with the preliminary investigation on WBT school program performed in junior high school (Ruini et al., 2006), where significant improvement in SQ physical well-being was shown. This aspect suggests that school-based WBT could have important clinical implications in view of the documented high prevalence of somatic symptoms in children and adolescents (Ginsburg, Riddle, & Davies, 2006; Muris, Vermeer, & Horselenberg, 2008). In literature, the efficacy of cognitive-behavioral school program in treating adolescents' psychological distress is well documented (Bernstein, Layne, Egan, & Tennison, 2005; Clarke, DeBar, & Lewinsohn, 2003; Kataoka et al., 2003; Lewinsohn, Clarke, Hops, & Andrews, 1990). In this protocol, CBT strategies were present, but the main ingredient was the promotion of well being, according to Ryff's model (Ryff, 1989). The results support previous data showing that changes in well-being may induce a decrease in distress and vice versa.

In the present investigation, the decreasing anxiety was sustained in the follow-up, demonstrating the potential preventing role of this school-based WBT intervention. This is according to previous data on WBT in adult clinical populations, where this approach was effective in treating affective disorders also in the long term (Fava et al., 2004). This long-term effect may probably be due to the fact that improving PWB and promoting optimal functioning could yield lasting personal changes which act as protective factors against stressful life events (Ryff & Singer, 1996). School-based interventions for preventing depression in youth (Clarke et al., 1995; Gillham et al., 2007; Merry, McDowell, Wild, Bir, & Cunliffe, 2004; Pössel, Horn, Groen, Hautzinger, 2004), until now, were mainly focused on reducing symptoms. The findings suggest their positive results, but their preventive efficacy in the long term is still controversial. Our hypothesis is that promoting positive functioning and building individual strengths could be more beneficial than simply addressing depressive or anxious symptoms especially in developmental settings.

Further, the results of this investigation show that WBT school program was effective also in improving personal growth and PWB in general (PWB total score), which are important domains for an adolescents' quality of life. On the contrary, in the attention-placebo group, symptomatology (particularly anxiety and somatization) tends to increase and PWB (total score and some dimensions) tends to remain stable or decrease after the intervention, documenting a possible iatrogenic effect of this nonstructured protocol. Good emotional and social climate has been shown to be associated with higher academic success, problem solving, and self-esteem of students, who present also less psychological and behavioral problems (Hoge, Smit, & Hanson, 1990; Roeser, 1998; Roeser, Eccles, & Sameroff, 1998; Roeser, Midgley, & Urdan, 1996). School organization should be implemented to promote student health by facilitating the realization of these capacities and thus student development and functioning.

This study has considerable limitations due to its preliminary nature: the limited number of sessions in each intervention (six sessions, once a week), the sample characteristics (self-selected school students, with no particular physical or mental problems) and the fact that assessment was based on self-rating scales only. However, we hope that future research with larger samples and longer follow-ups are necessary to confirm the efficacy of WBT, school-based intervention in improving PWB and decreasing adolescents' distress.

References

Beck, A. T., Rush, A. J., Shaw, B. F., & Emery, G. (1979). *Cognitive therapy of depression*. New York, NY: Guilford Press.

Bernstein, G. A., Layne, A. E., Egan, E. A., & Tennison, D. M. (2005). School-based interventions for anxious children. *Journal of the American Academy of Child and Adolescent Psychiatry, 44*, 1118–1127.

Brandon, C. M., & Cunningham, E. G. (1999). *Bright ideas manual*. Melbourne: OZ Child Australia.

Clarke, G. N., DeBar, L. L., & Lewinsohn, P. M. (2003). Cognitive-behavioral group treatment for adolescent depression. In A. E. Kazdin & J. R. Weisz (Eds.), *Evidence-based psychotherapies for children and adolescents* (pp. 120–134). New York, NY: Guilford Press.

Clarke, G. N., Hawkins, W., Murphy, M., Sheeber, L. B., Lewinsohn, P. M., & Seeley, J. R. (1995). Targeted prevention of unipolar depressive disorder in an at-risk sample of high school adolescents: A randomized trial of a group cognitive intervention. *Journal of the American Academy of Child and Adolescent Psychiatry, 34*, 312–321.

Fava, G. A., Rafanelli, C., Cazzaro, M., Conti, S., & Grandi, S. (1998). Well-being therapy. *Psychological Medicine, 28*, 475–480.

Fava, G. A., Rafanelli, C., Grandi, S., Conti, S., & Belluardo, P. (1998). Prevention of recurrent depression with cognitive behavioral therapy. *Archives of General Psychiatry, 55*, 816–820.

Fava, G. A., & Ruini, C. (2003). Development and characteristics of a well-being enhancing psychotherapy strategy: Well-being therapy. *Journal of Behavior Therapy and Experimental Psychiatry, 34*, 45–63.

Fava, G. A., Ruini, C., Rafanelli, C., Finos, L., Conti, S., & Grandi, S. (2004). Six year outcome of cognitive behavior therapy for prevention of recurrent depression. *The American Journal of Psychiatry, 161*, 1872–1876.

Fava, G. A., Ruini, C., Rafanelli, C., Finos, L., Salmaso, L., Mangelli, L., et al. (2005). Well-being therapy of generalized anxiety disorder. *Psychotherapy and Psychosomatics, 74*, 26–30.

Fava, G. A., Ruini, C., Rafanelli, C., & Grandi, S. (2002). Cognitive behavior approach to loss of clinical effect during long-term antidepressant treatment: A pilot study. *The American Journal of Psychiatry, 159*, 2094–2095.

Friedman, R. M. (2003). Improving outcomes for students through the application of a public health model to school psychology: A commentary. *Journal of School Psychology, 41*, 69–75.

Gillham, J. E., Reivich, K. J., Jaycox, L. I., & Seligman, M. E. P. (1995). Preventing depressive symptoms in school-children: two year follow-up. *Psychological Science, 6*, 343–351.

Gillham, J. E., Reivich, K. J., Freres, D. R., Chaplin, T. M., Shatté, A. J., Samuels, B., et al. (2007). School-based prevention of depressive symptoms: A randomized controlled study of the effectiveness and specificity of the Penn Resiliency Program. *Journal of Consulting and Clinical Psychology, 75*, 9–19.

Ginsburg, G. S., Riddle, M. A., & Davies, M. (2006). Somatic symptoms in children and adolescents with anxiety disorders. *Journal of the American Academy of Child and Adolescent Psychiatry, 45*, 1179–1187.

Hoge, D. R., Smit, E. K., & Hanson, S. L. (1990). School experiences predicting changes climate and difficulties in the social adjustment of middle school students. *Applied Developmental Science, 1*, 76–88.

Kam, C. M., Greenberg, M. T., & Walls, C. T. (2003). Examining the role of implementation quality in school-based prevention using the PATHS curriculum. *Promoting Alternative Thinking Skills Curriculum. Prevention Science: The official journal of the Society for Prevention Research, 4*, 55–63.

Kataoka, S. A., Stein, B. D., Jaycox, L. H., Wong, M., Escudero, P., Tu, W., et al. (2003). A school-based mental health program for traumatized Latino immigrant children. *Journal of the Academy of Child and Adolescent Psychiatry, 42*(3), 311–318.

Kelley, T. M. (2003). Health realization: A principle-based psychology of positive youth development. *Child and Youth Care Forum, 32*(1), 47–72.

Kellner, R. A. (1987). Symptom questionnaire. *The Journal of Clinical Psychiatry, 48*, 269–274.

Kendall, P. C. (1994). Treatment of anxiety disorders in children: A randomized clinical trial. *Journal of Consulting and Clinical Psychology, 62*, 100–110.

Lewinsohn, P. M., Clarke, G. N., Hops, H., & Andrews, J. (1990). Cognitive-behavioral group treatment for depressed adolescents. *Behaviour Therapy, 21*, 385–401.

McGrath, H., & Noble, T. (2003). *BOUNCE BACK: A classroom resiliency program for schools. Book 1: The teacher's handbook.* Sydney: Pearson Education.

Meichenbaum, D., & Deffenbacher, J. L. (1998). Stress inoculation training. *The Counseling Psychologist, 1*, 69–90.

Merry, S., McDowell, H., Wild, C. J., Bir, J., & Cunliffe, R. A. (2004). Randomized placebo-controlled trial of a school-based depression prevention program. *Journal of the American Academy of Child and Adolescent Psychiatry, 43*, 538–547.

Muris, P., Hoeve, I., Meesters, C., & Mayer, B. (2004). Children's perception and interpretation of anxiety-related physical symptoms. *Journal of Behavior Therapy and Experimental Psychiatry, 35*(3), 233–244.

Muris, P., Vermeer, E., & Horselenberg, R. (2008). Cognitive development and the interpretation of anxiety-related physical symptoms in 4–13-year-old non-clinical children. *Journal of Behavior Therapy and Experimental Psychiatry, 39*, 73–86.

Patton, G., Bond, L., Butler, H., & Glover, S. (2003). Changing schools, changing health? Design and implementation of the Gatehouse Project. *The Journal of Adolescent Health, 33*, 231–239.

Pössel, P., Horn, A. B., Groen, G., & Hautzinger, M. (2004). School-based prevention of depressive symptoms in adolescents: A 6-month follow-up. *Journal of the American Academy of Child and Adolescent Psychiatry, 43*, 1003–1010.

Reynolds, C. R., & Richmond, B. O. (1978). What I think and feel: A revised measure of children's manifest anxiety. *Journal of Abnormal Psychology, 6*(2), 271–280.

Roeser, R. W. (1998). On schooling and mental health: Issues, research, and future directions. *Educational Psychologist, 33*, 129–135.

Roeser, R. W., Eccles, J. S., & Sameroff, A. J. (1998). Academic and emotional functioning in early adolescence: Longitudinal relations, patterns, and prediction by experience in middle school. *Development and Psychopathology, 10*, 321–352.

Roeser, R. W., Midgley, C., & Urdan, T. C. (1996). Perceptions of the school psychological environment and early adolescent's psychological and behavioral functioning in school: The mediating role of goals and belonging. *Journal of Educational Psychology, 88*, 408–422.

Ruini, C., Belaise, C., Brombin, C., Caffo, E., & Fava, G. A. (2006). Well-being Therapy in school settings: A pilot study. *Psychotherapy and Psychosomatics, 75*, 331–336.
Ruini, C., Ottolini, F., Rafanelli, C., Ryff, C. D., & Fava, G. A. (2003). La validazione italiana delle psychological well-being scale (PWB) [The Italian validation of the psychological well-being scale (PWB)]. *Rivista di Psichiatria, 38*(3), 117–130.
Ryan, R. M., & Deci, E. L. (2001). On happiness and human potential: A review of research on hedonic and eudaimonic well-being. *Annual Review of Psychology, 52*, 141–166.
Ryff, C. D. (1989). Happiness is everything, or is it? Exploration on the meaning of psychological well-being. *Journal of Personality and Social Psychology, 57*(6), 1069–1083.
Ryff, C. D., & Singer, B. (1996). Psychological well-being: Meaning, measurement and implication for psychotherapy research. *Psychotherapy and Psychosomatics, 65*, 14–23.

Chapter 21
Applying Self-Determination Theory to Help Obese Portuguese Individuals

Sónia Mestre and José Pais-Ribeiro

Evidence shows that obesity is a multifactor disease, involving a complex network of genetic, metabolic and psychological factors, such as motivation (Lenfant, 2001). In a weight loss program, the main obstacle to success resides in the difficulty in maintaining weight stability. Therefore, it is essential to assess the patient's motivation (Devlin, Yanovski, & Wilson, 2000).

According to the World Health Organization (WHO, 2008), obesity has increased not only in high-income countries but also in low and middle-income countries, which is leading to a serious health problem within the population in general. Recent studies indicate that in Portugal, 50% of the adults are overweight and 15% are obese (Health Department, 2006).

In the current study, we will address the importance of motivation in sustaining a health behavior change, from a self-determination point of view.

Research on SDT (Deci & Ryan, 1985, 2002; Ryan & Deci, 2000) shows that the type of motivation (Deci & Ryan, 2008) is more important when pursuing an outcome, rather than the amount of motivation. In a continuum between autonomous and controlled motivation, the authors explain that people are autonomy regulated if they act according to their own choice and will; conversely, they are controlled motivated if they act as a result of external pressure and coercion. Moreover, this model clarifies the importance of social environment in sustaining people's basic need of autonomy, competence and relatedness. The positive effect of autonomous regulation is associated with more predisposition and effort to achieve positive health outcome (Pelletier, Dion, Slovinec-D'Angelo, & Reid, 2004), in the beginning and later with a dietary change program (Sheldon & Elliot, 1998). In addition, controlled regulation is a poor variable in predicting dietary change (Patterson, Kristal, & White, 1996).

S. Mestre (✉) • J. Pais-Ribeiro
Faculty of Psychology and Educational Sciences, University of Porto,
Porto, Portugal
e-mail: soniamest@gmail.com

I. Brdar (ed.), *The Human Pursuit of Well-Being: A Cultural Approach*,
DOI 10.1007/978-94-007-1375-8_21, © Springer Science+Business Media B.V. 2011

Losing weight is not typically a pleasurable action, but health care providers can help patients to identify and integrate the importance of a dieting behavior (Ryan, Patrick, Deci, & Williams, 2008). In fact, several studies show that if clinical providers were perceived as autonomous, individuals would be more autonomy regulated and have a better outcome in a dieting program for a period of 2 years (Williams, Grow, Freedman, Ryan, & Deci, 1996).

Similar to the concept of self-efficacy of Bandura (1989) is the notion of perceived competence that refers to a person's feelings of confidence to change (Ryan et al., 2008). Nevertheless, and contrary to Bandura's theory, SDT model considers that besides perceived competence, more is necessary for outcomes to occur. SDT considers that the basis of behavior change is a consequence of the relation between autonomy support, autonomous motivation and perceived competence.

Therefore, and based on SDT theory, the aim of the present study is to understand why obese individuals would enter and maintain confidence about being able to carry on the treatment regimen. We hypothesized that patients will be more autonomy regulated then controlled at the end of the program if they perceive their health care supporters with more autonomy. Additionally, a decrease in BMI would be a consequence of that support. We also expect that greater BMI will be positively associated with controlled regulation instead of with autonomous regulation, in both periods of the study. Moreover, negative association between the two subscales of the treatment self-regulation questionnaire (TRSQ) is expected.

Method

Participants

The participants in this study were severely obese individuals ($N=48$), who volunteered to complete the questionnaires twice for the investigation. The average age was 41 years, and 81% were female. The majority (60%) professionally active and had 8 years of education. Along 3 months treatment at a community hospital, the individuals followed a weight loss program that integrated psychological guidance, an individualized diet regiment and medical supervision. The inclusion criteria were: having a BMI above 30 kg/m^2, not taking any medication that could interfere with BMI, and in the beginning of the treatment, regardless of past attempts to lose weight.

Instruments

Treatment Self-regulation Questionnaire (TSRQ)

A Portuguese translation was made of this questionnaire (Mestre & Pais-Ribeiro, 2008) and was used to measure individual's autonomous and controlled reasons to engage and persist in a medical regiment concerning weight loss. The TSRQ was adapted to several areas of the study such as diabetes (Williams, Freedman, & Deci, 1998), smoking (Williams, Cox, Kouides, & Deci, 1999) and maintained weight loss (Williams et al., 1996). In this study, we used the 18 items version with four stems, such as: "I decided to enter this weight-loss program because..." or "If I remain in treatment, it will probably be because...". Each stem has several reasons that diverge in a seven-point scale ranging from "not at all true" (1) to "very true" (7). In an autonomous regulation (α=.88) to lose weight, we have reasons such as "I really want to make some changes in my life" or "Being overweight makes it hard to do many things". Controlled regulation (α=.92) appears with reasons such as: "I won't like myself very much until I lose weight" or "I want others to see that I am really trying to lose weight". Factor analysis of the questionnaire revealed two factors named "autonomous" (six items) and "controlling" (12 items). In the beginning of this study, we obtained subscales α values of .81 (autonomous regulation) and .82 (controlled regulation). In the end of the treatment, α reliabilities were .80 (autonomous regulation) and .85 (controlled regulation).

Perceived Competence Scale (PCS)

Patient's degree of personal confidence in maintaining a health diet was assessed by this short four-item scale (α=.90), formerly translated to Portuguese language (Mestre & Pais-Ribeiro, 2008). In a seven-point scale, participants scored items such as: "I feel confident in my ability to maintain a healthy diet" or "I am able to meet the challenge of maintaining a healthy diet". The total score on this scale is the average on the four items' responses. Factor analysis exposed one-factor solution. In this study, αreliabilities ranged from .92 (at baseline) and .93 (posttreatment).

Heath Care Climate Questionnaire (HCCQ)

This questionnaire quantifies the patients' perceptions of their health care providers, in terms of autonomy support. The original HCQQ is a 15-item measure, developed in non-health care field (Deci, Connell, & Ryan, 1989). In this investigation, we used a short form of six items, previously translated to Portuguese (Mestre & Pais-Ribeiro, 2008). The six items (α=.93) were scored on a seven-point scale ranging from "not at all true" (1), indicative of lower autonomy perception, to "very true" (7) indicative of high perceived support. Only one factor was extracted from the factor analyses, supporting SDT theory. The questionnaire included questions related to healthy diet, with items such as: "I feel my health care providers understand how I see things with respect to my diet" or "My health care practitioners encourage me to ask questions about my diet". The average of individual's response in the six items gives us the score of the questionnaire. High internal consistency was found in the present study for HCCQ (α=.92).

Procedure

Time 1

In the beginning of the treatment, participants completed the Portuguese version of the TSRQ, which concerns entering the weight loss program, and PCS, which concerns maintaining a healthy diet scale. BMI was also assessed and a demographic questionnaire was completed.

Time 2

After 3 months in treatment, all individuals were weighed, and they completed, once again, the Portuguese version of the TRSQ and PCS, and the HCCQ – healthy diet, Portuguese version.

Results

To test our hypotheses, we first examined psychometric properties, means and standards deviations for all four scales. Then the scores of the different scales were correlated using Pearson's correlation.

Weight Loss and Different Behavioral Regulatory Style through Treatment

Table 21.1 shows the means and standard deviations for the main variables and BMI. Overall, individuals were more autonomous than controlled regulated, in the

Table 21.1 Means and standard deviations of the variables in the study

Variable		M_1	M_2	t
Body mass index	M	46.27	44.98	4.13**
	SD	5.46	5.39	
Autonomous regulation	M	6.27	5.98	3.21**
	SD	0.73	0.76	
Controlled regulation	M	3.53	4.06	3.45**
	SD	1.09	1.12	
Perceived competence	M	4.98	5.07	0.58
	SD	1.34	1.17	
Perceived health care autonomy	M		5.22	–
	SD	-	1.08	

M_1 Time1 mean, M_2 Time 2 mean
** $p<.01$

two times of the study and had more perceived competence in maintaining a healthy diet at the end of the program. Moreover, and as predicted, there was also a decrease in the BMI during the 3 months of treatment.

Comparison between Time 1 and 3 months later shows statistically significant differences between initial autonomous motivation (3 months later, the value for 3 months was lower than at the beginning) and controlled regulation (with initial value lower than after 3 months).

Groups based on weight difference scores revealed significant mean differences between BMIs with higher value in Time 1 than in Time 2 of the study.

Relationship between Motivation Variables

In Table 21.2, we can verify the significant associations between all scales and BMI, in both phases of the study. The BMI was positively correlated with follow-up BMI and with autonomous motivation. Autonomous motivation was negatively associated with controlled motivation in the beginning and at the end of the investigation. The individuals showed better perceived competence when they were autonomously motivated only in the beginning of the treatment, and, at the end, it seems that this variable is associated with perceived support from health professionals. Controlled regulation showed significant regulation with controlled and autonomous motivation during the whole treatment. Neither autonomous nor controlled motivation was significantly associated with perceived support from health care providers.

Table 21.2 Correlations between scales

	Variable	2	3	4	5	6	7	8	9
Time 1	1. Body mass index	.18	.17	–.04	.92**	.08	.31*	–.26	.23
	2. Perceived competence	–	.26*	–.14	.12	.66**	.19	–.12	.23
	3. Autonomous regulation		–	–.44**	.15	.08	.65**	–.32*	.17
	4. Controlled regulation			–	–.01	–.02	–.18	.55**	.13
Time 2	5. Body mass index				–	–.09	.33*	–.25	.18
	6. Perceived competence					–	.21	.04	.28*
	7. Autonomous regulation						–	–.38*	.22
	8. Controlled regulation							–	–.06
	9. Perceived health care autonomy								–

*$p<.05$; ** $p<.01$

Comparison between Demographic and Motivation Variables

The correlation between weight difference and perceived competence at Time 1 was positive and moderate. We also found a negative association between the age and BMI in the beginning of the program (−.30) and after the 3 months (.29). Finally, a higher education seems to lead individuals to a controlled motivation in Time 1 (.29) and Time 2 (.32).

Discussion

This research examined the associations between different styles of motivation (autonomous and controlled) with perceived competence and perceived support in obese population.

In general, the results show that individuals are more autonomously motivated than controlled, over a 3-month period. This is an encouraging result for health professionals because autonomy motivation is associated with healthier behaviors (Pelletier et al., 2004) and better outcomes in psychotherapy (Zuroff et al., 2007) Our investigation underlines that autonomous motivation is not only important in pursuing the treatment's goal but also in weight management.

As hypothesized, at the end of the program, the individuals were more autonomously motivated than controlled. But, curiously, individuals seem to increase controlled motivation at the end of the weight loss program and decrease their autonomy regulation. As Vallerand, Pelletier, and Koestner (2008) point out, health behavior programs are not usually seen as pleasant activities and, therefore, not intrinsic (Ryan et al., 2008).

As SDT posits, there was a negative association between the two different forms of motivation. This indicates that peoples' behavior goes along a continuum of the most self-determined or autonomous to the least self-determined or controlled. Nowadays, though we still speak about intrinsic and extrinsic motivation, it is more correct to use terms such as autonomous and controlled. This theory explains that external and introjected regulations are controlled forms of motivation; identified and integrated regulations are autonomous forms of motivation (Deci & Ryan, 2008). Along this spectrum we still have amotivation which means lack of motivation and no intention to act. In the present research, we only investigated the two main forms of motivation (autonomous and controlled) for several reasons. The population in our study voluntarily sought medical help at the hospital to lose weight, and so they were not unmotivated. In addition, we wanted to use a questionnaire with good internal consistency and that, in terms of cultural context, would be similar to the Portuguese culture. The TSRQ had these properties. Moreover, we were more interested to assess autonomous and controlling reasons for participating in a weight loss program then to distinguish the different forms of autonomous and controlled regulation.

In the weight analysis, and as expected, there was a decrease in the BMI at the end of the treatment. Nevertheless and contrary to what was hypothesized, greater BMI was associated with autonomous motivation. SDT posits that the maintenance of health behavior requires the internalization of the importance of such behavior (Ryan et al., 2008). So, in this case, it seems that individuals did not internalize completely the importance of losing weight, because if they had, a greater BMI would be negatively correlated with autonomous and positively correlated with controlled motivation. However, we can consider that, in general, the goal was achieved because participants did decrease BMI after 3 months of treatment. Previous researches support this finding. For instance, Sheldon and Elliot (1998) fail to show the correlation between controlled regulation and outcome, and Judge, Bono, Erez, and Locke (2005) did not find a significant positive correlation between controlled motivation and work goals. Recently, Shahar, Kanitzki, Shulman, and Blatt (2006) did not demonstrate negative association between controlled motivation and goal progress.

Another important factor in the treatment of obese individuals is social support, namely from health care providers. In a recent study concerning physical activity by Fortier, Sweet, O'Sullivan, and Williams (2007), they found out that patients that had received more intensive interventions were more autonomously motivated and had a greater perceived competence. These results are consistence with our findings. The individuals felt more competent if they received greater autonomous support from health professionals. By providing choice and information about the guidelines of the treatment, supporters can increase a lasting self-determined action, which is one of the priorities in the treatment of obesity. Curiously, greater education was positively related with controlled motivation. This means, that although participants had information about the consequences of obesity, they adopted a poor internalized motivation. So, it is important that health care supporters understand that only providing more information on the patient's health condition is not sufficient; this has to be done in a friendly context.

As SDT highlights, individuals can move from a less intrinsic motivation to a more intrinsic regulation; however, the process itself is not known (Vallerand et al., 2008). The present research is also not clear on this process but shows that the two types of motivation and perceived competence seem to be dispositional motivational variables. This means that although it can be changed through time, it is relatively stable. In fact, the purpose of therapy is to change individuals' beliefs and help them to internalize and to value a behavior or an outcome, i.e., to become more autonomously motivated. Studies show that this is possible and that friends, family and professionals play an important role (Deci & Ryan, 2008).

As obesity continues to rise around the world, it is important to address the treatment for obesity in terms of dietary therapy, increased physical activity and behavioral therapy (Lang & Froelicher, 2006).

Limitations of the current investigation include that data were collected only in one community hospital and in a small number of individuals. Therefore, future research should examine this issue in a larger scale and even in other cultures. Furthermore, although we examined the motivation variables through a 3-month period, it might be important to investigate it in a longer period, because preventing weight regain is critical in a successful program.

Despite these limitations, overall, the findings from this study can help us to better understand how obese individuals feel in terms of motivation and how different types of motivation are related with other aspects of peoples' functioning.

Acknowledgments This study was support by the Science and Technology Foundation – Portuguese Government (FCT) grant SFRH/BD/23562/2005.

References

Bandura, A. (1989). Human agency in social cognitive theory. *The American Psychologist, 44*, 1175–1184.

Deci, E. L., Connell, J. P., & Ryan, R. M. (1989). Self-determination in a work organization. *The Journal of Applied Psychology, 74*, 580–590.

Deci, E. L., & Ryan, R. M. (1985). *Intrinsic motivation and self-determination in human behaviour*. New York: Plenum.

Deci, E. L., & Ryan, R. M. (2002). *Handbook of self-determination research*. Rochester: The University of Rochester Press.

Deci, E. L., & Ryan, R. M. (2008). Facilitating optimal motivation and psychological well-being across life's domains. *Canadian Psychology, 49*(1), 14–23.

Devlin, M. J., Yanovski, S. Z., & Wilson, G. T. (2000). Obesity: What mental health professional need to know. *The American Journal of Psychiatry, 157*(6), 854–866.

Fortier, M. S., Sweet, S. N., O'Sullivan, T. L., & Williams, G. C. (2007). A self-determination process model of physical activity adoption in the context of a randomized controlled trial. *Psychology of Sport and Exercise, 8*, 741–757.

Health Department (2006). *National health inquiry*. Retrieved September 6, 2006, from www.insa.pt/sites/INSA/Portugues/ComInf/Imprensa/ComNotas/ComunicadosNotas/INS-2005-2006_Principais%20Indicadores.pdf

Judge, T. A., Bono, J. E., Erez, A., & Locke, E. A. (2005). Core self-evaluation and job and life satisfaction: The role of self-concordance and goal attainment. *The Journal of Applied Psychology, 54*, 493–503.

Lang, A., & Froelicher, E. S. (2006). Management of overweight and obesity in adults: Behavioural intervention for long-term weight loss and maintenance. *European Journal of Cardiovascular Nursing, 5*, 102–114.

Lenfant, C. (2001). Physicians need practical tools to treat the complex problems of overweight and obesity. *American Family Physician, 63*(11), 2139–2145.

Mestre, S., & Pais-Ribeiro, J. L. (2008). Adaptação de três questionários para a população portuguesa baseados na Teoria de Auto-Determinação. *Actas do 7º Congresso Nacional de Psicologia da Saúde*, 623–625.

Patterson, R. E., Kristal, A. R., & White, E. (1996). Do beliefs, knowledge, and perceived norms about diet and cancer predict dietary change? *American Journal of Public Health, 86*, 1394–1500.

Pelletier, L. G., Dion, S. C., Slovinec-D'Angelo, M., & Reid, R. (2004). Why do you regulate what you eat? Relationships between forms of regulation, eating behaviours, sustained dietary behaviour change, and psychological adjustment. *Motivation and Emotion, 28*(3), 245–277.

Ryan, R. M., & Deci, E. L. (2000). Self-determination theory and the facilitation of intrinsic motivation, social development, and well-being. *The American Psychologist, 55*(1), 68–78.

Ryan, R. M., Patrick, H., Deci, E. L., & Williams, G. C. (2008). Facilitating health behaviour change and its maintenance: Interventions based on self-determination theory. *The European Health Psychologist, 10*, 2–5.

Shahar, G., Kanitzki, E., Shulman, S., & Blatt, S. J. (2006). Personality, motivation and the construction of goals during the transition to adulthood. *Personality and Individual Differences, 40*, 53–63.

Sheldon, K. M., & Elliott, A. J. (1998). Not all personal goals are personal: Comparing autonomous and controlled reasons for goals as predictors of effort and attainment. *Personality and Social Psychology Bulletin, 24*, 546–557.

Valerand, R. J., Pelletier, L. G., & Koestner, R. (2008). Reflections on self-determination theory. *Canadian Psychology, 49*(3), 257–262.

WHO. Retrieved August 20, 2008 from http://www.who.int/topics/obesity/en/

Williams, G. C., Cox, E. M., Koudines, R., & Deci, E. L. (1999). Presenting the facts about smoking to adolescent: Effects of an autonomy-supportive style. *Archives of Paediatrics and Adolescent Medicine, 153*, 959–964.

Williams, G. C., Freedman, Z. R., & Deci, E. L. (1998). Supporting autonomy to motivate glucose control in patients with diabetes. *Diabetes Care, 21*, 1644–1651.

Williams, G. C., Grow, V. M., Freedman, Z., Ryan, R. M., & Deci, E. L. (1996). Motivational predictors of weight-loss maintenance. *Journal of Personality and Social Psychology, 70*, 115–126.

Zuroff, D. C., Koestner, R., Moskowitz, D. S., McBridge, C., Bagby, M., & Marshall, M. (2007). Autonomous motivation for therapy: A new non-specific predictor of outcome in brief treatments of depression. *Psychotherapy Research, 17*, 137–148.

Chapter 22
A School-Based Intervention Involving Massage and Yoga for Disadvantaged Male Adolescents: An Exploratory Study on a Self-discovery Program*

Lesley Powell

Young people aged 10–20 years make up ~13–15% of the UK population (McDonald, 2006). Health issues are a concern among this age group and poor health behaviors established in adolescence can persist into adulthood, e.g., smoking, eating disorders, substance misuse, poor levels of physical activity and sexual risk taking (Currie, Elton, Todd, & Platt, 1997). In addition, young people who offend may experience abuse, neglect, and social exclusion (Hamilton, Falshaw, & Browne, 2002). Traditionally, interventions within educational settings, such as disciplinary techniques, detention, suspension, and expulsion, have been shown to be largely ineffective (Malloy, Cheney, Habner, Cormier, & Bernstein, 1998). In response to this, there has been a growth in the development of therapeutic interventions such as social skills training and relaxation (Lopata, 2003). The association between relaxation and physiological arousal reduction (Wolpe, 1958) underpins the rationale for incorporating relaxation as a component in interventions for disadvantaged young persons who may also experience emotional and behavioral difficulties (EBD). The following gives a brief overview of published literature regarding those interventions that comprise massage and yoga and that target young people, with EBD, attending education.

The Quiet Place Project (Spalding, 2000, 2001) aims to provide a holistic (including massage) client-led approach, where children attend six, weekly sessions. Renwick and Spalding (2002) examined the Quiet Place Project delivered to 172 children across seven schools compared to a control group ($n=54$) from three schools. Compared to the control group, pupils who took part in the Project were reported to display noticeable decreases in negative behaviors such as bullying,

* The study was supported by funding from the National Lottery Scheme: Awards for All Supporting Local Groups and Communities in England.

L. Powell (✉)
Applied Research Center in Health and Lifestyle Interventions,
University of Oxford, UK
e-mail: lpowell24@btinternet.com

I. Brdar (ed.), *The Human Pursuit of Well-Being: A Cultural Approach*,
DOI 10.1007/978-94-007-1375-8_22,

being disruptive, rule breaking and increases in positive behaviors such as obeying instructions, joining in with a group and asking for help in class.

In Germany, the Training of Relaxation with Elements of Yoga for Children program (*Torwe Y-C*; Stück & Gloeckner, 2005) was delivered to 48 pupils aged 11–12 years who showed "abnormal examination anxiety". The study involved the pupils meeting 15 times over 6 months and was divided into three parts: relaxation, yoga and an interactive type of game. The results from this study show that participating pupils were appreciative of the chance to learn the techniques, and feelings of helplessness and aggression were reduced. In the UK, Hallam and Price (1998) studied the value of playing calming music to a group of ten girls and boys aged 9–10 years attending an EBD Unit. The results showed improvements in both behavior and in mathematics performance.

Two USA studies have also utilized massage therapy for use with adolescents with developmental, emotional and behavioral difficulties and attention deficit hyperactivity disorder (ADHD), respectively (Diego et al., 2002; Khilnani, Field, Hernandez-Reif, & Schanberg, 2003). Both of these studies used relaxation as the control element. Results from both studies indicate less aggressive behavior, reduced hyperactivity, and improved attention span compared with the control groups that received relaxation only.

Although small, the evidence-base on interventions involving massage and yoga for young persons with EMD appears positive. Based on the available literature, and from the author's experience of developing and evaluating an intervention to teach massage techniques to parents and their children with life-long conditions and disability (Cullen-Powell, 2005; Powell, Barloe, & Cheshire, 2006; Powell & Cheshire, 2010), the author developed an SDP.

Self-Discovery Program

The purpose of the SDP (Powell, Barlow, & Bagh, 2005) is to take participating young people on a journey of self-discovery. The aims are to increase awareness of their physicality, cognitions, feelings and emotions, their behavior and how they respond or react to this awareness in the context of their environment/situation. In addition, the SDP aims to help develop a sense of self-worth. The theoretical framework that underpins the SDP is that of self-efficacy (Bandura, 1988). Strategies shown to enhance self-efficacy are mastery experience, role modeling, persuasion and reinterpretation of physiological and affective states (Bandura, 1988). In the context of the SDP, pupils are trained in relaxation techniques such as simple yoga stretches, hand massage, and deep breathing. The SDP provides them with a safe environment in which these techniques can be practiced (mastery experience), and each pupil can observe their peers also practicing the techniques (role modeling). The tutor is instrumental in providing clear instructions and explanations to why they may be helpful and help pupils to identify how the learned techniques can be used. Thus, pupils have a "self-help tool kit" that they can easily access and implement during times of stress. The aim is that pupils will be able to consider their response from a place of stillness rather than reacting automatically with aggression (persuasion). The relaxation techniques also provide a means of down-regulating physiological arousal and affective states (e.g., anger).

Earlier trials of the SDP (Cullen-Powell, 2005; Powell, Gilchrist, & Stapley, 2008; Powell et al., 2005) have shown the program to be of value in terms of improvements in self-control, being calmer in class and use of relaxation techniques (e.g., self-hand massage) during stressful situations in school. However, the SDP has not been tried in a school exclusively for disadvantaged male adolescents who also have a statement of special educational need (SEN).

The purpose of the exploratory study reported here was to determine the feasibility and value of providing the SDP for male pupils attending a school exclusively for adolescents aged 11–16 years with SEN, EBD, autism spectrum disorder, and severe and mild learning disabilities. Ethical approval was granted by Coventry University's Ethics Committee. As this was an exploratory study, a combination of quantitative and qualitative data collected using a simple pretest–posttest design. However, data from this and previous studies will help inform a wider, randomized controlled trial in the future.

Method

Sample

Of the 52 pupils attending the school, 98% were working with the child and adolescent mental health team, 68% were working with the youth offending team, 12% were working with the community and safety team for acceptable behavior and 62% received free school meals. Of these 52 pupils, a purposeful sample of 36 was identified by the head teacher to take part in the study. Inclusion criteria used were based on age (i.e., 11–15 years), those who were engaged in the school learning program (i.e., pupils with a minimum of 70% attendance rate). The research team provided the school with 36 information sheets about the SDP and the study and parental consent/pupil assent forms to take part in the study. These forms were distributed to parents and pupils. In addition, prepaid envelopes were provided for completed forms to be returned to the research team.

Of the 36 pupils invited to take part, consent was received from 23 parents and assent received from 23 boys giving a response rate of 64%. Thirteen parents failed to return the consent form and, therefore, 13 pupils were unable to take part in the study. Although no pupils withdrew from the study, complete sets of data are available for 21 pupils only and form the basis of all analyses. Thus, although 23 pupils took part in the SDP, the results are based on complete data sets for 21 pupils.

Pupils were aged 11–15 years, 18 were described as "White British", two were "Black/Afro-Caribbean" and one was "mixed race". Of the 21 pupils, six were diagnosed with an EBD alone, two were diagnosed with EBD and ADHD, two were diagnosed with ADHD alone, one was reported by teachers to have ADHD and epilepsy and one pupil had a diagnosis of "global delay". The remaining nine pupils had mild-to-severe learning disability. Six pupils were reported to be receiving additional help, such as play therapy, during school hours.

The Self-discovery Program Adapted for Male Pupils

The SDP consisted of 12 sessions spread over two school terms (spring and summer). The primary themes of the SDP included sensory awareness, massage (where pupils learnt to massage their own hands), yoga stretches, meditation/visualization and relaxation. A range of topics were covered within the themes and a range of activities were implemented. These involved a handshake at the start and finish of the sessions (positive touch), music and color, sports massage, breath work, positive thinking, choices, and reflections.

For the massage sessions, a guest speaker was invited to introduce the topic of massage to pupils. The guest speaker was a male sports massage therapist with experience of working within schools. The purpose of this was (a) to help pupils to overcome any sensitive issues they may have about touch, (b) to give pupils some insight of how massage can be used as a career, and (c) to provide a male role model as a professional sports massage therapist.

Two tutors (one was qualified in the field of complementary therapy and one was an ex-teacher with experience of working with adolescents with EBD) were employed to deliver the SDP throughout the duration of the project to ensure consistency in delivery. The tutors received additional training (half day) by Dr. Powell in the delivery and format of the SDP and the associated research requirements. A teaching assistant (TA) also attended each SDP session. The TA's role was to support the tutor, to ensure the safety of the pupils and the tutor and to maintain the discipline expected within school.

Procedure

On receipt, by the research team, of the consent and assent forms, baseline questionnaires were posted at the school for completion by teachers and pupils, respectively. Once baseline questionnaires were returned to the research team, using the prepaid envelopes provided, the school was informed and pupils were then divided into five groups (four to five children in each group), according to class (chronological age), ready to commence the SDP.

Quantitative data were collected by questionnaires completed by teachers and pupils at two points in time: immediately before commencing the SDP and immediately after completing the SDP.

Qualitative data were collected on completion of the SDP by open questions on the questionnaires and verbal feedback from the pupils about their experience of the SDP. In addition, tutor monitoring forms were completed for the duration of the SDP.

Measures

Basic demographic information, including each pupil's class year and age, level of attainment, medical diagnoses (if applicable), ethnic origin and support received from school and/or outside agencies was collected at baseline only.

Teachers

A behavioral profile was developed specifically for the study and included information on pupils' self and social confidence, communication, self-control within the school/classroom and attention span. The behavioral profile is a nonstandardized measure consisting of nine questions, each rated 1–7, with low scores indicating no confidence, great difficulty in communication, no eye contact and no contribution in class. Scores are reported for each subscale and summed to give a total behavioral score (minimum 7, maximum 63).

A *strengths and difficulties questionnaire* (Goodman, 1997, 2001) is a measure of aggressive behavior and is used in schools. It consists of 25 items divided between five scales: emotional symptoms, conduct problems, hyperactivity, peer relationship problems and prosocial behavior. Some statements are negative and some are positive. Statements are anchored from "not true", "somewhat true" to "certainly true". Each subscale consisted of five questions, and each question scored between 1 and 3 points. Scores are banded from "normal " through "borderline" and "abnormal" in order to identify individuals likely to have mental health disorders. Low scores generally indicate "normal" behavior, whilst high scores indicate abnormal behavior.

Children

The *strengths and difficulties questionnaire*, as reported above. *Qualitative data* were collected via *open-ended questions* immediately after the SDP. Pupils answered the following questions:

- Did you enjoy taking part in the SDP?
- Name one activity or skill learnt on the SDP that you liked.
- Name one activity or skill that you learnt on the SDP that you disliked.
- Have you used any of the techniques learnt on the SDP in class/school?

It was considered that some pupils may experience difficulty in articulating their experiences in written form; thus, informal *verbal feedback* was gained from the pupils on completion of the SDP. Pupils were seen in their respective SDP group and written notes taken.

In addition, tutor *monitoring forms* provided information on the tutors' experiences of the sessions on a weekly basis and an overall reflection of their experience of the SDP in terms of delivery and content.

Results

Quantitative Data

Teacher and pupil ratings of the pupils' behaviors did not differ, either before or after the SDP. Thus, the teachers' views of the behavior of the pupils changed in the same direction as the pupils themselves reported.

Behavior Profiles Completed by Teachers

The total mean behavioral score before commencing the SDP was 36.10 (SD 10.85) and 38.40 (SD 10.20) on completion of the SDP, indicating an overall improvement in behavior. Specifically, improvements were noted for self-confidence, social confidence with peers and with teachers, communication with peers and with teachers, self control, attention span and eye contact with teachers. Contribution in class showed no improvement.

Table 22.1 shows the mean scores on each subscale of the SDQ for both teacher ratings of students and student ratings both before and after the SDP. The general

Table 22.1 Comparison of teachers' and students' ratings on strengths and difficulties questionnaire before and after the self-discovery programme

	Scale	Before SDP	After SDP	t
TEACHER	Emotional symptoms	4.90	5.00	0.84
	Conduct problems	3.81	4.52	0.00
	Hyperactivity scale	6.32	5.72	2.48*
	Peer problems	4.70	4.30	1.01
	Total difficulties	20.10	19.50	0.98
	Pro-social score	4.50	5.00	1.50
PUPIL	Emotional symptoms	4.90	5.00	0.84
	Conduct problems	3.81	4.52	0.00
	Hyperactivity scale	6.32	5.72	2.48*
	Peer problems	4.70	4.30	1.01
	Total difficulties	20.10	19.50	0.98
	Pro-social score	5.30	5.20	0.26

SDP self-discovery programme
* $p<.05$

overall trend is toward improvement, and even where there are no significant responses, the range of responses narrowed, indicating less extremes of response. The prosocial score, i.e., the extent to which pupils were actively kind and helpful toward other pupils, also indicated improvement (Table 22.1). However, none of the changes in scores on the SDQ were of statistical significance with the exception of hyperactivity, as rated by the teachers.

Qualitative Data

Pupils (Questionnaire Responses)

Nineteen pupils responded to the open questions on the questionnaire on completion of the SDP. Of these 19 responses, 16 pupils indicated that they had enjoyed taking part in the SDP. Of the three pupils who stated they had not enjoyed the SDP, two gave no further clarification as to why, and one pupil found it "*a bit boring*", which may be a combination of both content and experience of the tutor. These three pupils also reported that they had enjoyed the massage.

The most enjoyed features of the SDP were the meditations/visualizations and the massage, with eight boys commenting that the massage was the most enjoyable part of the program. Yoga was the most disliked activity, although in at least one case, the boy who disliked yoga the most, cited Tai Chi as the most enjoyable part (basic Tai-Chi movements were used by one tutor as an alternative to Yoga).

Thirteen pupils reported they had used some of the skills (breathing [3], self hand massage [3], meditation [1]) learnt on the SDP in class. Six pupils referred to these skills as just "techniques" without clarification as to what these techniques were.

Pupils (Verbal Feedback)

On the whole, pupils appeared to have enjoyed taking part in the SDP. They particularly liked some of the activities, especially the topic on "unusual and healthy" foods (incorporating sensory awareness and color), massage, breath, and meditation. One pupil did not like the oil used for the massage, but alternatives were, at this time, offered (such as a moisturizing cream). Five pupils suggested that they had used some of the techniques, particularly massage, breath techniques and meditation at home as well as in school. One pupil liked the breathing techniques and suggested that it did help to keep him calm during demanding situations. Interestingly, two pupils found the meditations were repeated too many times. It was explained that this was the purpose of meditation to become "master" of one's own ability to problem solve and of "quieting the mind".

In terms of the timing and length of the sessions and the overall SDP, this was reported to be "*okay*". In terms of improving the SDP, it was felt that there was not enough time for all the activities to be completed during one session; thus, perhaps, longer sessions, or more weeks, would be better. The pupils also liked the tutors who were described as "*always pleasant and calm*", "*they never got angry*".

Teachers

Teachers reported that they had noticed changes in pupils during the SDP such as increased attention in class. In particular, two pupils who reported to use "techniques" learnt on the SDP in class were also noted by their respective teachers to have global changes (more self-control and concentration skills, appeared less worried, had better communication skills, higher contribution levels in class) and had observed these same pupils using breathing and hand massage techniques. One pupil, who reported that he does not employ any of the skills learnt on the SDP, had nevertheless been noted by his teacher to be calmer and more relaxed in stressful situations.

The teacher of one pupil noted that whilst the SDP had been in progress, the pupil had experienced a "*very unsettling time in his home life*" which in turn affected his behavior in a negative manner. It is possible, that given the chaotic nature of these pupils' lives, that there was more than one pupil experiencing an unsettling time, but this information was not recorded.

Tutors' Experiences

Reflections from the tutors who delivered the SDP show that the experience of delivering the program had been very positive and had enhanced their own personal growth and development. However, it was felt by both tutors that it had been very challenging on their own ability to keep pupils motivated and actively engaged in activities. Both tutors felt that they would have liked to have received more intense training in the delivery of the SDP and on some of the mandatory activities required (i.e., massage, yoga, meditations, and relaxation techniques).

Discussion

The purpose of this study was to determine the feasibility and the value of providing an SDP for male pupils aged 11–15 years with a statement of special educational needs, who have EBD (emotional and behavioural disorders) as the primary issue and are attending a school exclusively for disadvantaged boys. Overall, the SDP was well received by pupils. Important was the positive change in pupils' reduced hyperactivity as reported by teachers. This change is important in terms of social behavior, group working, concentration and integration into school life. Although no other statistically significant changes were noted, there were trends (i.e., scores moving in the right direction) toward improvements in pupils' emotional symptoms and conduct, self and social confidence, communication with peers and teachers, self-control, attention span, and eye contact with teachers.

It is unlikely that statistically significant changes would occur in such a short time among pupils who are excluded from mainstream education, experiencing EBD, ADHD, autism spectrum disorder, have a statement of SEN, come from socially disadvantaged backgrounds and require additional support during the school day. The pupils in our study live in a chaotic and unstable environment outside of school that often filters into school life. It is more likely that the small incremental steps demonstrated in our findings are important over longer periods of time. For pupils with SEN, these small steps may be far more productive in the longer term than any immediate, sudden change that may be difficult to accommodate and assimilate.

The qualitative data demonstrates that pupils enjoyed attending the SDP with many pupils using the "techniques" learnt on the SDP that they felt comfortable with. They valued having the opportunity to take part in a program that was "fun" and gave them practical, pragmatic skills that are easily implemented into their daily life, as well as being something "different" for them to do. Of interest was the pupils liking of massage, breath work and meditation. The introduction of massage via a male sports therapist may have contributed to the popularity of the massage.

Challenges and Limitations

The response rate was 64%. Even though parents initially indicated verbally to the head teacher that their son could participate in the SDP, it became apparent that the lives of the children and parents were too chaotic to give time to reading and filling in "nonessential" forms (i.e., reading information sheets and signing consent forms). Thus, gaining consent and assent from parents and pupils, respectively, was both a challenge and a limitation of the study. It may be that the use of a "nonconsent" form may have given a higher rate of return. Woods & White (2005) studied bullying and aggression levels in adolescents. They made use of a nonconsent form, whereby parents and guardians were sent a form and asked to sign it only if they did not want their child to participate. This clearly would be for consideration in any future studies.

The small number of participants and the lack of a control group, blind scoring (i.e., teachers knew which pupils were taking part and, when necessary, helped pupils complete their questionnaire) and randomization suggest the results of this study should be treated with caution. However, the results do suggest that the SDP may be a valuable intervention for this group of pupils. Although our findings do not show large amounts of change, they do show trends toward improvement, both with positive overall changes and a lessening of ranges (i.e., extreme responses). Pupils in this study have very chaotic and difficult social backgrounds, have a statement of SEN, and some experience ADHD and autism, and, therefore, change may take longer to surface than can be expected in one 12-week program.

However, it is important to "sow the seeds" for positive change and provide this group of young people with a range of practical, pragmatic skills that they can implement and use easily and comfortably as and when they feel a need. In this way, pupils become self-empowered. In addition, providing such skills may serve to enhance their sense of self-worth and confidence in finding solutions to their often negative situations and emotions. Extending the length of the program may not be feasible, taking into account the demands of an academic year. Providing a rolling program and/or refresher or review program may be future options to explore. Further, tutor training needs to be refined and improved with an accreditation to a continued professional development standard with a recognized professional body. These refinements will be explored prior to future delivery. However, our findings do add support to the literature in general on complementary therapy-based programs for young people with extra needs and EBD.

In conclusion, the SDP appears to be of value to this group of adolescents and with refinement of both content and tutor recruitment and training could provide a useful intervention for similar cohorts. It is now necessary to conduct a larger, wider, randomized study or tracker study to validate the efficacy of the SDP and ensure that the SDP is a cost-effective intervention available to pupils and schools nationwide.

References

Bandura, A. (1988). Perceived self- efficacy: Exercise of control through self-belief. In J. P. Dauwalder, M. Perrez, & V. Hobbi (Eds.), *Annual series of European research in behaviour therapy* (Vol. 2, pp. 27–59). The Netherlands: Lisse.

Cullen-Powell, L. (2005). Promoting inner stillness; the value of a self discovery programme for children with social, emotional and behavioural difficulties. *British Journal of Special Education, 32*(3), 137–143.

Currie, C. E., Elton, R. A., Todd, J., & Platt, S. (1997). Indicators of socio-economic status of adolescents: The WHO health behaviour in school aged children survey. *Health Education Research, 12*(3), 385–397.

Diego, M. A., Field, T., Hernandez-Reif, M., Shaw, J. A., Rothe, E. M., Castellanos, D., et al. (2002). Aggressive adolescents benefit from massage therapy. *Adolescence, 37*(147), 597–607.

Goodman, R. (1997). The strengths & difficulties questionnaire: A research note. *Journal of Child Psychology, Psychiatry, and Allied Disciplines, 40*(5), 791–799.

Goodman, R. (2001). Psychometric properties of the strengths and difficulties questionnaire. *Journal of the American Academy of Child and Adolescent Psychiatry, 40*(11), 1337–1345.

Hallam, S., & Price, J. (1998). Can the use of background music improve the behaviour and academic performance of children with emotional and behavioural difficulties? *British Journal of Special Education, 25*(2), 88–91.

Hamilton, C. E., Falshaw, L., & Browne, K. D. (2002). The link between recurrent maltreatment and offending behaviour. *International Journal of Offender Therapy and Comparative Criminology, 46*(1), 75–94.

Khilnani, S., Field, T., Hernandez-Reif, M., & Schanberg, S. (2003). Massage therapy improves mood and behaviour of students with attention-deficit/hyperactivity disorder. *Adolescence, 38*, 623–638.

Lopata, C. (2003). Progressive muscle relaxation and aggression among elementary students with emotional or behavioural disorders. *Behavioural Disorders, 28*(2), 162–172.

Malloy, J., Cheney, D., Habner, D., Cormier, G., & Bernsten, S. (1998). Personal futures planning for youth and young adults with emotional and behavioural disorders. *Reaching Today's Youth, 2*, 2–30.

McDonald, W. (2006). *The health needs of young offenders*. National Primary Care Research and Development Centre, University of Manchester. Retrieved from www.ohrn.nhs.uk/resource/Research/PCSysRevYO.pdf

Powell, L. A., Barlow, J. H., & Bagh, J. (2005). The Self-Discovery Programme for children with special educational needs in mainstream primary and secondary schools: An exploratory study. *Emotional and Behaviour Difficulties, 10*(3), 189–201.

Powell, L., Barlow, J. H., & Cheshire, A. (2006). The Training and Support Programme for parents of children with cerebral palsy: A process evaluation. *Complementary Therapies in Practice, 12*(3), 192–199.

Powell, L. A., & Cheshire, A. (2010). Evaluation of a massage programme for children who have been sexually abused and their non-abusing mothers. *Child Abuse and Neglect, 19*, 141–155.

Powell, L. A., Gilchrist, M., & Stapley, J. (2008). A journey of self-discovery: An intervention involving massage, yoga and relaxation for children with emotional and behavioural difficulties attending primary schools. *Journal Emotional and Behavioural Difficulties, 13*(3), 193–199.

Renwick, F., & Spalding, B. (2002). 'A Quiet Place' project: An of early therapeutic intervention within mainstream schools. *British Journal of Special Education, 29*(3), 144–150.

Spalding, B. (2000). The contribution of a 'Quiet Place' to early intervention strategies for children with emotional and behavioural difficulties in mainstream schools. *British Journal of Special Education, 27*(3), 129–134.

Spalding, B. (2001). A quiet place: A healing environment. *Support for Learning, 16*(2), 69–73.

Stück, M., & Gloeckner, N. (2005). Yoga for children in the mirror of the science: Working spectrum and practice fields of the training of relaxation with elements of yoga for children. *Early Child Development and Care, 175*(4), 371–377.

Wolpe, J. (1958). *Psychotherapy by reciprocal inhibition*. Stanford, CA: Stanford University Press.

Woods, S., & White, E. (2005). The association between bullying behaviour, arousal levels and behaviour problems. *Journal of Adolescence, 28*(3), 381–395.

Index

I. Brdar (ed.), *The Human Pursuit of Well-Being: A Cultural Approach*,
DOI 10.1007/978-94-007-1375-8, © Springer Science+Business Media B.V. 2011

MIX
Papier aus verantwortungsvollen Quellen
Paper from responsible sources
FSC® C105338

If you have any concerns about our products,
you can contact us on
ProductSafety@springernature.com

In case Publisher is established outside the EU,
the EU authorized representative is:
Springer Nature Customer Service Center GmbH
Europaplatz 3, 69115 Heidelberg, Germany

Printed by Libri Plureos GmbH
in Hamburg, Germany